CHILD CARE AND CHILD DEVELOPMENT

Child Care
and Child Development

*Results from the NICHD Study
of Early Child Care and Youth Development*

Edited by
THE NICHD EARLY CHILD CARE RESEARCH NETWORK

Foreword by Duane F. Alexander

THE GUILFORD PRESS
New York   London

© 2005 The Guilford Press
A Division of Guilford Publications, Inc.
72 Spring Street, New York, NY 10012
www.guilford.com

Printed in the United States of America

This book is printed on acid-free paper.

Last digit is print number: 9 8 7 6 5 4 3 2 1

Library of Congress Cataloging-in-Publication Data
Child care and child development: results from the NICHD study of early
child care and youth development / edited by NICHD Early Child Care
Research Network.
    p. cm.
  Includes bibliographical references and index.
  ISBN 1-59385-138-3 (hardcover)
  1. Child care—United States—Longitudinal studies. 2. Child development—
United States—Longitudinal studies. I. NICHD Early Child Care Research
Network.
  HQ778.63.C515 2005
  362.7′071′073—dc22

                                                          2004022874

Editors and Contributors

MEMBERS OF THE NICHD EARLY CHILD CARE RESEARCH NETWORK (2004)

Virginia Allhusen, PhD, Department of Psychology and Social Behavior, University of California, Irvine, California

Jay Belsky, PhD, School of Psychology, Birkbeck College, University of London, London, United Kingdom

Cathryn Booth-LaForce, PhD, Departments of Family and Child Nursing and Psychology, University of Washington, Seattle, Washington

Robert Bradley, PhD, Center for Applied Studies in Education, College of Education, University of Arkansas, Little Rock, Arkansas

Celia A. Brownell, PhD, Department of Psychology, University of Pittsburgh, Pittsburgh, Pennsylvania

Margaret Burchinal, PhD, Center for Developmental Science, University of North Carolina, Chapel Hill, North Carolina

Susan B. Campbell, PhD, Department of Psychology, University of Pittsburgh, Pittsburgh, Pennsylvania

K. Alison Clarke-Stewart, PhD, Department of Psychology and Social Behavior, University of California, Irvine, California

Martha Cox, PhD, Center for Developmental Science and Department of Psychology, University of North Carolina, Chapel Hill, North Carolina

Sarah L. Friedman, PhD, National Institute of Child Health and Human Development, Bethesda, Maryland

Willard W. Hartup, EdD, Institute of Child Development, University of Minnesota, Minneapolis, Minnesota

Kathryn Hirsh-Pasek, PhD, Department of Psychology, Temple University, Philadelphia, Pennsylvania

Aletha C. Huston, PhD, Department of Human Ecology, University of Texas at Austin, Austin, Texas

Deborah Johnson, PhD, Department of Family and Child Ecology, Michigan State University, East Lansing, Michigan

Bonnie Knoke, MS, RTI International, Research Triangle Park, North Carolina

Nancy Marshall, EdD, Center for Research on Women, Wellesley College, Wellesley, Massachusetts

Kathleen McCartney, PhD, Harvard Graduate School of Education, Harvard University, Cambridge, Massachusetts

Frederick J. Morrison, PhD, Department of Psychology and School of Education, University of Michigan, Ann Arbor, Michigan

Philip Nader, MD, Department of Pediatrics, School of Medicine, University of California, San Diego, California

Marion O'Brien, PhD, Department of Human Development and Family Studies, University of North Carolina, Greensboro, North Carolina

Margaret Tresch Owen, PhD, School of Human Development, University of Texas at Dallas, Dallas, Texas

Ross D. Parke, PhD, Department of Psychology, University of California, Riverside, California

Deborah Phillips, PhD, Department of Psychology, Georgetown University, Washington, DC

Robert Pianta, PhD, Department of Human Services, Curry School of Education, University of Virginia, Charlottesville, Virginia

A. Vijaya Rao, PhD, RTI International, Research Triangle Park, North Carolina

Wendy W. Robeson, EdD, Center for Research on Women, Wellesley College, Wellesley, Massachusetts

Carolyn Roy, PhD, Department of Human Development and Family Life, University of Kansas, Lawrence, Kansas

Susan Spieker, PhD, Department of Family and Child Nursing, School of Nursing, University of Washington, Seattle, Washington

Deborah Lowe Vandell, PhD, Departments of Educational Psychology and Human Development and Family Studies, University of Wisconsin, Madison, Wisconsin

Marsha Weinraub, PhD, Department of Psychology, Temple University, Philadelphia, Pennsylvania

ADDITIONAL CONTRIBUTORS

Mark Appelbaum, PhD, Department of Psychology, University of California, San Diego, California

Bill Barfoot, PhD, The Winston School, Dallas, Texas

Dee Ann Batten, PhD, U.S. Merit Systems Protection Board, Washington, DC

Kimberly Boller, PhD, National Institute of Child Health and Human Development, Bethesda, Maryland

Donna Bryant, PhD, School of Education, University of North Carolina, Chapel Hill, North Carolina

Yvonne Caldera, PhD, Department of Human Development and Family Studies, Texas Tech University, Lubbock, Texas

Bettye Caldwell, PhD, Department of Pediatrics, University of Arkansas for Medical Sciences, and College of Education, University of Arkansas, Little Rock, Arkansas

Jeffrey Cohn, PhD, Departments of Psychology and Psychiatry, University of Pittsburgh, Pittsburgh, Pennsylvania

Eric Dearing, PhD, Department of Psychology, University of Wyoming, Laramie, Wyoming

Ganie DeHart, PhD, Department of Psychology, State University of New York at Geneseo, Geneseo, New York

Kaye Fendt, MA, National Institute of Child Health and Human Development, Bethesda, Maryland

Wendy Goldberg, PhD, Department of Psychology and Social Behavior, University of California, Irvine, California

Ellen Greenberger, PhD, Department of Psychology and Social Behavior, University of California, Irvine, California

Elizabeth Jaeger, PhD, Department of Psychology, St. Joseph's University, Philadelphia, Pennsylvania

Jean F. Kelly, PhD, Department of Family and Child Nursing, University of Washington, Seattle, Washington

Lori McLeod, PhD, RTI International, Research Triangle Park, North Carolina

Lauren Nelson, MA, Frank P. Graham Child Development Institute, University of North Carolina, Chapel Hill, North Carolina

Mary Overpeck, DrPH, National Institute of Child Health and Human Development, Bethesda, Maryland

Kenneth Poole, PhD, RTI International, Research Triangle Park, North Carolina

Sharon Landesman Ramey, PhD, School of Nursing and Health Studies and Center on Health and Education, Georgetown University, Washington, DC

Suzanne Randolph, PhD, Department of Family Studies, University of Maryland, College Park, Maryland

David Redden, PhD, RTI International, Research Triangle Park, North Carolina

Henry Ricciuti, PhD, National Institute of Child Health and Human Development, Bethesda, Maryland, and Department of Human Development, Cornell University, Ithaca, New York

Peter Scheidt, MD, Children's National Medical Center, Washington, DC

Anne Stright, PhD, Department of Counseling and Educational Psychology, School of Education, Indiana University, Bloomington, Indiana

Louisa B. Tarullo, PhD, Administration for Children and Families, Washington, DC

Beck A. Taylor, PhD, Department of Economics, Baylor University, Waco, Texas

Kathleen E. Wallner-Allen, PhD, RTI International, Research Triangle Park, North Carolina

Anne M. Ware, PhD, Fort Worth Independent School District, Fort Worth, Texas

Foreword

In 1987, participants in a conference on early child care, organized by the Zero to Three National Center for Infants, Toddlers, and Families and hosted by the National Academy of Sciences, called to the attention of the National Institute of Child Health and Human Development (NICHD) that the scientific knowledge about child care and its effects on the development of children was less than entirely coherent due to scientific design limitations. As indicated elsewhere in this volume, previous studies had small numbers of subjects and short follow-up. The samples from the population were mostly those that researchers could get easy access to ("samples of convenience"). Many studies did not control for child and family factors that could explain the findings either fully or in part. Different studies focused on different aspects of the child care experience without controlling for variations in the aspects of child care not under scrutiny. These scientific design limitations might have led to the conflicting results that were reported in the scientific literature and disseminated to an understandably confused public and to policymakers.

In the absence of authoritative scientific guidance, parents continued to wonder if it was safe to place infants and toddlers in child care. When parents heard findings suggesting that child care was safe, they wanted to know at what age they could leave their child with other caregivers while they were at work. They asked for how many hours per week they could be separated from their infant or toddler without ill effects, and whether there might be developmental benefits from day care for their child. They wondered if they should choose an unstructured, family-like environment or a more structured, academically oriented environment. Finally, they wanted to know how to determine that the child care they selected was of sufficient quality. More or less at the same time, lawmakers who heard about extreme cases of neglect by caregivers were calling for hearings about the availability, cost, and quality of child care and about the development of children who were in child care. Congress considered passing laws and appropriating funds that would ensure the safety and health of infants and toddlers who were in child care, and sought some guidance from scientists. Likewise, local government administrators who needed to determine how best to allocate local government resources for social programs that support families and children asked questions about the return on their investment in child care. They asked if children's language, cognition, achievement, and psychosocial adjustment were better when child care was of higher quality.

To respond to the public need for authoritative information, NICHD planned to embark on designing, with the scientific community, one large, comprehensive, and in-depth longitudinal study of child care and the development of children. Children were to be assessed in terms of their social adjustment and family relationships, their cognitive and linguistic school readiness, and their growth and health. The planned study was to be conducted by a large team of investigators from across the nation. The selected investigators were asked to work collaboratively among themselves and with NICHD staff on conducting one study across research sites. They were also asked to follow up a geographically diverse sample of families from all walks of life. To achieve its goal, NICHD provided funds to be distributed equivalently among the participating grantees. The funds were expected to allow for frequent face-to-face meetings among the investigators, for face-to-face centralized training of data collectors, and for face-to-face meetings of the staff coordinating the data collection at the site level. Funds were also provided for staying in contact with families that moved away from the geographical location of the data collection sites. To ensure the high quality of the data, and to facilitate data analyses and the production of scientific papers, NICHD augmented the team of developmental investigators with data management and analytical expertise from a data center. The data center received the data from the collection sites, monitored their completeness and accuracy, and analyzed them in collaboration with the study investigators. As the study children were growing older, NICHD required that age-appropriate developmental expertise would be added to the team of investigators and that the data would be shared with other interested and qualified investigators in the scientific community.

The investigators who were selected through peer review to participate in this study, together with the NICHD partners and the staff of the data center, adopted organizational structures that supported collaboration. Together, they demonstrated remarkable collegiality in their planning and implementation of the study as well as in writing scientific papers. They developed the study hypotheses, designed the specific methods of the study, and designed detailed scientific plans for the implementation of the study. They made sure that the data obtained across the 10 data collection sites would be collected in a consistent manner and be of very high quality, and they documented the study methods, data collection procedures, and the variables in the data sets. They collaborated effectively on the publication of influential scientific papers and are currently engaged in training others in the use of the data sets.

At the time of the writing of this foreword, the NICHD Study of Early Child Care and Youth Development has produced 116 scientific publications by investigators affiliated with NICHD, with 10 grantee institutions, and with a data center. Twenty-two additional scientific papers by the study investigators are in press. The study investigators also made numerous oral presentations aimed at the dissemination of their findings to practitioners, media, and public policymakers. Affiliated investigators, who conducted secondary data analyses, have already published 20 papers.

For this volume, the NICHD Early Child Care Research Network, comprising the research team and the chair of its Steering Committee, collated and abridged some of the most important scientific papers based on data from the first 4½ years of the children's lives. I commend the Network for making the major findings from the early phases of the study easily accessible. I expect that the Network will do the same with the findings pertaining to the effects of family and school on children's development during middle childhood and early adolescence.

DUANE F. ALEXANDER, MD
Director, National Institute
of Child Health and Human Development

Preface

Nonmaternal child care, either as a supplement to maternal care or as a substitute for it, has been a part of human activity for as long as there have been accounts of family life. Mothers are believed to have cared exclusively for their babies only briefly in the oldest hunter–gatherer societies; siblings and child caretakers were also major care providers. The situation is thought to have been little different in early subsistence economies in which complex caretaker combinations often supplemented or replaced exclusive maternal care. Since these early times, historical changes in almost every society known have been momentous, including the increasing use of child care purchased from nonrelatives whose social connection to the child's family are of limited scope and duration. But both historically and cross-culturally, the exclusive care of infants and young children by mothers is the exception rather than the rule.

Child care by grandparents or by other relatives, care by a non-relative in the child's home, family child care (i.e., care by a nonrelative away from the child's home), and child center care increased especially rapidly in the United States during World War II and the decades following. These changes occurred partly as a result of increased use of nonmaternal care for infants and young children during the war when women entered the workforce to take over positions of men who served in the armed forces. Both economic need and social changes in the aspirations of women led to the increased participation of women in the labor force in the postwar years, giving rise to further increases in the use of nonmaternal child care. Currently, child care by individuals other than mothers is used extensively but varies enormously from family to family in terms of who is involved, the kinds of care provided, and the circumstances under which it occurs.

At the same time, disagreements about the wisdom (indeed, the morality) of nonmaternal child care for very young children remain. Scholars of child development began to write many years ago about the ways in which the attachment bond between mother and child is formed in early infancy through mother–child interaction and about the centrality of this bond for the healthy psychological development of children. Other scholars drew analogies between child care, mother–child separation, and the institutionalization of children in hospitals when children had prolonged illnesses. Still others stressed similarities between placement of children in certain care situations and the placement of healthy children in orphanages. In many instances, the case was made that the development of children suffers when they are separated from their mothers in early infancy and placed in child care. Other experts assumed, however, that nonmaternal care of high quality can make positive contributions to the development of low-income children. In addition, researchers have recommended for many years that enrollment in nursery school or other early care for preschool-age children is a positive contribution to children's development.

Not surprisingly, given these considerations, consensus in public attitudes has never materialized. Unfortunately, social policies concerning the best ways to care for young children have become politicized: In many countries, both public support for nonmaternal forms of child care and regulatory legislation vary according to broader ideology. Conflicts about modes of early child care remain bitter and unresolved.

In the United States, as well as in many other Western countries, such conflicts sometimes drive parents and policymakers to turn to science in an effort to guide decision making. Some scientists, in turn, are eager to use their methods to provide valid information to answer the questions on the minds of parents and policymakers. Usually, the consumers ask scientists simple questions about the effects of child care on human development, for example, "Is child care good or bad for the child's development?" But the answers tend not to be simple because the developmental processes by which child care experience relates to child development are extraordinarily complex and must be examined in conjunction with child characteristics, family experience, and other aspects of the social context.

The initial investigations of early child care generally addressed what today appear to be relatively unsophisticated research questions about child care and its developmental consequences. As a result, most of the research preceding the 1990s failed to yield convincing answers to such common questions as whether infant and child care is deleterious or whether "other care" is not as good for the child as "mother care." Samples were small, the measurement base restricted, developmental and societal consequences were not studied for sufficient lengths of time, and analytic methods were simplistic.

Against this background, the National Institute of Child Health and Human Development (NICHD) began in 1987 to make plans for a study that would overcome some of the methodological limitations that existed in earlier studies. The study that was designed over 18 months turned out to be the most ambitious one ever undertaken of early child care and its consequences. At the same time skepticism remained about the possibility that social science was in a position to tackle such a difficult subject, but theoretical, methodological, and quantitative advances during the last half of the 20th century promised that an investment in such an investigation would be likely to provide better answers to certain questions than those provided in earlier studies.

This volume is a collection of research reports selected from those published by the NICHD Early Child Care Research Network since the study began. Because members of the Network believed that it is important to present findings to a broad audience, these chapters were originally published in a large number of different scholarly journals. Although this strategy did, indeed, help to reach a broad audience, results of the NICHD Study of Early Child Care are, as a consequence, scattered across the scientific literature. In some cases, articles are difficult for readers to locate even by electronic means. Our intent, now, is to bring together the most important findings from the NICHD Study of Early Child Care in one volume, including findings from the time that the children were born until they reached the age of 4½ (and in one case, in Chapter 21, into kindergarten).

To use space efficiently, to reduce redundancy in describing our methods and in reviewing relevant literature, and to report our findings with a minimum of repetition, all but two of the chapters in this volume were abridged before being reprinted. No further changes were made in either the data or the language of the original publications. Citations not surviving the abridgement process were also eliminated and a common reference list was generated. We believe that these changes make the volume easier to use. In addition, the volume includes a commentary by Sharon Landesman Ramey, an investigator who has had no connection to the NICHD study itself, and who writes about issues that she herself chose.

Although many individuals contributed as authors to the chapters included in this compilation, the "corporate banner" attached to each of the originals is not reproduced here. Interested readers should consult the original publications for these rosters. It can be said, however, that the NICHD Early Child Care Research Network has included a sizable number of individuals who contributed to all the chapters collected in this volume as well as a number of individuals who contributed to only one or two. The NICHD Network as it existed in 2004 bears responsibility for this volume. The names of Network members are given in "Editors and Contributors." Jeanette Renaud and James Teufel provided logistical support for the work on this volume.

It goes without saying that a study of the magnitude and complexity of this one requires a substantial investment of time, energy, and capital. Working under a cooperative agreement, the investigators from participating universities and from NICHD collaborated for more than 10 years to produce the results collected in this volume. More than 1,200 families contributed time and effort to the project. We cannot overstate the importance of their contributions or our gratitude in being able to work with them. And, finally, we wish to acknowledge our thanks to NICHD, its Director, Duane Alexander, and its Council for their continuing support.

Contents

I

Overview

At the end of 1987, in response to a scientific debate about the important public health questions surrounding maternal employment and the growing use of child care, especially when it begins in infancy, Dr. Duane Alexander, Director of the National Institute of Child Health and Human Development (NICHD), decided to invest public resources in a collaborative study between multiple grantees and NICHD aimed at answering questions about the effects of child care on the development of infants and toddlers. Later, NICHD extended the study to allow the evaluation of the effects of child care during the preschool years and beyond.

This study, which followed 1,364 children born in 1991 from infancy through elementary school and collected information about family, child, child care, and other aspects of context, was not the first one designed to answer questions about the effects of child care. As a matter of fact, research was believed to be sufficient to justify the publication in 1990, by the National Academy Press, of a scholarly book titled *Who Cares for America's Children?* (Hayes, Palmer, & Zaslow, 1990). But most of the evidence cited in that book was derived from three waves of small studies, and the methods employed in them were relatively unsophisticated by today's standards: These earliest studies consisted mostly of comparisons between children in child care and those who were not. Later studies examined the effects of child care characteristics (especially quality) on child development, but typically only one at a time rather than together (see below). Most, however, did not statistically control for other factors that might predict enrollment in child care or children's performance and adjustment. For example, even though family characteristics forecast both the selection of child care arrangements for children and developmental outcomes, the majority of investigators either did not control for family characteristics or took only demographic characteristics into account, not parental character-

1

istics or the quality of the home environment. A few studies preceding the initiation of the NICHD Study of Early Child Care controlled for a wide range of family factors in considering the effects of child care quality, but they have not considered the links between child care and parenting. For example, they have not examined how child care affects mother–child interaction.

Prior to the initiation of the NICHD Study of Early Child Care investigators also tended to assess information about one or another aspect of child care while neglecting others that are theoretically important to the prediction of developmental outcomes. Information was thus collected about the quality of child care or the type of child care (e.g. family day care and center care) or the number of hours children spend in child care—but not all three simultaneously. Consequently, scholars could not evaluate the unique contribution of quality of care or of the number of hours spent in care to children's behavior and development—or the interaction of the many features of the child care experience.

Another limitation of the earlier studies was that in assessing child care, researchers often relied on indirect measures of quality, for example the ratio of children to adults or the educational training of the child care providers. Rare studies of qualitative processes, including the actual behavior of the child care providers, assessed the quality of the setting as a whole rather than the quality of individual children's experiences in spite of the fact that different children have different experiences in the same child care setting, depending on their own characteristics and biases of the providers. And, finally, studies of the effects of child care on children's development did not focus on multiple domains of outcome, thereby restricting the opportunity for finding that effects of a specific feature of child care (e.g., hours or quality) may appear in one domain and not in another.

Taken together, these limitations (along with sampling restrictions and the use of limited time frames) produced conflicting results about child care and its relation to child development. The investigators who designed the NICHD Study of Early Child Care set out to conduct a study that would overcome many of the shortcomings of earlier research. The first chapter of this volume is an unabridged work published in 2001 that describes the research methods and objectives of the study used from the birth of the study children until they reached 54 months of age. The chapter provides an overview of the research, including some early findings, and provides the conceptual framework necessary for a full appreciation of the remainder of the book. As one can see, this study is much more than a study of child care but, rather, is a comprehensive longitudinal study of development with detailed information about the various contexts in which children spend their time.

For further information pertaining to the study's research methods, see the manuals of operation, instrument documents, and data reports at *http:// secc.rti.org/*.

1

Nonmaternal Care and Family Factors in Early Development
An Overview of the NICHD Study of Early Child Care

NICHD EARLY CHILD CARE RESEARCH NETWORK

During the past 25 years, a dramatic change has taken place in the early experiences of the youngest children in the United States. In 1975, 37% of married women with children under age 6 were employed; by 1998, the rate of employment for that group of women had risen to 64%. Employment rates for married mothers of infants under age 2 have increased even more sharply, from 31% in 1975 to 62% in 1998 (U.S. Bureau of the Census, 1999c). These changes in maternal employment have brought changes in patterns of child care as well. About 5% of preschoolers with employed mothers are cared for by their mothers at work, but the remainder regularly spend time being cared for by someone other than their mothers (U.S. Bureau of the Census, 1997).

The dramatic increase in the number of infants and preschoolers receiving nonmaternal care has generated scientific and social policy questions about the effects of early child care experiences on children's development (Booth, 1992; Fox & Fein, 1990). Some writers have argued that all nonmaternal care poses risks for infants because healthy development requires continuous caregiving by one person, usually the mother (Hojat,

From *Journal of Applied Developmental Psychology*, 2001, Vol. 22, pp. 457–492. Copyright 2001 by Elsevier. Reprinted by permission.

1990; Leach, 1994; White, 1985). Others have contended that child care, as experienced in the United States, is problematic primarily when it is extensive—more than 20–30 hours/week (Belsky, 1988, 1990b). Still others have asserted that very young children can thrive in child care arrangements as long as the quality of care is high (Clarke-Stewart, 1987; Field, 1991; McGurk, Caplan, Hennessy, Martin, & Moss, 1993; Phillips & Howes, 1987). Finally, some have argued that early experience alters developmental trajectories only if it involves extreme deprivation, as in the case of abuse and neglect (Scarr, 1992).

In response to the need for data to address these scientific and policy issues, the National Institute of Child Health and Human Development (NICHD) initiated a large-scale prospective longitudinal study of the effects of early child care arrangements on children's development. In its initial phase (1991–1994), the NICHD Study of Early Child Care followed the development of over 1,300 children at 10 sites in the United States from birth through age 3. Phase II of the study (1995–1999) followed the same children's development through first grade; in Phase III (2000–2004), their development during middle childhood is being tracked.[1]

In late 1999, the members of the NICHD Early Child Care Research Network completed their major analyses of the data from Phase I of the study.[2] On January 1, 2000, protocol documentation and data sets from Phase I, covering the period from birth to 36 months, were released for further analysis by other members of the scientific community. Details about the procedures for gaining access to the data are available at the study's website (*http://www.nichd.nih.gov/od/secc/index.htm*). Data from subsequent phases will also be released for use by other researchers, as the study's planned data analyses for each phase are completed.

STUDY RATIONALE AND GOALS

The primary purpose of the NICHD Study of Early Child Care is to examine how variations in nonmaternal care are related to children's social-emotional adjustment, cognitive and linguistic development, and physical growth and health. For the purposes of the study, nonmaternal care is defined as regularly occurring care by anyone other than a child's mother, including the child's father, other relatives, and nonrelatives. Nonmaternal care may be provided in the child's home, in someone else's home, or in a child care center or preschool.

Major constructs in the study are developmental outcomes and trajectories in three major domains (cognitive, social–emotional, and physical growth and health), the contexts that influence and are influenced by these outcomes and trajectories, and time. The study is guided by two conceptual frameworks—Bronfenbrenner's ecological framework (Bronfenbrenner, 1979, 1995, 1999; Bronfenbrenner & Morris, 1998) and life course theory, exemplified by the work of Elder (1998, 1999). Both approaches emphasize the importance of time in understanding variations in psychological outcomes, necessitating a longitudinal approach. Together, they provide a framework for conceptualizing the ways normative and individual contextual influences are related to developmental outcomes and trajectories over time.

The ecological framework takes into account the complex interactions between nonmaternal care experiences, family circumstances, and child characteristics and places individuals and families in social, cultural, and economic context. Based on this framework, family and home environment, child care settings, school, out-of-school settings, parents' work, and socioeconomic factors are all included in the study as contexts with potential influences on development. Bronfenbrenner's recent addition of time to his ecological model, the *chronosystem*, emphasizes the importance of tracking developmental outcomes and trajectories over time and in historical context.

The life course approach also focuses attention on the timing of events and transitions in the lives of children and their families. Some experiences are normative in that they occur at particular, predictable ages for most people (e.g., school entry), and some are nonnormative in that they are not associated with a specific age and are often unexpected (e.g., parental divorce, changes in child care arrangements, and family relocation). The timing of both normative and nonnormative events and transitions can make a difference in their influence on children's development—for example, the impact of divorce on children depends in part on the age at which it is experienced. On a larger scale, the historical time—and even the particular year—in which a child is born can affect development. For example, the impact of the Great Depression on children's development depended in part on how old they were during the period of maximum economic hardship (Elder, 1999).

A central focus of the study is the interplay between early and concurrent experience in varied contexts and developmental trajectories from birth to later points in development. Data from the study can also be used to examine relations between child care experiences and concurrent psychological and physical outcomes. Because it is prospective and longitudinal, the study provides an opportunity to test several competing hypotheses about connections between early child care experiences and development.

According to the *primacy of early experience* hypothesis, the contexts to which a child is exposed early in development have continuous and long-term influences that outweigh many of the influences of contexts encountered later in development. In other words, the developmental effects of early child care would be expected to endure over time, despite later changes in the care a child receives.

The *contemporaneous effects* hypothesis suggests that, at any point in development, current contexts have a stronger influence on developmental status than early experience does. As a result, the effects of early child care on developmental outcomes would be expected to be transient and to fade over time.

Other hypotheses incorporate contemporaneous influences with the early experiences the child brings to a context. According to the *incremental* hypothesis, early experience produces effects on development that are maintained, enhanced, or deflected by exposure to later contexts. Changes in contexts add incrementally and independently to the prediction of developmental outcomes. Based on this hypothesis, child care would be expected to contribute cumulatively to developmental outcomes, its effects increasing gradually with continued exposure.

A variation on the incremental hypothesis posits the *magnification of small differences*: The initial effects of early environments may be small, but they are magnified as children get older. This hypothesis has been used to explain socioeconomic status–related discrepancies in school performance that increase over time (Entwisle, Alexander, & Olson, 1997). One prediction based on this hypothesis would be that early child care's effects on development may not be immediately obvious but will appear at a later point in time.

Finally, the *sensitive periods* hypothesis posits that contexts have especially important effects at particular ages or junctures in development. For example, events or contextual changes associated with major transitions may be more important than those that occur at other times. Based on this hypothesis, nonmaternal care during the first 12 months of life might be expected to have particularly far-reaching effects on development because of the importance of that period for attachment formation. Changes in care arrangements that coincide with major developmental transitions, such as entering toddlerhood or starting school, might also have a particularly strong impact.

In addition to its major focus on relations between early child care and children's subsequent development, the study has several secondary goals:

- To examine how the home environment influences child outcomes, focusing on issues such as quality of parenting and quality and stability of home environment;
- To examine demographic and family characteristics associated with different patterns of child care usage;
- To provide a longitudinal description of the variety, stability, and changes in children's care experiences over time, including quantity and quality of care;
- To provide information about patterns of maternal employment and experiences of parents with nonmaternal care over time; and
- To examine relations between children's experiences in child care and parent–child interactions.

METHOD

The NICHD Study of Early Child Care is distinguished by its breadth, detail, and complexity of design. Its unique features include (1) sites located across major regions of the country in urban, suburban, and rural areas, representing different populations and widely varying state child care regulations; (2) inclusion of ethnic-minority, single-parent, and low-education families at every site; (3) a sample large enough to permit reasonably precise estimation of effect sizes; (4) children followed from birth through a wide range of child care experiences rather than being recruited after child care arrangements were already made; (5) assessment of combinations and changes in child care arrangements over time; (6) extensive direct observation of home, child care, and school experiences; (7) multiple measures of social–emotional development, cognitive and language development, achievement, and physical growth and health; and (8) use of multiple quality-of-care indices: individual children's observed experiences, observed global quality of the care setting, and structural features such as caregiver training and child–caregiver ratios.

Sample

Enrollment

The study's sampling procedures were designed to include families from diverse geographic regions, economic backgrounds, and ethnic groups, with diverse plans for maternal employment during the child's first year of life. Participants in the study were recruited from 24 hospitals in the vicinity of 10 data collection sites (Charlottesville, VA; Irvine, CA; Lawrence, KS; Little Rock, AR; Madison, WI; Morganton, NC; Philadelphia, PA; Pittsburgh, PA; Seattle, WA; and Wellesley, MA). Factors such as location, availability, previous working relationships with site investigators, and patient population contributed to the selection of hospitals at each site.

A total of 1,364 families with healthy newborns were enrolled in the study, with approximately equal numbers of families at each site. Approximately half (53%) of the mothers planned to work full time during their child's first year of life, 23% planned to work part time, and 24% not at all. The enrolled families varied in socioeconomic level, sociocultural background, and family composition; for example, 25% of the families belonged to ethnic minorities, just over 10% of the mothers did not complete high school, and 14% of the mothers were single. Table 1.1 provides additional demographic characteristics of the sample.

Based on U.S. Census Tract data, on most demographic variables the study sample reflects the population of families with young infants residing in the communities from which research participants were recruited. However, as shown in Table 1.1, there are some differences in education level

TABLE 1.1. Demographic Characteristics of Families in Study
Sample, Study Site Census Tracts, and Entire United States

	Study sample	Census tract	United States
Race/ethnicity[a]			
White, non-Hispanic	75.0%	N/A	64.9%
Black, non-Hispanic	12.8%	N/A	15.7%
Hispanic	6.6%	3.4%	15.3%
Asian	1.5%	3.1%	3.6%
Native American	0.4%	0.6%	0.9%
Other (primarily biracial)	3.7%	4.7%	N/A
Mother's education			
< 12th grade	10.4%	20.1%	24.6%
High school graduate	21.1%	27.8%	30.1%
Some college	33.2%	27.5%	26.7%
Bachelor's degree	20.8%	16.1%	12.3%
Graduate/professional degree	14.5%	8.5%	6.3%
Mean household income	$37,781.28	$39,264.12	$36,875.31
% on public assistance	18.8%	6.0%	7.5%

[a]Source for U.S. data: 1991 births by race and Hispanic origin (U.S. Bureau of the Census, 1993).

and income. Parents in the study had higher than average education levels for their census tracts. At the same time, families in the study were more likely to be on public assistance and had slightly lower household incomes than the average for their census tracts.

Enrollment in the study involved three steps: (1) a hospital screening of mother–newborn dyads within 48 hours after birth; (2) a 2-week phone call to mothers found to be eligible at screening; and (3) a 1-month interview with families that remained eligible after the 2-week phone call, agreed to the 1-month interview, and kept the interview appointment. Recruitment took place during the first 11 months of 1991.

Hospital Screening. A total of 8,986 mother–newborn dyads were screened in the hospital. Each site was expected to screen a minimum of 20 mother–newborn dyads in the participating hospitals per week, netting 10 or more eligible dyads for a 2-week phone call. To identify dyads for screening, 24-hour birthing intervals were selected for each hospital and all babies born during those intervals were screened. Up to four 24-hour birthing intervals across the site's hospitals could be selected per week to accomplish the screening goals. Over the course of recruitment, birthing intervals were to cover the days of the week and the participating hospitals within a site somewhat uniformly. Sites were encouraged to screen many more dyads than the minimum required.

The hospital screening was a two-stage process. First, information available from the hospital, without contact with the mother, was reviewed. If the information available from the hospital did not indicate a reason for exclusion, the mother was visited in the hospital for further screening. Mother–newborn dyads were excluded from the study if: (1) the mother was under 18 years old; (2) the mother did not speak English; (3) the family planned to move from the area within 1 year; (4) the infant had serious medical complications or was born to a mother with known or acknowledged substance abuse; (5) the mother was too ill; (6) the mother was placing her infant for adoption; (7) the mother refused to do the 2-week phone call; (8) the mother lived more than 1 hour's drive from the lab site; (9) the family was enrolled in another study; (10) the mother lived in a neighborhood deemed by police too unsafe for visitation (generally high-rise public housing projects); or (11) the mother refused the hospital interview. During the hospital visit with the mother, the following additional background information was collected: infant's gender, weight, and gestational age; mother's age, ethnic/racial identification, education, employment status during the past 6 months, and plans to return to work or school in the child's first year; whether mother's partner was present in the home; and partner's education.

Two-Week Phone Calls. Each week the results of the hospital screenings were used to generate calling lists of eligible families for the 2-week phone calls. For the first 3–4 months of the 11-month enrollment period, the calling list for each site was simply the list of eligible families arranged in random order. For the remainder of the enrollment period, specific family characteristics were monitored, and the order of the calling list for each site was adjusted to increase representation of various subgroups. Each site was expected to enroll at least 10% single-parent households, 10% mothers with less than a high school education, and 10% ethnic minority mothers. Some sites added another hospital to help meet these constraints. In addition, enrolled families at each site were to split approximately 60%, 20%, and 20% on the mothers' plans to return to work full time, part time, and not at all during the child's first year, respectively. This approximate distribution occurred naturally without adjusting the calling list order.

The sites were instructed to follow each week's calling list in sequential order until four calls were completed to families that were eligible for and consented to the 1-month interview. Families were excluded at this stage if (1) the infant had been hospitalized for more than 7 days; (2) the family planned to move from the area within 3 years; (3) there were three unsuccessful calls to reach the family; or (4) the mother refused to participate.

One-Month Interview. Families were officially enrolled in the study upon successful completion of all data collection through the 1-month interview.

If a family that had agreed to the interview did not keep the interview appointment, another family was selected from the current week's calling list. Figure 1.1 portrays the screening process and the number of families excluded and retained at each stage.

Retention

Subject retention has been high compared to other large-sample, multisite longitudinal studies. Of the original 1,364 families, only 131 families (9.6%) had dropped out of the study at the end of Phase I. By the end of data collection for Phase II (when most of the children had finished second grade), 133 additional families had dropped out, leaving a sample of 1,100 families. This translates to a retention rate of 80.6% from the time of recruitment 8 years earlier. As shown in Table 1.2, retention varied somewhat across racial and ethnic categories.

Sample Limitations

Although the families in the study represent a range of socioeconomic and sociocultural backgrounds, the sample is not nationally representative. Compared to Census Bureau figures for all births in the United States in 1991, white, non-Hispanic children are somewhat overrepresented in the sample, and children from ethnic minority groups are somewhat underrepresented (see Table 1.1). The sample does include a sizable black, non-Hispanic subgroup, but the numbers of Hispanic, Asian, and Native American children involved are too small to allow separate analyses of developmental trajectories for all groups included in the study. As shown in Table 1.1, the sample also differs from national patterns for several other demographic characteristics. Mean household income and maternal education level in study families were both higher than the U.S. average. However, sample families were also more likely to receive public assistance than U.S. families in general.

Assessments

Table 1.3 outlines the data collection schedule for Phases I and II of the study. Specifics of the procedures can be found in the study's operation manuals (Phase I: NICHD Early Child Care Research Network, 1993; Phase II: obtainable from NICHD).

Face-to-face assessments during Phases I and II occurred when the children were 1, 6, 15, 24, 36, and 54 months of age, and when they were in first grade. Children were observed in the home, laboratory, child care setting (for those in care more than 10 hours/week), and in school (first grade). Between face-to-face assessments, data were obtained using telephone interviews and questionnaires. During Phase I (birth–36 months), phone calls

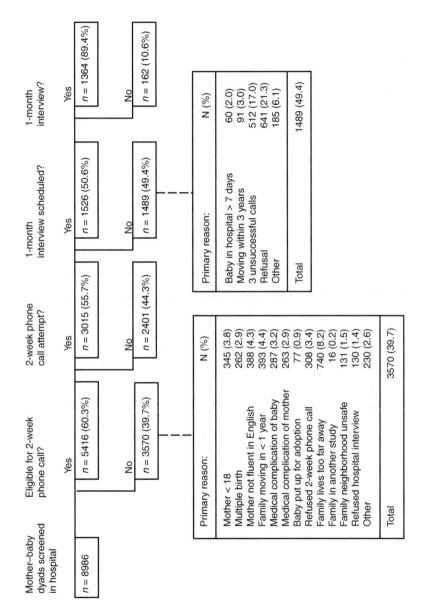

FIGURE 1.1. Overview of NICHD Study of Early Child Care enrollment process.

11

TABLE 1.2. Number of Study Families over Time, by Race/Ethnicity

	Enrollment	End of Phase II	Retention rate
White, non-Hispanic	1,023	840	82.1%
Black, non-Hispanic	175	129	73.7%
Hispanic	90	70	77.8%
Asian	20	15	75.0%
Native American	5	4	80.0%
Other (primarily biracial)	51	42	82.4%
Total	1,364	1,100	80.6%

were made to families every 3 months. During Phase II (37 months–first grade), calls were made every 4 months until the children entered school. Starting in kindergarten, calls were made approximately every 6 months, once during fall semester and once during spring semester.

Throughout the study, research assistants from all sites have been trained and certified on each procedure to ensure the reliable administration of all measures and to guard against variability in practices from site to site. Procedures to ensure uniformity have included:

1. Receiving identical training materials and manuals;
2. Meeting as a group for centralized training workshops;
3. Submitting videotaped examples of several administrations of each measure for certification;
4. Receiving telephone and e-mail feedback on questions that arise before and during data collection; and
5. Participating in careful evaluations of reliability during data collection.

TABLE 1.3. Timing and Location of Assessments for Phases I and II

Assessments	\multicolumn{8}{c}{Time of measurement}

Assessments	1 mo	6 mo	15 mo	24 mo	36 mo	54 mo	K	1st grade
Home	X	X	X	X	X	X	M[a]	X
Laboratory			X	X	X	X		X
Child care		X	X	X	X	X		M[a]
School							M[a]	X
Phone[b]	X	XX	XXX	XXX	XXXX	XXXX	XXX	XX

[a]Mail contacts only.
[b]Multiple Xs indicate the number of contacts since the previous major assessment point.

In most of the families in the study, the mother was the parent primarily involved in assessments of family factors during Phase I. With additional funding from the U.S. Department of Health and Human Services, 6 of the 10 sites (Arkansas, California, Kansas, North Carolina, Pittsburgh, and Wisconsin) expanded Phase I to include direct measures of fathers' attitudes and perceptions. This added component was designed to examine (1) how marital quality and paternal attitudes contribute to families' child care choices and to time use during nonworking family time in families with employed and nonemployed mothers; (2) how marital quality and paternal attitudes influence the quality of mother–child relationships in families with employed and nonemployed mothers; (3) the extent to which maternal employment and reliance on child care may affect the quality of the marital relationship; and (4) the direct and indirect influences of father involvement on children's development, in households with employed and nonemployed mothers.

Measures

Reflecting the ecological and life course frameworks on which the study is based, the child care environment, the home environment, and the child's characteristics are conceptualized as interdependent and evolving over developmental periods and contextual changes. Rather than merely examining child care as an isolated predictor of children's development, the study attempts to untangle the conditions and processes that mediate or moderate connections between child care and developmental outcomes. These include family circumstances, parental characteristics, child characteristics, and experiences of the child both inside and outside the family.

Experience during early development was assessed through a diverse array of measures designed to capture the child's experiences in the contexts of home and family, child care, and school. Measures of social-emotional, cognitive, linguistic, and academic development and physical growth and health were used to assess children's developmental status. In selecting measures, we considered (1) developmental level; (2) psychometric properties of the measure; (3) applicability of measures to children and families of varying ethnicity and socioeconomic status; (4) time needed to complete the measure; (5) relations among measures planned for each visit; and (6) results of pilot testing.

Two criteria were considered in selecting specific child outcomes for assessment. First, the developmental importance of the outcome had to be well documented in previous research and theory. Second, there had to be reasonable support for hypotheses that children's development in the particular domain involved would be affected by early childrearing environments.

Insofar as possible, each construct was evaluated with multiple measures at each assessment point, to increase the reliability and validity of the findings. For example, child care quality was measured by both structural indicators, such as child–caregiver ratio, and process variables, such as frequency and quality of caregiver–child interactions. This approach allows the investigation of the empirical connections between theoretically related measures, some of which are easy to employ for regulation and accreditation of child care settings.

Table 1.4 presents an overview of the child care, school, home, family, and child outcome constructs, along with the ages at which they were assessed.[3] Information on some of the constructs presented in Table 1.4 was also collected during the periodic telephone interviews with the mother.

TABLE 1.4. Constructs for Phases I and II

	Time of measurement							
	1 mo	6 mo	15 mo	24 mo	36 mo	54 mo	K	1st grade
Child care environment								
Structural regularities	X	X	X	X	X	X	X	X
Quantity	X	X	X	X	X	X	X	X
Stability	X	X	X	X	X	X		X
Quality	X	X	X	X	X	X		X
Caregiver characteristics	X	X	X	X	X	X		X
School environment								
Structural context							X	X
School curriculum							X	X
Child's perceptions								X
Home/family environment								
Structural context	X	X	X	X	X	X	X	X
Quality of home life		X	X	X	X	X		X
Parent characteristics	X	X	X	X	X	X	X	X
Social–Emotional								
Quality of relationships		X	X	X	X	X	X	X
Adjustment		X	X	X	X	X	X	X
Self-concept and identity								X
Cognitive development								
Global intellectual functioning			X	X		X		X
Knowledge and achievement					X	X	X	X
Cognitive processes			X	X	X	X	X	X
Language development			X	X	X	X	X	X
Health	X	X	X	X	X	X	X	X

Child Care Environment

At each major assessment point, children who were in child care for 10 or more hours per week during Phase I or 8 or more hours per week during Phase II were observed in their primary child care setting. During Phase I, the primary setting was the one in which the child spent the most time; if the child spent equal time in two settings, the more formal of the two was regarded as the primary setting. During Phase II, the primary setting was, in general, the most formal setting in which the child spent time. Priority was given to settings in which there were other 2- to 6-year-olds who were not siblings of the target child and the caregiver was not the child's mother or father.

Both proximal and distal characteristics of the child care environment were assessed with observations, interviews, and questionnaires. Proximal characteristics include (1) features of the setting experienced directly by the children (e.g., cleanliness and safety, degree to which learning materials were available, number of adults per child, group size) and (2) aspects of individual children's experiences (e.g., age of entry into child care, number of hours per week in child care, number of child care arrangements experienced, and interactions between target children and their caregivers). Distal characteristics are those that are not experienced directly by the children but are believed to influence their day-to-day experiences in child care (e.g., caregivers' education level, years of experience in providing care, attitudes about raising children, and wages and fees). These proximal and distal characteristics provided information about both structural and human interaction dimensions of child care. Data on these characteristics were collected through interviews with caregivers and parents and through observations in the child care settings.

Quantity and Stability of Child Care Experiences. Information on (1) number of hours per week each child spent in child care (quantity) and (2) stability of care (number of child care arrangements started and stopped) was obtained during periodic phone calls to the mother.

Characteristics of Caregivers. Caregivers were asked to provide basic demographic data such as age, education, and ethnic identity, as well as information about length of experience as child care providers, training, and wages. Caregivers' professionalism was assessed in a brief interview concerning attitudes toward the job, reasons for providing care, plans for the future, and participation in professional activities. Caregivers' attitudes toward childrearing were measured using the Modernity Scale (Schaefer & Edgerton, 1985), which provides an estimate of how traditional (strict, conservative) versus modern (progressive) adults' attitudes toward childrearing are.

Characteristics of the Child Care Environment. Type of care, group size, and adult–child ratio were observed in the child care settings that were visited. When access to child care could not be arranged, the information was obtained through an interview with the mother or, in the case of center care, with the center director. Data about other child care features, such as staffing patterns, number and ethnicity of children in the care setting, wages, and fees, were obtained from caregiver and director interviews.

The child care environment was observed and coded using instruments that describe aspects of the setting available to all children in it and instruments that focus on specific interactions of target children with their caregivers. During Phase I, observations of the settings were coded with a child care version of the Home Observation for Measurement of the Environment (HOME) Inventory (Caldwell & Bradley, 1984) developed for the current project and with an adaptation of the Assessment Profile for Early Childhood Programs (Profile; Abbott-Shim & Sibley, 1987, 1993; Abbott-Shim, Sibley, & Neel, 1992). The HOME Inventory was used in all home-based settings (i.e., the target child's home or another person's home) and was designed to measure the quality and quantity of stimulation and support available to a child in the child care environment. Two different versions of the Profile were used, one for centers and one for home settings (care in a home that was not the child's residence). In Phase II (when the children were 54 months old), the Profile was replaced with a new Physical Environment Checklist developed for the study to reflect such aspects of the setting as health and hygiene practices, safety, organization, and stimulation.

To assess interactions between caregivers and children, the study investigators developed the Observational Record of the Caregiving Environment (ORCE; NICHD Early Child Care Research Network, 1996, 2000a). This instrument provides two types of data: (1) frequency counts (called behavior scales) of specific caregiver and child behaviors and (2) ratings (called qualitative ratings) of caregivers' behaviors that take into account the quality of the caregiver's behavior in relation to the child's behaviors. The ORCE can be used in a variety of child care settings, including centers, child care homes, and less formal settings. Because the characteristics of positive caregiving differ by age, the ORCE was systematically adapted to the various ages at which the children were observed.

For the 54-month assessment, the Classroom Practices Inventory (CPI; Hyson, Hirsh-Pasek, & Rescorla, 1990) was also used to assess quality of child care centers or formal preschool settings. The CPI is an observational instrument based on the National Association for the Education of Young Children (NAEYC) guidelines for developmentally appropriate practices for 4- and 5-year-old children. It consists of items that index both the academic activity focus and the emotional climate of the program. The items are rated based on several hours of direct observation.

Characteristics of the Before/After-School Child Care Environment. In first grade, the child's primary before-school or after-school care arrangement was evaluated using questionnaires to the care provider and interviews with the mother and the child. The child's primary arrangement was any nonparental arrangement (including self-care) in which he or she spent at least 5 hours/week. If time spent in two different arrangements was similar, the primary arrangement was the one that was more formal. If there was no nonparental arrangement of at least 5 hours/week, then parental care was the primary arrangement. Information was collected on type of care, quantity and stability of care, caregiver characteristics, and perceptions of care quality and satisfaction. Measures of the mother's and child's satisfaction with care were used because they have been found to be related to observed quality of care. The mother's satisfaction with the child's primary before/after-school arrangement was assessed using a scale developed for the study based on scales by O'Connor (1991) and Rosenthal and Vandell (1996). The child's satisfaction was assessed using a modification of the After School Questionnaire (ASQ; Rosenthal & Vandell, 1996). This questionnaire, given in the form of an interview, focuses on children's feelings of support from peers and caregivers in their after-school settings, as well as their general feelings about the arrangement.

School Environment

Kindergarten. When children were in kindergarten, teachers completed a questionnaire pertaining to the child's classroom, the instructional program, and the supports and challenges individual teachers experienced within the school. Included were questions about the teacher's background and the background of any aide present in the classroom. The teacher also completed a questionnaire on the student–teacher relationship (Pianta, 1992). Items in this questionnaire are derived from attachment theory and the Attachment Q-Set (Waters & Deane, 1985), as well as from a review of the literature on teacher–child relationships. The items address the teacher's feelings and beliefs about his or her relationship with the child and about the child's behavior toward the teacher.

First Grade. In first grade, the school environment was assessed through a classroom observation, a recess observation, teacher-completed questionnaires, and school records. Information was obtained on school and teacher characteristics, teacher–student relationships, and parental involvement.

An observation system called the First Grade Classroom Observation System (COS-1) was developed for the study. The COS-1 is a multiconstruct, multilevel observational system that includes both behavior frequencies and global rating scales. The frequency data are focused on four categories: (1) *activity*, the situation or activity in which the target child is involved; (2) *con-*

tent, the content of the activity; (3) *teacher behavior*, behavior directed at the target child; and (4) *child behavior*, child engagement and behavior toward the teacher and peers. The global ratings capture classroom-level factors, such as climate and classroom management strategies, and aspects of the teacher's behavior toward individual children, such as sensitivity and intrusiveness/overcontrol.

A recess observation to assess peer interaction was conducted using the First Grade Unstructured Peer Interaction Observation System, a measure modeled on the ORCE and the COS-1. Behavior frequencies were recorded in the areas of activity, teacher behavior, child's behavior with peers, and child engagement, along with information about the settings in which behaviors were seen. Qualitative rating scales were used to record the child's negative affect, positive affect, prosocial behavior, and assertiveness, as well as the teacher's monitoring and involvement.

Home Environment

Measures of the home/family context were designed to assess structural characteristics of the family, quality of home life, and parent characteristics.

Structural Characteristics of the Family.   In phone and face-to-face interviews, information was collected regularly and frequently about who lived in the child's household. Mothers were also asked if the child had formal or informal alternate custodial arrangements. Household structure (nuclear two-parent family, extended two-parent family, single-parent family, extended single-parent family, blended two-parent family, etc.) and the stability/fluidity of the composition of the child's household were coded. Information was obtained about the child's father and/or the mother's partner and, when the father was not in the home, the child's contact with him.

Mothers reported on both maternal and paternal employment. Mothers were asked whether they were working for pay and whether they were on leave from a job. Because many mothers and fathers had multiple jobs, information was collected about each job currently held by each parent, including the number of hours, income, start and stop dates, times of day worked, and hours of the paid job worked at home. Occupation codes from the U.S. Census Bureau were used to describe jobs, and these 13 codes were later collapsed into three occupational levels: executive/professional, white collar, and blue collar. Mothers were asked to rate how satisfied they and their partners were with their family's current employment situation and to identify what employment situation they would ideally prefer. Information about parents' school enrollment, hours devoted to school, and class schedules was also obtained.

Quality of the Home Environment.   The quality of the home environment was assessed using information about (1) parental attitudes and perceptions of socialization; (2) observed parental sensitivity, stimulation, and quality of assistance; and (3) observed parental involvement.

During Phase I, parenting style was assessed by asking parents about their attitudes toward raising children, using the Modernity Scale (Schaefer & Edgerton, 1985). This instrument is designed to measure parents' traditional authoritarian and progressive democratic beliefs. During Phase II, parents were asked about parental discipline strategies using a scale called Raising Children (Posner & Vandell, 1994), which was modified from the Raising Children Checklist (Greenberger & Goldberg, 1989). This scale measures three dimensions of parental control: firm responsiveness, harshness, and laxness. Parents also completed a modified version of the Maturity Demands Scale (Greenberger & Goldberg, 1989), which measures parental demands for mature behavior from the child.

Sensitivity, stimulation, and quality of assistance were observed using ratings of the quality of parents' interaction with their children during videotaped mother–child and father–child tasks. The tasks provided a context for assessing age-appropriate qualities of supportiveness, intrusiveness, positive regard, hostility, and quality of instruction in both mother–child and father–child interaction.

The HOME Inventory (Caldwell & Bradley, 1984) was used to assess the quality of the family environment. The HOME Inventory consists of direct observation and a semistructured interview with the mother and is designed to measure the quality and quantity of stimulation and support available to a child at home. The focus is on the child in the environment, as a recipient of inputs from objects, events, and interactions.

Parental involvement was assessed with questionnaires focusing on the relative roles of father and mother in caring for the target child, the extent of each parent's contact with caregivers or teachers, and each parent's level of involvement in the child's schooling.

Parental Characteristics. Mothers' and fathers' health, depression, social support, life stress, job stress, financial stress, and marital quality were measured in interviews and questionnaires at multiple points throughout the study. During the telephone interviews, mothers were asked about their general health status and were asked to describe the health of their husband/partner. During the home visits, mothers who had referred to a medical problem at an earlier contact were asked additional questions about their medical problems and contacts with physicians. Mothers and fathers/partners completed the Center for Epidemiological Studies–Depression (CES-D) scale, a self-report measure designed to measure depressive symptomatology (Radloff, 1977). Mothers completed the Relationships with Other People Questionnaire, designed to assess their general perception of availability of social support (Marshall & Barnett, 1993). To assess life stress, mothers completed the Life Experiences Survey (LES; Sarason, Johnson, & Siegel, 1978). The LES lists a number of stressful life events, and respondents report which ones have occurred in their lives over the last year and rate the degree of stress associated with the event. The Job Experience Scale (modified from the Job Role Quality Scale; Barnett & Marshall, 1991) was used to measure mothers' and fathers' job stress. On this scale, parents rate conditions on their jobs, the level of reward or concern associated with these conditions, and how rewarding or stressful their job situations are overall. Family financial stress was measured at every assessment period, using a self-report instrument developed for the study, with items on parents' satisfaction with their financial situation, worry about financial matters, and predictability of income. To assess marital quality, both mothers and fathers/partners completed the emotional intimacy subscale from the Personal Assessment of Intimacy in Relationships (PAIR) Inventory (Schaefer & Olson, 1981). Mothers also completed the love, conflict, and ambivalence subscales of a measure by Braiker and Kelly (1979).

Child Outcomes

Measures of child outcome were designed to assess social–emotional functioning, cognitive development, and health and physical development. Social–emotional constructs included (1) quality of relationships (with mother, father, friends, caregivers, and teachers); (2) adjustment (emotional adjustment, social competence, behavior problems, and self-regulation); and (3) self-concept and identity. Cognitive constructs included (1) global intellectual functioning; (2) knowledge and achievement (school readiness and literacy); (3) cognitive processes (attention, problem solving, and memory); and (4) language development. Constructs from the health domain included health (status, illnesses, injuries, and health care usage) and growth (height and weight).

Table 1.5 and Table 1.6 list the outcome measures collected when the children were 1, 6, 15, 24, 36, and 54 months of age and when they were in kindergarten and first grade. In addition to the measures shown in the tables, information was also collected about school attendance, referral to special services (e.g., speech/language, tutoring, and gifted/talented), and retention in grade.

Units of Analysis

The NICHD Study of Early Child Care was designed as a study of the development of children in contexts over time. Multiple assessments of the target children's families, child care settings, schools, and after-school settings were collected to provide information about the contexts in which the children were reared. Some measures focused on the experiences of the target children in these settings, including interaction with others. Other assessments focused on household characteristics (e.g., income and number of people), parents (e.g., education, employment, and attitudes), the home

TABLE 1.5. Phase I Child Outcome Measures

	Source(s) of data at each assessment point[a]					Data type	Reference
	1 mo	6 mo	15 mo	24 mo	36 mo		
Social–emotional constructs							
Quality of relationships							
Mother–child interaction		M, C	M, C	M, C	M, C	Observation	NICHD ECCRN (1993)
Child care separation/reunion scale (attachment)		Cg	Cg	Cg		Questionnaire	NICHD ECCRN (1993)
Strange Situation (attachment)			C			Observation	Ainsworth and Wittig (1969)
Attachment Q-Set				C		Observation	Waters and Deane (1985)
Separation–reunion					C	Observation	Cassidy et al. (1992)
Peer observation					C	Observation	NICHD ECCRN (1993)
ORCE behavior scales (Frequency of Child's Activity, Child's Interaction with Other Children)		C	C	C	C	Observation	NICHD ECCRN (1993, 1996)
ORCE qualitative ratings (sociability with peers)		C	C	C	C	Observation	NICHD ECCRN (1993, 1996)
Adjustment							
Early Infant Temperament Questionnaire (EITQ)	M					Questionnaire	Medoff-Cooper, Carey, and McDevitt (1993)
Revised Infant Temperament Questionnaire (ITQ-R)		M, Cg				Questionnaire	Carey and McDevitt (1978)
Child Behavior Checklist (CBCL)				M, Cg	M	Questionnaire	Achenbach, Edelbrock, and Howell (1987)
ORCE behavior scales (Frequency of Says "No"/Refuses Adult, Acts Defiant to Adult)			C	C	C	Observation	NICHD ECCRN (1993, 2000a)

(continued)

21

TABLE 1.5. *(continued)*

	Source(s) of data at each assessment point[a]						Data type	Reference
	1 mo	6 mo	15 mo	24 mo	36 mo			
Social–emotional constructs *(cont.)*								
Adjustment (cont.)								
ORCE Behavior Scales (Frequency of Prosocial Acts, Negative Acts [Nonaggressive], Verbal Aggression, Physical Aggression, Complies with Adult)				C	C		Observation	NICHD ECCRN (1993, 2000a)
ORCE qualitative ratings (positive mood, negative mood, activity level)		C	C	C	C		Observation	NICHD ECCRN (1993, 1996, 2000a)
Compliance: Bayley				C			Observation	NICHD ECCRN (2000a)
Compliance: Lab clean-up				C	C		Observation	NICHD ECCRN (2000a)
Compliance: Growth					C		Observation	NICHD ECCRN (1993)
Resistance to temptation/Self-control (forbidden toy)					C		Observation	NICHD ECCRN (2000a)
Cognitive constructs								
Global intellectual functioning								
Bayley MDI			C	C			Child test	Bayley (1969, 1993)
Knowledge and achievement								
Bracken Test of Basic Concepts (school readiness)					C		Child test	Bracken (1984)

22

Cognitive processes

Measure					Method	Source
Play complexity (solitary play)			C	C	Observation	Belsky and Most (1981)
Attention (solitary play)			C	C	Observation	NICHD ECCRN (1993)
Attention (CBCL)			M, Cg	M	Questionnaire	Achenbach, Edelbrock, and Howell (1987)
ORCE qualitative ratings (sustained attention)		C	C	C	Observation	NICHD ECCRN (1993, 1996)

Language development

Measure					Method	Source
MacArthur Communicative Development Inventory			M	M	Questionnaire	Fenson et al. (1994)
Reynell Developmental Language Scales				C	Child test	Reynell (1991)

Health constructs

Measure					Method	Source
Growth (height and weight)		C	C	C	Observation	NICHD ECCRN (1993)
Health status[b]	M	M	M	M	Interview	NICHD ECCRN (1993)
Ear infections[b,c]	M	M	M	M	Interview	NICHD ECCRN (1993)
Respiratory infections[b]	M	M	M	M	Interview	NICHD ECCRN (1993)
Gastrointestinal illnesses[b]	M	M	M	M	Interview	NICHD ECCRN (1993)
Chronic illnesses	M	M	M	M	Interview	NICHD ECCRN (1993)
Injury		M	M	M	Interview	NICHD ECCRN (1993)
Sleep	M	M	M	M	Interview	NICHD ECCRN (1993)

[a]M, mother; Cg, caregiver; C, child.
[b]Information also collected from phone calls every 3 months.
[c]Information also obtained from medical records at physician's office or clinic where child received primary medical care.

TABLE 1.6. Phase II Child Outcome Measures

	Source(s) of data at each assessment point[a]			Data type	Reference
	54 mo	K	Grade 1		
Social–emotional constructs					
Quality of relationships					
Adult–child interaction	M, F, C		M, F, C	Observation	NICHD ECCRN[b]
Playmates	M	M	M	Questionnaire	NICHD ECCRN[b]
Friendship/peer observation	C		C	Observation	NICHD ECCRN[b]
Friends or foes	Cg	T	T, Cg	Questionnaire	Ladd (1983)
STRS (my child's relationship with me; with caregiver/teacher)	M, F, Cg	M, T	M, F, T	Questionnaire	Pianta (1992, 1994)
Classroom Observation System (frequency of child behavior toward teacher, child behavior toward peers)			C	Observation	NICHD ECCRN[b]
Sociometric rating system		T	T, Cg	Questionnaire	Cillessen, Terry, Coie, and Lochman (1998)
After-school Questionnaire			C	Questionnaire	Rosenthal and Vandell (1996)
ORCE qualitative ratings (social withdrawal from peers)	C			Observation	NICHD ECCRN[b]
Adjustment					
Social Skills Rating Scale	M, F	M, T	M, F, T, Cg	Questionnaire	Gresham and Elliott (1990)
Social Problem Solving Task	C			Child test	Rubin (1983)
Delay of Gratification	C			Child test	Mischel, Ebbesen, and Zeiss (1972)
Child Behavior Checklist	M, F, Cg	M, T	M, F, T, Cg	Questionnaire	Achenbach (1991a, 1991c)
Child Behavior Questionnaire (temperament)	M, Cg			Questionnaire	Rothbart, Ahadi, and Hershey (1994)

Measure	Reporter	Method	Source
ORCE behavior scales (Frequency of Prosocial, Complies with Adult, Says "No"/Refuses Adult, Acts Defiant to Adult)	C	Observation	NICHD ECCRN [b]
ORCE qualitative ratings (self-reliance, aggression/angry affect, positive affect/mood, activity level)	C	Observation	NICHD ECCRN [b]
California Preschool Social Competency Scale	Cg	Questionnaire	Levine, Elzey, and Lewis (1969)
Attribution Biases	C	Child interview	Feshbach (1989)
Loneliness and Social Dissatisfaction Questionnaire	C	Child questionnaire	Asher, Hymel, and Renshaw (1984)
Classroom Observation System (qualitative ratings of self-reliance, positive affect, activity level/restlessness; frequency of disruptive behavior)	C	Observation	NICHD ECCRN [b]
Getting ready for school (adjustment to school)	M, T	Questionnaire	Pianta (1995)
Attendance, referrals, retention	T	Questionnaire	NICHD ECCRN [b]
Self-concept and identity			
Ethnic preference and identity	C	Child test	Johnson, Chung, and Levy (1998)
Cognitive constructs			
Knowledge and achievement			
Woodcock–Johnson–Revised (achievement, tests 22, 25: reading, mathematics)	C	Child test	Woodcock and Johnson (1989)
Woodcock–Johnson–Revised (achievement, test 31: reading)	C	Child test	Woodcock and Johnson (1989)
Teacher Questionnaire (academic skills)	T	Questionnaire	Nicholson, Atkins-Burnett, and Meisels (1997)
Child Evaluation (mock report card)	T	Questionnaire	Pierce, Hamm, and Vandell (1999)

(continued)

25

TABLE 1.6. *(continued)*

	Source(s) of Data at Each Assessment Point[a]				
	54 mo	K	Grade 1	Data Type	Reference
Cognitive constructs *(cont.)*					
Cognitive processes					
Woodcock–Johnson–Revised (cognitive ability, tests 2, 4, 6; short-term memory, auditory processing, comprehension–knowledge)	C		C	Child test	Woodcock and Johnson (1989)
Woodcock–Johnson–Revised (cognitive ability, test 1: long-term retrieval)			C	Child test	Woodcock and Johnson (1989)
Stroop Task (impulsivity)	C			Child test	Gerstadt, Hong, and Diamond (1994)
Continuous performance test (CPT) (attention)	C		C	Child test	Rosvold, Mirsky, Sarason, Bransome, and Beck (1956)
Child Behavior Checklist (attention)	M, F, Cg	M, T	M, F, T, Cg	Questionnaire	Achenbach (1991a, 1991c)
Tower of Hanoi (planning/problem solving)			C	Child test	Welsh (1991)
ORCE qualitative ratings (attention)	C			Observation	NICHD ECCRN[b]
Classroom Observation System (frequency of child engagement–attention)			C	Observation	NICHD ECCRN[b]

Language development

Measure			Method	Source
Preschool Language Scale	C		Child test	Zimmerman, Steiner, and Pond (1979)
Adaptive Language Inventory	Cg		Questionnaire	Feagans and Farran (1983, 1995)
ORCE Behaviorals (Frequency of asks adult question, child other talk)	C		Observation	NICHD ECCRN[b]
Health Constructs				
Growth (height and weight)[c]	C	C	Observation	NICHD ECCRN[b]
Health status[c]	M	M	Interview	NICHD ECCRN[b]
Ear infections[c]	M	M	Interview	NICHD ECCRN[b]
Respiratory infections[c]	M	M	Interview	NICHD ECCRN[b]
Gastrointestinal illnesses[c]	M	M	Interview	NICHD ECCRN[b]
Chronic illnesses	M	M	Interview	NICHD ECCRN[b]
Injury	M	M	Interview	NICHD ECCRN[b]

[a]M, mother; F, father; Cg, caregiver; T, teacher; C, child.
[b]Procedural manuals for Phase II may be obtained from the NICHD Study of Early Child Care, NICHD, 6100 Executive Boulevard, Room 2C01, Bethesda, MD 20892-7510.
[c]Information also collected from phone calls every 4 months.

environment (e.g., availability of books), child care providers (e.g., education, experience, and attitudes), child care environments (e.g., adult–child ratio, group size, and licensing), teachers, and school environments. Because data were collected about the children from multiple contexts (home, child care setting, and school) and varied people (parents, child care providers, and teachers), data can be analyzed without regard to target child in order to answer questions about these contexts and categories of people. However, in most analyses conducted to date, the unit of analysis is the individual child.

SUMMARY OF MAJOR RESULTS

To date, results have been published from Phase I of the study, covering the period from birth to 36 months. Major analyses have focused on characterizing the early nonmaternal care experiences of the children in the study and examining how early care experiences and family factors are associated with child outcomes.

Early Nonmaternal Care Experiences

Amount and Nature of Nonmaternal Care

During their first year of life, the children in the study experienced high rates of nonmaternal care, with early entry into care, relatively long hours of care, and frequent changes in care arrangements. The average age at which the children entered nonmaternal care was just over 3 months (NICHD Early Child Care Research Network, 1997a). At 12 months, 68.6% of the children were regularly receiving nonmaternal care, and 80% had experienced some form of regularly scheduled nonmaternal care by that time.

When the children first entered care, their primary care arrangement was most often with their father or their mother's partner (25%), with grandparents or other relatives (25%), or with nonrelatives in child care homes (24%); only about 13% were cared for in their homes by nonrelatives (i.e., nannies or babysitters) and 13% were enrolled in child care centers. By age 1, children had become somewhat less likely to be cared for by fathers/partners (23%), grandparents/other relatives (21%), or nannies/babysitters (12%), and more likely to be cared for in child care homes (27%) and child care centers (17%). Over the first year of life, the majority of children in nonparental care experienced more than two different child care arrangements, and more than one-third experienced three or more arrangements (NICHD Early Child Care Research Network, 1997a).

At their first entry into nonmaternal care, the children averaged 29 hours of care per week (NICHD Early Child Care Research Network, 1997a); by age 12 months, children in care averaged 33.9 hours/week. As

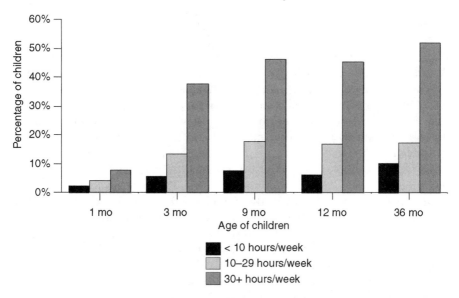

FIGURE 1.2. Children in nonmaternal care during first 3 years of life.

shown in Figure 1.2, from the first month of life, a majority of the children who were in nonmaternal care spent 30 or more hours a week there. At 12 months, nearly half of all the children in the study (45.3%) were in care for 30 or more hours a week.

By the time they were 36 months old, 92% of the children had experienced some form of regular nonmaternal care, 80% were presently in nonmaternal care, and 52% were regularly spending 30 or more hours a week in care. As shown in Figure 1.2, the amount of time the children spent in care had risen only slightly from the first year of life; children in care at 36 months averaged 34.4 hours/week. However, the type of care had changed considerably, with 44% in center care, 25% in child care homes, 12% cared for by their father or their mother's partner, 10% cared for by in-home nannies or babysitters, and 9% cared for by grandparents (NICHD Early Child Care Research Network, 2000a).

It is difficult to compare the prevalence of various care arrangements in the study sample with figures reported in nationwide surveys because of differences in data collection and reporting across studies. However, when care by father or mother's partner is excluded, the overall proportion of children in nonparental care in the NICHD Study of Early Child Care (53% at 12 months, 70% at 36 months) is comparable to proportions reported for 1-year-olds (50%) and 3-year-olds (68%) in the 1995 National Household Education Survey (National Center for Education Statistics, 1995).

Economic factors accounted for much of the variability in the amount and nature of infants' nonmaternal care, but family characteristics and mothers' attitudes and beliefs played a role as well, as shown in Table 1.7 (NICHD Early Child Care Research Network, 1997c). Family and maternal income were involved in every aspect of the children's care experiences, including the age at which they entered care, hours spent in care, and type of care received. Families with the lowest nonmaternal income were the most likely to place infants in care before age 3 months, probably because they were the most dependent on the mother's income. In contrast, infants from families with the highest maternal and nonmaternal incomes tended to start care between 3 and 5 months. Infants who started care after 5 months most often came from families with income between the two extremes. The higher their mothers' earnings, the more hours infants spent in nonmaternal care; however, the higher the *nonmaternal* earnings in their family, the *fewer* hours they spent in care. Families with low maternal and nonmaternal earnings were the most likely to rely on fathers or other relatives for child care, whereas families and mothers with high incomes were the most likely to use in-home care provided by nonrelatives.

Family characteristics other than income did not seem to influence the age at which infants entered care, but they were involved in the number of hours infants spent in care and the type of care they received. For example, infants with more siblings spent less time in care than other infants and were more likely to be cared for by their fathers and to receive in-home care. Maternal education was associated with both hours and type of care; the more education mothers had, the fewer hours the infants spent in care, the less likely they were to be cared for by fathers or grandparents, and the more likely they were to receive in-home care from a nonrelative.

TABLE 1.7. Factors Associated with Use of Nonmaternal Care in the First 15 Months of Life

	Age at entry	Hours of care	Type of care
Economic factors			
Maternal income	*	+	*
Nonmaternal income	*	–	*
Family characteristics			
Family size		–	*
Maternal education		–	*
Maternal attitudes and beliefs			
Benefits of work	–	+	
Risks of work		–	*
Nonauthoritarian childrearing		+	

Note. +, positive relationship; –, negative relationship; *, nonlinear relationship. Source: NICHD Early Child Care Research Network (1997c).

Finally, maternal attitudes and beliefs contributed to the age at which infants entered care and the hours and type of care they received. Mothers who believed their children benefited from their employment tended to place their infants in care earlier and for more hours. Nonauthoritarian childrearing attitudes were also associated with a higher number of hours in nonmaternal care. In contrast, mothers who believed maternal employment carried high risks for children tended to put their infants in care for fewer hours and were especially likely to rely on their infant's father for child care.

Quality of Nonmaternal Care

Observations of quality of nonmaternal care received by the children in the study at 6 months indicated that more positive caregiving occurred when children were in smaller groups, child–adult ratios were lower, caregivers held less authoritarian beliefs about childrearing, and physical environments were safe, clean, and stimulating (NICHD Early Child Care Research Network, 1996, 1997e). Observed quality of care for poor children was generally lower than for nonpoor children when they were cared for by an unrelated caregiver, with one exception: Poor children in centers received better quality care than did near-poor children, perhaps because they were more likely to be in subsidized settings, which tend to be more regulated.

However, when the child care center classes attended by children in the study at ages 6, 15, 24, and 36 months were evaluated against guidelines of the American Public Health Association and the American Academy of Pediatrics (1992), the results were not encouraging. These guidelines include standards for child–staff ratio (3:1 at 6 and 15 months, 4:1 at 24 months, 7:1 at 36 months), group size (6 at 6 and 15 months, 8 at 24 months, 14 at 36 months), and caregiver training (formal, post-high school training in child development, early childhood education, or a related field at all four ages). An additional higher education standard (caregivers with at least some college) was also included in the evaluation. As shown in Table 1.8, most classes observed in the study did not meet all four of these guidelines.

TABLE 1.8. Percentage of Child Care Classes Meeting Recommended Guidelines at Ages 6–36 Months

	6 mo	15 mo	24 mo	36 mo
Child–staff ratio	36%	20%	26%	56%
Observed group size	35%	25%	28%	63%
Caregiver training	56%	60%	65%	75%
Caregiver education	65%	69%	77%	80%

Early Care Experiences and Child Outcomes

Several aspects of early nonmaternal care experiences were found to be associated with social–emotional, cognitive, and health-related child outcomes in the first 3 years of life. Table 1.9 provides an overview of the results for quality, amount, type, and stability of nonmaternal care.

Quality of Care

After controlling for nonrandom use of child care by families of different socioeconomic backgrounds, the observed quality of nonmaternal care emerged as a consistent predictor of child outcomes during the first 3 years of life. Observed quality of caregivers' behavior—particularly the amount of language stimulation provided—was positively related to children's performance on measures of cognitive and linguistic abilities at ages 15, 24, and 36 months (NICHD Early Child Care Research Network, 2000b).

Quality of care was also related to measures of social and emotional development. At 24 months, children who had experienced higher-quality care were reported to have fewer behavior problems by both their mothers and their caregivers and were rated higher on social competence by their mothers (NICHD Early Child Care Research Network, 1998a). At 36 months, higher-quality care was associated with greater compliance and less negative behavior during mother–child interactions and fewer caregiver-reported behavior problems.

Over the first 3 years of life, higher-quality child care was also associated with greater maternal sensitivity during mother–child interaction among the families that used nonmaternal care (NICHD Early Child Care Research Network, 1999a). In addition, poor-quality child care was related to an increased incidence of insecure infant–mother attachment at 15 months, but only when the mother was also relatively low in sensitivity and responsiveness (NICHD Early Child Care Research Network, 1997b).

TABLE 1.9. Summary of Findings: Aspects of Child Care and Developmental Outcomes[a]

	Attachment	Parent–child relationships	Non-compliance in child care	Problem behaviors	Cognitive development and school readiness	Language development
Quality	*	*		+	+	+
Amount	*	*		*		
Type			*	*	+	+
Stability	*		*			

Note. +, consistent effects; *, effects under some conditions.
[a] After controlling for child and family variables.

The extent to which children's child care center classes met professional guidelines was related to developmental outcomes at 24 and 36 months (NICHD Early Child Care Research Network, 1999b). Children in classes that met the guidelines for child–staff ratio had fewer behavior problems and more positive social behaviors at both ages. Three-year-olds in classes that met the standards for caregiver training and higher education showed greater school readiness, better language comprehension, and fewer behavior problems. The *number* of standards met did not seem to make a difference for 2-year-olds. In 3-year-old classes, however, the higher the number of standards met, the better the children scored on measures of school readiness, language comprehension, and behavior problems.

Preliminary results from Phase II of the study indicate that quality of care continued to be associated with developmental outcomes throughout the preschool years. At age 54 months, overall quality of child care experienced since infancy retained its positive association with children's performance on tests of preacademic skills and language (NICHD Early Child Care Research Network, 2001f). In addition, structural measures of quality (child–staff ratio and caregiver training) were associated with proximal measures of caregiving quality, which in turn were associated with measures of children's cognitive and social competence (NICHD Early Child Care Research Network, 2002b).

Quantity of Care

The quantity of nonmaternal care was also a statistically significant predictor of some child outcomes. When children spent more hours in child care, mothers were less sensitive in their interactions with their children (at 6, 15, 24, and 36 months) and children were less positively engaged with their mothers (at 15, 24, and 36 months) (NICHD Early Child Care Research Network, 1999a). In addition, analyses of attachment at 15 months showed that children who spent more hours in child care *and* had mothers who were relatively insensitive and unresponsive were at heightened risk for insecure infant–mother attachments (NICHD Early Child Care Research Network, 1997c). At 24 months, spending more hours in care was associated with mothers' reports of lower social competence and caregivers' reports of more problem behaviors (NICHD Early Child Care Research Network, 1998b). These associations were not seen at 36 months, but preliminary results from Phase II show a reappearance of quantity effects later in the preschool years. At 54 months, quantity of care was once again positively associated with caregiver-reported behavior problems (NICHD Early Child Care Research Network, 2001f). At the kindergarten assessment, quantity of care was associated with both teacher and mother ratings of problem behaviors (NICHD Early Child Care Research Network, 2001d).

Type of Care

Type of child care was clearly associated with rates of early communicable illnesses (NICHD Early Child Care Research Network, 2001a). Children attending child care centers and child care homes had more ear infections and upper respiratory illnesses than did children cared for at home, especially during the first 2 years of life. The number of other children in the child care setting was also positively related to frequency of upper respiratory illnesses and gastrointestinal illnesses through age 3. However, these heightened rates of illness did not seem to have significant adverse developmental consequences over the first 3 years of life.

Otherwise, type of care by itself seemed to have a relatively low impact on child outcomes. At age 2, children who were being cared for in child care centers and child care homes did better on measures of cognitive and language development than did children in other forms of care. By age 3, greater *cumulative* experience in center care and *early* experience in child care homes were both associated with better performance on cognitive and language measures than other forms of care, assuming comparable quality of caregiving environment (NICHD Early Child Care Research Network, 2000a). Based on preliminary results from Phase II, at 54 months cumulative experience in center care continued to be positively associated with performance on cognitive and linguistic measures; at this age, cumulative center care experience was also associated with caregiver reports of externalizing behavior problems (NICHD Early Child Care Research Network, 2001h).

Experience with group care (settings with at least three other children, not counting siblings), whether in centers or child care homes, made some difference in several social–emotional outcomes at ages 2 and 3 (NICHD Early Child Care Research Network, 1998a). Children with more cumulative experience in group care showed more cooperation with their mothers in the laboratory at age 2, less negative laboratory interaction with their mothers at age 3, and fewer caregiver-reported behavior problems at both ages. However, greater group experience before 12 months was associated with more mother-reported behavior problems at age 3, suggesting that benefits from group care may begin in the second year of life.

Stability of Care

Stability of care—the number of times children changed care arrangements—appeared to have a limited impact on child outcomes. At 15 months, children who had experienced more changes in care arrangements *and* maternal insensitivity were at heightened risk of insecure attachment (NICHD Early Child Care Research Network, 1997b). At age 2, experience with more child care arrangements was associated with a higher number of behavior problems, as reported by mothers and observed in the child care setting.

However, this relation was not found at age 3, suggesting that stability of care may be particularly salient during developmentally significant transitions (NICHD Early Child Care Research Network, 1998a).

Family Factors and Child Outcomes

Analyses of the effects of child care experiences and family factors on child outcomes indicated that family characteristics were more consistent predictors of both social–emotional and cognitive child outcomes through age 3 than were child care factors. In addition, family factors predicted child outcomes similarly for children who spent many hours in child care and for children in exclusive maternal care (NICHD Early Child Care Research Network, 1998b).

In the social–emotional domain, mothers' sensitivity, responsiveness, and overall psychological adjustment predicted infant–mother attachment security at 15 months, but observed quality and amount of nonmaternal care, age at entry into care, and frequency of changes in care arrangements did not (NICHD Early Child Care Research Network, 1997b). However, low-quality nonmaternal care, spending more than 10 hours/week in care, and changes in care arrangements did increase the risk of insecure attachment when combined with low maternal sensitivity.

Secure infant–mother attachment at 15 months in turn predicted more positive mother–infant interaction at 24 months and fewer mother-reported behavior problems at 36 months. In addition, maternal sensitivity during the first 2 years of life was a better predictor of self-control, compliance, and problem behaviors at 24 and 36 months than any aspect of children's early nonmaternal care experiences (NICHD Early Child Care Research Network, 1998a).

In the cognitive domain, family factors accounted for a much larger share of the variance in cognitive and linguistic outcomes across the first 3 years of life than child care factors did (NICHD Early Child Care Research Network, 2000b). Maternal vocabulary and quality of home environment were significant predictors of cognitive and language development at 15, 24, and 36 months. Family income-to-needs ratio and observed maternal cognitive stimulation predicted performance on cognitive measures at 24 and 36 months and on language measures at 36 months.

To help provide a comprehensive picture of children's early developmental contexts, connections between family factors and child outcomes have also been examined without regard to early child care experiences. For example, maternal depressive symptoms were found to be linked to mother–child interaction and child outcomes in several ways (NICHD Early Child Care Research Network, 1999c). Mothers who chronically reported feelings of depression showed less sensitivity in play with their children during the first 3 years of life than mothers who sometimes or never reported depressive symptoms. In turn, children of women with depressive symptoms performed more poorly on measures of cognitive–linguistic functioning, cooperation, and problem behavior at 36 months. For some measures, differences in maternal sensitivity accounted for the poorer outcomes among children of depressed women; for others, maternal sensitivity appeared to act as a buffer.

CONCLUSION

The NICHD Study of Early Child Care provides an exceptionally rich data set for addressing questions about the significance of varying contexts of development from infancy through middle childhood. The fine-grained information collected about children's experiences at home, in child care settings, and at school facilitates examination of the interplay among familial and extrafamilial influences on development. Results from Phase I of the study, covering the first 3 years of life, make it clear that the impact of early child care experiences cannot be adequately assessed without reference to children's experiences in their families. In both cognitive and social-emotional domains, quality and type of child care have a clear impact on child outcomes even after controlling for family factors. However, family influences are consistently better predictors of children's outcomes than early child care experiences alone. This is not to say that children's experiences with nonmaternal care are not significant but simply that the impact of those experiences often depends on other factors in a child's life. For example, the quality of child care can make a particular difference in social-emotional outcomes for children who do not experience sensitive care at home. All these findings have potential implications for public policy and for families making decisions about care arrangements for their children.

NOTES

1. Additional details about the history and current status of the study can be found at the study's website, *http://www.nichd.nih.gov/od/secc/index.htm*.
2. A list of publications from the NICHD Study of Early Child Care is available at the study's website, *http://www.nichd.nih.gov/od/secc/index.htm*.
3. A list of the specific measures used in Phase I of the study is available on the study's website, *http://www.nichd.nih.gov/od/secc/index.htm*; a list of measures used in Phase II can be obtained by writing to NICHD.

II

—

Child Care Use and Quality

The chapters included in this section describe child care in the United States in the early 1990s, with a special emphasis on child care quality. The National Institute of Child Health and Human Development (NICHD) investigators collected information about the whole range of child care settings used by parents, including care by relatives and nonrelatives in the child's home or elsewhere and care in centers and licensed family child care homes. The information collected in the study pertains to age of entry into care, the number of hours per week that children spend in child care, the stability of care, the type of care, and the quality of care. Quality of care is assessed in terms of standards that can be regulated and in terms of the quality of the experiences of the children participating in the study. Standards of quality that can be regulated include adult–child ratio, the education level and professional experience of child care providers, and the group size in settings in which several children receive care. These standards are often referred to as the structural aspects of child care. The experience of children in child care is assessed during lengthy and repeated visits to the settings. During these sessions observers use time sampling methods and rating scales to assess the quality of the study child experiences with the child care provider and with peers.

The 10 sites comprising the NICHD investigation examined information concerning the use, patterning, and stability of nonmaternal child care during the first year of life for 1,281 families. Chapter 2 presents the results, which reveal high reliance on nonmaternal infant care, very rapid entry into such care postbirth, and substantial instability in child care arrangements.

Chapter 3 reports results from observations of 576 6-month-old infants and their nonmaternal caregivers. Babies were observed in five types of nonmaternal child care (centers, child care homes, in-home "sitter" arrangements, grandparents, and fathers). An overall measure of "positive caregiving," based on extensive observations of care providers' interactions with the study children, was developed by the investigators who then studied it in relation to type of care, group size, adult–child ratio, the physical environment, and attitudes of the care providers. Positive caregiving is more frequent when group size and child–adult ratios are small rather than large, when caregivers have nonauthoritarian beliefs about childrearing, and when physical environments are safe and stimulating.

Children with special needs frequently require nonmaternal care. Consequently, Chapter 4 describes and compares maternal employment patterns, child care characteristics, and maternal concerns of a group of 166 children with special needs with those of typically developing children and their mothers. The target babies in this case were diagnosed (chiefly with developmental delay or Down syndrome) or were at risk for developing some form of developmental disability. Special needs were an important concern in making employment decisions and finding child care for one-third of the sample. Mothers of children with special needs returned to the workforce at a slower rate than did mothers of typically developing children, and the children themselves entered child care later and for fewer hours per week.

Child care is a multidimensional phenomenon: It comes in many varieties or types; children attend for different amounts of time, attendance may be stable across time or variable, and the experience itself may vary in quality. Because quality of care is considered a central aspect of child care, considerable time was spent in the development and validation of a new instrument for assessing this construct—the Observational Record of the Caregiving Environment (ORCE). One of the important features of this instrument is that it assesses the quality of the caregiving experienced by each individual child. Chapter 5 describes the instrument in detail.

The final chapter in this section, Chapter 6 describes the structural features of the care giving environment that are related to positive caregiving when the study children were 6, 15, 24, and 36 months of age. Across ages and types of care, positive caregiving is more likely when child–adult ratios and group sizes are smaller; caregivers are more educated, hold more child-oriented beliefs about childrearing, and have more experience in child care; and environments are safer and more stimulating. By 36 months of age, the significance of child–adult ratio decreases and in-home arrangements become less positive. Perhaps the most important data included in this manuscript, however, are the extrapolations to the quality of care in the United States as a whole by applying the NICHD observational parameters, stratified by maternal education, child age, and care type, to the distribution of U.S. families documented in the National Household Education Survey (Hofferth, Shauman, Henke, & West, 1998). The reported results show that a only a small percentage of children experience either very high quality or very low quality care; the largest group of children experience child care where positive caregiving is somewhat uncharacteristic.

2

Child Care in the First Year of Life

NICHD Early Child Care Research Network

Reliance on nonmaternal child care during the first year of life has become a normative aspect of rearing children in the United States (U.S. Bureau of the Census, 1992). The rates of increase in labor force participation of mothers have been most dramatic for mothers of infants (Hofferth, Brayfield, Deich, & Holcomb, 1991).

The growth of infant child care has been accompanied by research on the effects of nonmaternal care arrangements on children's development (Belsky, 1988; Clarke-Stewart, 1988; Field, 1991; Howes, 1990). Yet, none of the available data sets provides prospective or repeated reports of care during the first year of life and, consequently, the basic demographics of infant child care are virtually unknown. When do families first initiate child care? For how many hours? In what types of arrangements? At what cost? With what degree of stability over time?

This chapter provides information on child care during the first 12 months of life, specifically the initiation and amount of infant child care; child care history patterns during the first year; and the types, multiplicity, and stability of care used by parents of infants over the course of the first year. Child care is broadly defined to include all regular, nonmaternal care, including care by fathers, grandparents, and in-home sitters as well as care in centers and child care homes. However, where useful, we provide supplemental information that is specific to father care or nonparental care.

From *Merrill-Palmer Quarterly*, 1997, Vol. 43, No. 3 pp. 340–360. Copyright 1997 by Wayne State University Press. Reprinted by permission.

METHOD

Participants and Sample Representativeness

For a detailed description of the recruitment, enrollment, retention, and demographic characteristics of the sample participating in the National Institute of Child Health and Human Development (NICHD) Study of Early Child Care, see Chapter 1 of this volume.

Data for the analyses presented in this chapter focus on the 1,089 children whose nonmaternal child care began before their first birthday. Table 2.1 provides demographic characteristics of the participating families as measured at the 1-month enrollment interview and of the 1,089 children and their parents.

When the infants were 1 month old, 1,364 families (58% of those contacted) with healthy newborns were enrolled in the study. Of the mothers, 53% were planning to work (or attend school) full time, 23% were planning to work part time (10 to 30 hours per week), and 24% were planning to be at home in the child's first year. By age 6 months, actual employment patterns differed somewhat from the mothers' stated plans: 46% were employed or in school for 30 or more hours per week, 17% were employed/in school for 10–30 hours, 4% were employed or in school for less than 10 hours, and 33% were neither employed nor in school.

The enrolled sample is distinctly nonrepresentative. In 1990, in the United States, 52.8% of women ages 15–44 who had had a child in the last year were in the labor force (U.S. Bureau of the Census, 1995); and 52% of mothers in the National Child Care Survey (1990) were employed 1 year after birth (Hofferth et al., 1991). In this study, when the children were 12 months of age, 65.5% of the participating mothers were employed (excluding school hours) more than 0 hours.

Data Collection Procedures

Mothers were interviewed in their homes when the children were 1 month old and families were telephoned when the infant was 3, 5, 9, and 12 months of age to update information about child care and family characteristics.

In these interviews mothers were asked to indicate whether "anyone other than yourself is caring for [CHILD'S NAME] on a regular basis." Use of child care could be for any reason and for any number of hours as long as the infant was in the arrangement on a regular basis; occasional care was excluded. Care provided by fathers and partners was included if it was regularly scheduled when the mother was not present. Care provided by the mother herself was included as a child care arrangement when the mother provided care for the infant at her workplace; this included care, for example, by mothers who cared for their own infants while they worked as child care providers.

TABLE 2.1. Demographic Characteristics of the Enrolled Families and Those Using Nonmaternal Infant Child Care

	Enrolled sample (n = 1,364)		Child care sample (n = 1,089)	
	n	%	n	%
Child ethnicity				
White, non-Hispanic	1,042	76.4	835	76.7
Black, non-Hispanic	173	12.7	133	12.2
Hispanic	83	6.1	67	6.2
Other	66	4.8	54	5.0
Maternal education				
< 12th grade	139	10.2	97	8.9
High school graduate/GED	287	21.0	207	19.0
Some college	455	33.4	372	34.2
Bachelor's degree	284	20.8	238	21.9
Postgraduate work	198	14.5	175	16.1
Husband/partner at home				
Yes	1,166	85.5	935	85.9
No	198	14.5	154	14.1
Number of children in family				
1	559	41.0	487	44.7
2	498	36.5	397	36.5
3	214	15.7	145	13.3
4	62	4.5	41	3.8
5	17	1.2	10	0.9
6 or more	14	1.1	9	0.8
Maternal employment status (6 months)				
Full time	490	35.9	485	44.5
Part time	316	23.2	286	26.3
None	471	34.5	275	25.3
Maternal work hours (6 months)				
Daytime	641	47.0	616	56.6
Nondaytime	76	5.6	68	6.2
Varies	105	7.7	103	9.5
Monthly family income (6 months)				
< $1,250	164	12.0	111	10.2
$1,250–$2,499	238	17.4	187	17.2
$2,500–$3,749	304	22.3	242	22.2
$3,750 or more	564	41.3	500	45.9
Receipt of public assistance (6 months)				
Yes	314	23.0	235	21.6
No	965	70.7	813	74.7

Measuring Patterns and Features of Child Care

Five aspects of child care were examined for this report:

Age of Entry

Age of entry was the child's age (in months) at the time he or she first entered nonmaternal care.

Amount of Care

At each assessment period, mothers reported the number of hours per week that their infant was in nonmaternal care on a regular basis.

Type of Care

Children's primary child care arrangements were classified into one of 10 categories: (1) mother at work, (2) father/partner, (3) grandparent in child's home, (4) grandparent in grandparent's home, (5) other relative in child's home, (6) other relative in the relative's home, (7) nonrelative in the child's home, (8) nonrelative in a child care home, (9) child care center, and (10) other (e.g., sibling care). For children in multiple child care settings, the type of care in which the child spent the most time was considered primary.

History of Care

Children were divided into six unique history patterns: (1) exclusive maternal care throughout the first year of life; (2) some child care from the father or mother's partner, but no other nonmaternal arrangement; (3) one continuous nonparental care arrangement; (4) one nonparental arrangement and then a return to exclusive maternal care; (5) more than one continuous child care arrangement; and (6) more than one arrangement with at least one termination. Mothers who cared for their infants at work are not reflected in these six history categories.

Multiplicity and Stability of Care

Two measures were used: (1) multiplicity of care arrangements—the total number of arrangements used at entry into child care; and (2) stability of care—the total number of arrangements (simultaneous and sequential) used over the course of the first year of life.

Maternal Employment

In addition to assessing these characteristics of child care, we collected information about maternal employment and related this information to the families' use of child care. Child care experiences were examined separately for subgroups of children defined by maternal employment status and work schedule. Maternal employment was defined as full time (35 or more hours per week), part time (greater than 0, but less than 35 hours per week), or none. These hours included hours at work and/or hours in school. Work schedule was defined as daytime (day or day and evening), not daytime (evening, night, day and night, evening and night, or day and evening and night), or variable. Table 2.2 presents descriptive data on these variables for all families with any entry into child care, entry for 10 or more hours, and entry for 30 or more hours when the infants were 6 months of age.

RESULTS

Age of Entry

Of the 1,364 infants enrolled in the study, 1,089 (80%) experienced some regular nonmaternal child care during the first 12 months of life. Using as a base the number of infants who remained in the study for 12 months (n = 1,291), 84% experienced nonmaternal care during the first year. The average age at which these infants first entered child care was 3.11 months (see Figure 2.1). About three-quarters (72%) entered care prior to 4 months of age, 24% entered between 4 and 8 months, and fewer than 5% entered between 9 and 12 months of age. Excluding father/partner care, 72% of the infants experienced some child care with an average age at entry of 3.31 months.

Using 10 hours of care per week—a more stringent criterion for entry—74% of the infants experienced some nonmaternal child care (average age at entry was 3.27 months). Using 30 hours of care per week as the criterion

TABLE 2.2. Descriptive Data on Maternal Employment Status and Work Hours at Age 6 Months for Families Using Nonmaternal Child Care

	Total sample		Children in any care		Children in 10+ hr care		Children in 30+ hr care	
	n	%	n	%	n	%	n	%
Maternal employment status at 6 months								
Full time	490	35.9	485	44.5	480	47.9	465	59.0
Part time	316	23.2	286	25.3	265	26.4	152	19.3
None	471	34.5	275	25.3	217	21.6	139	17.6
Maternal work schedule at 6 months								
Day	641	47.0	616	56.6	601	59.9	519	65.9
Nonday	76	5.6	68	6.2	64	6.4	43	5.5
Varies	105	7.7	103	9.5	96	9.6	70	8.9

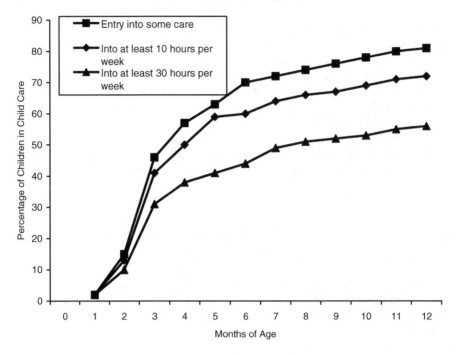

FIGURE 2.1. Age of entry into nonmaternal child care shown as percentages of children who have entered into some care, into at least 10 hours of care per week, and into at least 30 hours of care per week for each month of age during the first year.

for entry, 58% of the infants experienced some nonmaternal care (average age at entry was 3.57 months). Thus, regardless of the criterion used, the majority of infants in the study experienced some nonmaternal care during the first year of life and most care was initiated very early during the first year. From the history analyses (see "History of Care" section below), we know that about 10% of these infants (*n* = 115) returned to exclusive maternal care after having begun child care.

Maternal employment status was a significant predictor of age at onset of child care (all *F* values > 10.00; *p*'s < .001). Both full-time employed and nonemployed mothers initiated infant care at earlier ages than did part-time employed mothers. Although employed mothers (including those attending school) were substantially more likely to use child care than were nonemployed mothers, a sizable share of nonemployed mothers also relied on child care. Of the infants who experienced nonmaternal care during the first year of life (any hours), 24% (*n* = 234) had nonemployed mothers. It is important to note that of the mothers who were not employed at the time they initiated infant child care, 71% became employed or attended school at some point later during their child's first year.

Amount of Care

At the time of first entry into nonmaternal child care, infants were in care for 29 hours per week, on average. Excluding father care, the average number of hours of care per week was 28. For infants who entered into 10 or more hours of care per week, the average number of hours was 33, and for infants who entered into 30 or more hours per week, the average number of hours was 42.

Maternal employment status was a significant predictor of hours of care at entry (all F values > 10.00; p's < .001). Part-time employed mothers used fewer hours of care than did full-time employed and nonemployed mothers; nonemployed mothers used fewer hours of care than did full-time employed mothers, with one exception. Once an infant entered care for 30 hours or more per week, both full-time ($n = 482$) and nonemployed ($n = 138$) mothers used the same amount (43 hours per week).

Type of Care

At entry, the most common forms of care were father/partner care (25%), care in a child care home by a nonrelative (24%), and care by relatives, including grandparents, in either the child's or the relative's home (23%). Care in a child care center (12%) or in-home care by a nonrelative (12%) was less common.

This distribution of infants across different types of arrangements did not change substantially over the course of the first year. The only notable shift was that by 12 months of age, care by fathers/partners and grandparents had decreased and care in centers and in child care homes had increased.

Mothers' employment status and work schedule significantly predicted the type of child care used during the first year. Distinct patterns were revealed for each of the three employment groups and each of the three groups defined by maternal work schedules.

At entry, fathers/partners were more likely to be primary care providers when mothers were employed part time (35%) or, to a lesser extent, were not employed (22%), than when mothers were employed full time (17%), $\chi^2 = 85.48$, p < .001. Full-time employed mothers, in contrast, were more likely to have children in child care homes (31%) and center care (18%) than were other mothers (17% and 7%, respectively, for part-time employed mothers; 16% and 10% for nonemployed mothers). Nonemployed mothers more often used care by grandparents (in either the child's home or the grandparent's home) and by nonrelatives in the child's home than did the other mothers.

When mothers worked nondaytime hours, children were more likely to be cared for by fathers (50%) than when mothers worked varying schedules (33%) or daytime hours (19%), $\chi^2 = 80.33$, $p < .001$. Other relatives, however, were used equally by mothers with different work schedules; about one in four children received care by grandparents and other relatives. In-home care by a nonrelative was used almost twice as much when mothers' work schedules varied as when schedules were stable (20% vs. 11–12%) and care in child care homes and centers was used primarily when mothers worked daytime hours (45% vs. 24% of mothers with varying hours and 15% of mothers with nondaytime hours).

The types of care used by families with full-time employed mothers did not change between the initiation of care and the infants' 12-month birthdays. For families with nonworking mothers, however, care by fathers and other relatives declined by half and care by in-home providers who were not related to the child and in centers doubled. Families with part-time employed mothers reduced their reliance on relatives (other than fathers) somewhat and showed a corresponding modest increase in use of child care homes and centers.

By 12 months of age, infants whose mothers had daytime work schedules received less father care and more center-based care. When mothers had varying work schedules, use of father care declined somewhat, as did use of in-home care by nonrelatives, whereas the use of child care homes (also with providers who were not relatives of the child) increased. The largest shifts in care over the first year of life were seen among mothers with nondaytime work hours. In those families, father care increased notably and use of other relatives and nonrelative in-home care dropped substantially. They also increased their use of child care homes.

History of Care

Figure 2.2 illustrates patterns of care for the 1,291 children who remained in the study through their 12-month birthday.

Multiplicity and Stability of Care

At entry (any hours) into nonparental child care, 90% of the infants were enrolled in a single child care arrangement. Of those who started child care for at least 10 hours a week, 82% were in a single arrangement, and of infants starting care for 30 hours or more per week, only 74% were in a single arrangement. Interestingly, the families with part-time employed mothers were much more likely than either the full-time employed or nonemployed mothers to layer together more than one arrangement over the course of a week if 10 or more hours of care were required.

Over the course of the first year, infants who experienced nonparental child care were in more than two such arrangements, on average; over one-third (36.5%) had at least three different nonparental arrangements. Mothers' work schedules were closely linked to stability of care. Infants of mothers who worked variable hours were much more likely to have experi-

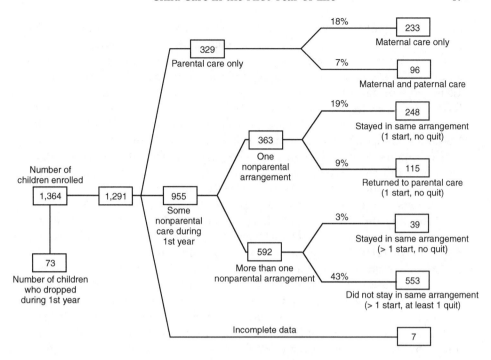

FIGURE 2.2. History of infant child care. The figure illustrates patterns of care for children who remained in the study through their 12-month birthday.

enced three or more arrangements (45%) than were infants of mothers with daytime (36%) or nondaytime (34%) work schedules. In contrast, maternal employment status had only a modest relation to the number of nonparental arrangements infants experienced over the first year. Forty percent of infants of full-time employed mothers and 34% of infants of both part-time employed and nonemployed mothers were in three or more arrangements during the first year of life.

DISCUSSION

The description of infant care experiences provided by the NICHD sample must be considered in the context of the relatively high proportion of employed mothers who were studied. The exclusion of adolescent mothers, mothers who did not speak English, mothers living in very unsafe areas, and mothers who planned to move within the year may have eliminated from the sample women who are less likely to be employed.

    We found that over 80% of infants received regular nonmaternal care and 70% received care from someone other than their parents. Only 18% of the infants spent the entire first year at home with mother without supple-mental child care. These high rates of reliance on infant child care exceed prior estimates from national surveys that include employed and non-employed mothers, which have indicated that about half of all infants under 12 months of age receive regular nonparental care (Hofferth et al., 1991; National Center for Education Statistics, 1995). However, they match quite closely national estimates based on subsamples of employed mothers. The National Child Care Survey, for example, conducted in 1990, found that 63% of infants of employed mothers received nonparental care (Hofferth et al., 1991) and the comparable figure from the Survey of Income and Pro-gram Participation for Fall, 1991 is 71% (Casper, Hawkins, & O'Connell, 1994). This figure rose to 76% by 1993 (see Casper, 1996).

Not only did the vast majority of infants in the NICHD study spend time in nonmaternal care, but they were first enrolled in care at very young ages and for relatively long hours. Once in child care, few infants returned to exclusive maternal care. Moreover, extensive, early child care use was not unique to employed mothers but characterized over one-third of infants of mothers not employed (or in school) in the infant's first year.

Long-standing evidence that parents attempt to keep the care of infants within the family was confirmed by our findings. Close to half of the infants received primary care from their fathers or other relatives—mostly grandparents—at entry into child care. Nationally, as of fall 1993, 17.5% of infants under 1 year of age with an employed mother were in the care of their fathers (M. O'Connell, personal communication, January 1997). Fam-ilies in the NICHD study who used parental care (exclusive maternal care or use of fathers when mother worked) had more children and fewer eco-nomic resources, which would constrain their use of higher cost nonfamilial arrangements. Mothers in these families also had more traditional child-rearing beliefs, including concerns about the effects of maternal employ-ment on their infants.

Over the first 12 months of life, the increase in use of more formal or public care settings that has been well documented over the course of the preschool years had already begun. By 12 months of age, 43% of the infants were in child care homes or centers, compared with 36% at first entry into nonmaternal care. Reliance on center-based care in particular, even for infants, has grown dramatically over the past 25 years (Casper, 1995, 1996; Hofferth et al., 1991).

The stability of care for infants has been found to predict developmen-tal outcomes. Children with more child care changes are more frequently classified as insecurely attached (Suwalsky, Zaslow, Klein, & Rabinovich, 1986), are less competent with peers as toddlers (Howes & Stewart, 1987), are more withdrawn and aggressive in preschool (Howes & Hamilton, 1993), and have more problems in school as first graders (Howes, 1988b). Our findings that infants in care typically experienced more than two nonparental arrangements during the first year of life are, accordingly, of concern. Over one-third of the infants who began nonparental care before their first birthday experienced three or more different arrangements with providers other than their parents. Moreover, the minority of families that had stable arrangements were relatively more advantaged compared with families that relied on multiple providers. Prior studies have documented inequities linked to income in access to high-quality child care (Phillips, Voran, Kisker, Howes, & Whitebook, 1994). The NICHD Study of Early Child Care suggests that similar inequities characterize parents' ability to arrange stable child care.

The restriction of child care options available to mothers whose employment entails nonstandard hours has been well documented (Brayfield, Deich, & Hofferth, 1993; Phillips, 1995). The children of mothers in the NICHD Study of Early Child Care with variable work hours were significantly less likely than other children to be in child care homes, center-based arrangements, or father care arrangements that are likely to be relatively stable. Instead, they were likely to receive care from nonrelative, in-home providers, or grandparents. Interrelations between the conditions of maternal employment, access to various child care options, and stability of care, particularly with regard to implications for child well-being, warrant further examination. If parents with nonstandard work hours are unable to avail themselves of stable child care arrangements, a serious work–family conflict exists.

3

Characteristics of Infant Child Care
Factors Contributing to Positive Caregiving

NICHD EARLY CHILD CARE RESEARCH NETWORK

In response to what they identified as "a quiet crisis" confronting infants and their families, the Carnegie Corporation (1994) called for strong and immediate changes to improve the quality of nonparental infant care in the United States. In particular, they called for efforts to adopt, support, and monitor nationwide child care standards for children under 3 years of age. But what should these standards be, and what impact will they have on the emotional and intellectual well-being of children?

Most existing child care research has not included infants or has combined infant and toddler care in ways that cannot be disentangled. Thus, there is an assumption, essentially untested, that high-quality care for infants can be defined in the same terms as care for older children, that is, by child–adult ratios, group sizes, and caregivers' qualifications. But do these dimensions influence the kinds of caregiving experiences that infants have, and do these experiences ultimately contribute to children's development?

In this investigation, observations from the National Institute of Child Health and Human Development (NICHD) Study of Early Child Care are used to examine associations between structural and caregiver characteris-

From *Early Childhood Research Quarterly*, 1996, Vol. 11, No. 3, pp. 296–306. Copyright 1996 by Elsevier. Reprinted by permission.

tics as they apply to infants' experiences with their caregivers. At 6 months, infants who were in a nonmaternal care arrangement for 10 or more hours per week were observed in that arrangement. Covering the gamut of contemporary child care, these nonmaternal care arrangements included care by fathers, grandparents, and in-home sitters as well as in centers and child care homes.

To evaluate these different arrangements, an observational instrument, the Observational Record of the Caregiving Environment (ORCE), was developed to record caregivers' behaviors, identified in the research literature as contributing to children's social and intellectual development, such as responding promptly to the infant's social signals and distress, expressing positive feelings toward the infant, and stimulating the infant's cognitive development. These caregivers' behaviors are examined in relation to the child care standards suggested by the experts—child–adult ratios, group sizes, and caregivers' formal education and specialized training. Other possible standards such as caregivers' experience and beliefs about childrearing and the safety of the physical environment also are examined.

STRUCTURAL AND CAREGIVER CHARACTERISTICS ASSOCIATED WITH OBSERVED CAREGIVING BEHAVIORS

One of our goals is to identify the structural characteristics and caregivers' qualifications that are associated with caregiving behaviors that are sensitive, warm, and responsive to infants. We expect that such caregiving will be compromised by large group sizes. We also hypothesize that caregivers' training and education are positively related to the quality of their interactions with the study infants and that having fewer children to care for in a safe and physically stimulating environment allows caregivers to provide the most attentive and positive care. We do not make a prediction about how caregivers' experience is related to these interactions.

CHARACTERISTICS OF DIFFERENT TYPES OF CHILD CARE

Our second goal is to examine variations in structural and caregivers' characteristics as a function of the type of care. Previous studies have compared two types of care settings: home based (typically child care homes) and center based. The NICHD study extends the comparison of child care settings beyond these two types of care to include care by fathers, grandparents, and in-home sitters. This broad, inclusionary strategy was followed so that we might investigate the full range of nonmaternal child care arrangements experienced by infants.

Caregivers' behaviors are expected to vary in these different types of care. Previous research would lead to the prediction that centers and child care homes would provide more stimulating care than fathers, grandparents, or in-home sitters. However, the intensity of infants' needs may be more difficult to meet when group sizes and ratios are larger or when caregivers are unrelated to the child and, therefore, less emotionally involved. If this is the case, fathers, grandparents, and in-home sitters might provide more sensitive, responsive, and positive care for infants. Information from the NICHD study affords the opportunity to test these rival predictions.

DESCRIPTION OF INFANT CARE

Our third purpose is to provide descriptive data about nonmaternal infant care in the United States. Several recent reports have suggested that child care for many children in the United States is inadequate. These previous reports of poor or minimally adequate child care for toddlers underscore the need for a large-scale investigation to answer the following questions: What are the structural characteristics of infant child care settings? What are the characteristics and qualifications of infant caregivers? Are caregivers' behaviors related to these structural characteristics and caregiver qualifications? Do caregivers' behaviors vary in different types of settings? Because of the developmental needs and vulnerabilities of infants, it is particularly urgent that we address these issues.

METHOD

Participants

Families were recruited for the study (approximately 136 families per site) during 1991. The 1,364 recruited families closely approximated the demographic characteristics of the "population" defined as the 5,416 eligible families in the designated locations. For additional details of the recruitment plan see Chapter 1.

Data Collection and Creation of Variables

Visits to the families began when the infants were 1 month old. At 5 months, mothers were telephoned and asked about their current child care arrangements and if changes were anticipated in the next month. If no changes were anticipated, information about the child care setting was obtained. If a mother anticipated changes, she was called back 1 month later to find out about the infant's current child care arrangement. Five types of nonmaternal care were identified: father care, grandparent care, in-home sitter (in the child's home), child care home (care provided in the care-giver's home, 27% were licensed), and child care center.

At 6 months of age, 879 infants were in a nonmaternal care arrange-ment. Of these infants, 198 were in more than one care arrangement. For children in more than one arrangement, a primary arrangement was identi-fied. A primary arrangement was operationally defined as the one in which the infant spent the most time or, if the child spent equal time in two arrangements, the more "formal" or institutional arrangement. For all chil-dren in a single arrangement for 10 or more hours per week, providers (n = 734) were contacted and asked to participate in the study.

Observations were not conducted for 113 infants who qualified for observation but whose providers refused to be observed. Eleven (or 11%) of the eligible fathers contacted, 15 (or 13%) of eligible grandmothers, 11 (or 11%) of eligible in-home sitters, 73 (or 27%) of the eligible child care home providers, and 3 (or 3%) of the eligible centers refused observation. An additional 24 children were not observed because the visits could not be scheduled within the assessment window. A total of 597 infants thus were visited and observed in their primary nonmaternal child care arrangement; of these, 576 could be classified as being in one of our five types of care. These child care observations were evenly distributed across the research sites.

There are some differences in those families in which eligible child care was observed and those families in which eligible care was not observed. Mothers' and fathers' levels of education were higher in those families whose eligible child care was observed, $t(241) = 4.26$, $p < .001$, and $t(199) = 3.37$, $p < .001$, respectively. Income-to-needs ratios also were higher for those families whose eligible child care was observed, $t(212) = 2.56$, $p < .01$. Children from single-parent households and those with minority race status were more likely to be in eligible but nonobserved child care, $\chi^2(1) = 11.47$, $p < .001$, and $\chi^2(1) = 5.01$, $p < .03$, respectively.

Two half-day visits to observe and assess the infants' child care experi-ences were scheduled to occur within a period of 2 weeks. The first of these visits was within 2 weeks of the infant's 6-month birthday, and at this visit observers typically completed two ORCE observation cycles (see below) and the appropriate Assessment Profile scale. At the second visit, two additional ORCE observations were made, and the Child Care Home Observation for Measurement of the Environment (HOME) Inventory (Caldwell & Bradley, 1984) evaluation was completed for home-based care. Interviews were held with caregivers and questionnaires were admin-istered to them at the end of the visit. This data collection plan served two methodological purposes: It provided the assurance that data were not collected on a single, possibly atypical, occasion, and it permitted observers to be blind to caregivers' views and background while observing their behavior.

Observational Assessments

A major innovation in this study was the development of an observational instrument, the ORCE, to assess the characteristics of caregiving for an individual child. This instrument is particularly valuable because it can be used to assess children's experiences in different types of settings. Other measures are applicable only for center-based care or only for home-based care. Also, in contrast to other instruments, the ORCE focuses on caregivers' behaviors with a specific child (in this case, the study child) rather than on what happens in the classroom at large. A third feature of the ORCE is that it provides both frequency counts (called behavior scales) and ratings (called qualitative ratings) of caregivers' behaviors. The behavior scales provide a record of the occurrence (or quantity) of specific acts, whereas the qualitative scales take into account quality (and nuances) of the caregiver's behaviors in relation to the child's behaviors.

The ORCE format consists of 44-minute cycles, each broken into four 10-minute observation periods. In each 10-minute period observers alternate between 30-second observe and record frames. During the observe intervals observers focus on the study child's behavior, activities, and interaction with the caregiver or other people. During the record intervals the observer completes the frequency checklist. At the end of the 10-minute period the observer makes brief notes and tentative qualitative ratings of behaviors for 2 minutes. This process is repeated for three 10-minute periods. In the final 10-minute period the observer makes observations exclusively for the qualitative ratings. At the end of the 44 minutes the observer makes final qualitative ratings using 4-point scales that range from not at all characteristic to highly characteristic based on all four 10-minute periods. Typically, four 44-minute ORCE cycles, distributed over 2 days, were completed for each infant. For the 576 children in this report, the average number of complete 44-minute cycles was 3.9.

Although most infants (79%) were observed with the same caregiver across the four observation cycles, some were observed with two (11%), three (7%), or more (3%) caregivers. Our qualitative ratings are based on the caregiver for whom we had the most complete data. The behavior scales included frequencies of acts for all available caregivers.

A composite variable based on the ORCE behavior scales called positive caregiving frequencies was created by averaging three standardized behavioral summary scores that included nine of the original behavior categories: positive behavior (shared positive affect + positive physical contact), responsive behavior (responds to vocalization + facilitates infant behavior), and stimulating behavior (stimulates cognitive development + stimulates social development + asks question + other talk + reads); Cronbach's alpha = .81. This *a priori* combination, which the investigators believed best reflected positive caregiving for infants, was supported by a confirmatory factor analysis.

A composite variable based on the ORCE qualitative ratings was constructed by summing five of the qualitative ratings: sensitivity or responsiveness to nondistressed communication, positive regard, stimulation of cognitive development, detachment (reflected), and flat affect (reflected). This composite was labeled positive caregiving ratings. Scores varied from 5 to 20 (*M* = 14.8, *SD* = 3.0; Cronbach's alpha = .89). The first principal component of a confirmatory factor analysis corresponded to this *a priori* conceptually constructed composite variable.

At the beginning and end of each ORCE cycle observers recorded the composition of the group of adults and children in the care setting. Variables derived from these records included group size, representing the average across ORCE cycles of the number of children under 13 years observed in infant's group; child–adult ratio, representing the average across the ORCE cycles of the number of awake children observed per caregiver; and age mix of children (1 = study child alone, 2 = infants only, 3 = infants and toddlers only, 4 = children beyond age 2 present, in at least 75% of the observed cycles).

In addition to the ORCE assessments, two other observational instruments were used. Caldwell and Bradley's (1984) HOME Inventory (with the wording of some items modified by Caldwell and Bradley to make them more appropriate for child care situations) was completed in all home care arrangements. The Child Care HOME employs an interview and observation format to assess caregivers' responsivity, acceptance, and involvement with the child; the organization and learning materials in the home environment; and the variety of experiences offered the child. The 45 items, scored yes or no, had a Cronbach's alpha of .81.

The other observation instrument was the Assessment Profile for Early Childhood Programs (Abbott-Shim & Sibley, 1987). This instrument provided a classroom-level assessment and was available in two versions, for centers and for homes. Three additional items from Wachs (1991) were added to assess quiet, crowding, and clutter. For the purposes of this investigation, a subset of items was selected from this instrument to provide a measure of the physical environment of the child care setting. These items evaluated the extent to which the space and equipment were clean and safe, the environment was uncrowded and uncluttered, a variety of developmentally appropriate toys was available, and the infant had a play area that was protected and quiet (17 items in the center scale, Cronbach's alpha = .64, and 29 items in the home scale, Cronbach's alpha = .74).

Caregiver Interviews and Questionnaires

Structured interviews with the caregivers administered at the end of the second child care visit formed the basis for the following variables: caregiver's formal education (scored as 1 = less than high school graduation, 2 = high school diploma or GED, 3 = some college, 4 = bachelor's degree, 5 = some graduate work, including master's degree, 6 = EdD, PhD, or other post-master's degree); specialized training in child development or early education (scored as 0 = none, 1 = high school courses, 2 = adult or vocational courses, 3 = college courses, 4 = college or graduate degree); caregiving experience (years of providing child care or working in a child care or early childhood center); caregiver's own children present during the time that the study infant is in care (0 = absent; 1 = present). Caregivers' beliefs about childrearing were assessed using a 30-item questionnaire that discriminates between "modern" and "traditional" childrearing beliefs (Schaefer & Edgerton, 1985). A principal component factor analysis yielded a single dimension of nonauthoritarian childrearing beliefs.

Training and Reliability

The 24 child care observers first studied the extensive manuals prepared by the investigators, which detailed each assessment procedure, and then they were trained in all observation and interview procedures at a 1-week group session. This training consisted of viewing master-coded videotapes, conducting "live" observations in centers and home-based child care settings, completing written tests, and participating in question-and-answer sessions pertaining to each procedure. Further training and practice were conducted at each site using videotaped and live examples and instruction. Then, questions that arose in the course of collecting the observational data were answered by the instrument developers via e-mail sent to all observers.

To ensure cross-site reliability on the ORCE observations, before any data collection was initiated, observers coded six tapes, each containing one 44-minute ORCE cycle. These tapes had been master coded by the investigators who developed the ORCE. The tapes represented all five types of care and captured a range of quality. To be certified as data collectors, each observer had to achieve exact agreement with the master codes of the behavior scales at a level of 70% or better and with the qualitative ratings at a level of 60% or better. After certification, reliability was checked across the 10 months of data collection with three further rounds of videotape testing, each consisting of six new master-coded 44-minute ORCE cycles. To remain certified, observers had to maintain exact agreement with the master codes of the behavior scales at a level of 70% or better and with the qualitative ratings at a level of 60% or better. In fact, agreement was typically much higher.

In addition to using master-coded videotapes, which ensured that sites were applying similar standards to their ORCE assessments, pairs of observers at each site completed qualitative ratings and behavior checklists during visits to child care settings. These "live" observations occurred across the 10-month data collection period. At each site, all possible pairs of observers were required to visit both home-based and center-based child care. Pearson correlations and repeated-measures analyses of variance (ANOVA) (Winer,

1971) were used to estimate reliability at the variable level. With few exceptions, reliability estimates were acceptable (see NICHD Early Child Care Research Network, 1996).

Interobserver reliabilities also were determined for the composite variables derived from the qualitative ratings and the behavior categories. The median reliability (Pearson correlation) for the positive caregiving rating composite was .94 for the master-coded videotapes and .90 for the live observations. Reliability for the positive caregiving frequency composite was .98 for the videotapes and .86 for the live observations.

Training and certification on the Child Care HOME procedure involved a combination of videotaped and live experiences analogous to those used for the ORCE. To be certified, observers had to obtain 90% agreement (41 out of 45 items correctly scored) with a master-coded videotape of a Child Care HOME. In addition, an observer at each site was responsible for conducting a Child Care HOME interview that was videotaped and assessed by the scale developers for appropriateness of administration and accuracy of scoring (90% agreement with the master coders). The site videotape also was scored by others at the site, with 90% agreement being required. The observer whose Child Care HOME administration was certified was then responsible for accompanying all other child care observers at the site to verify their approach to administering the Child Care HOME.

Approximately 3 and 6 months after data collection began, sites were sent two additional sets of master-coded videotapes. Observers had to maintain 90% agreement with the master codes to retain certification.

Observers were trained on the home and center versions of the Assessment Profile by developers of that instrument. (These were different investigators than those responsible for the ORCE and the Child Care HOME.) The scale developers accompanied the observers on visits to both home- and center-based settings. Observers' agreement with the scale developers and with other observers who had extensive experience with the scales were assessed during these live visits. Overall agreement across items and observers was 80%.

RESULTS

Four sets of analyses are presented: (1) descriptive analyses pertaining to structural features, caregivers' characteristics, and caregivers' behaviors for care that we observed; (2) analyses showing the associations between these structural features and caregivers' characteristics and our observations of positive caregiving for the sample as a whole; (3) analyses showing the differences in structure, caregivers' characteristics, and positive caregiving associated with type of care arrangement; and (4) analyses examining the predictors of positive caregiving in different types of care.

Characteristics of Observed Infant Care

Infants' nonmaternal child care arrangements varied widely in structural and caregivers' characteristics (see Table 3.1 for information about the number and percent of children in child care arrangements varying in terms of type, group size, child–adult ratio, caregiver's education, caregiver specialized training, and years of caregiving experience). Other analyses show that, as expected, observed group size and child–adult ratio were strongly and positively related. In addition, providers who cared for more children had worked longer in child care and had more specialized training pertaining to children. The number of children cared for was not strongly related to caregivers' level of formal education, nonauthoritarian beliefs, or the extent to which the physical environment was highly rated.

Caregivers with more formal education had more specialized training pertaining to children (r = .17; p < .0001), held less authoritarian child-rearing beliefs (r = .47; p < .0001), and were in settings that were rated as more safe, clean, and stimulating (for home care settings r = .23, p < .01; for centers r = .22, p < .05). Caregivers with less authoritarian beliefs had more specialized training (r = .32, p < .0001) and experience in child care (r = .13, p < .001), as well as more formal education (r = .47, p < .0001), and provided safe, clean, and stimulating physical settings (for child care homes r = .24, p < .001 and for center care r = .36, p < .001). Still other observers' ratings of caregivers, averaged across the four 44-minute observation cycles, show that most caregivers were rated as moderately or highly positive to the infant (74% on the Sensitivity to Nondistress scale; 80% on the Positive Regard scale). The majority (81%) of caregivers appeared either minimally or not at all detached, and explicit negative regard for the infant was rare (.1%). Cognitive stimulation was not a major aspect of caregivers' interactions with 6-month-olds: the majority of caregivers were rated as either not at all stimulating (26%) or somewhat unstimulating (49%).

Mean percentages for the individual behavior scales across all available ORCE cycles show that, on average, infants were involved with the caregiver in some kind of activity, beyond simple physical caretaking, for nearly half of the time they were observed. Warm, physical contact and helpful or entertaining interactions with the caregiver were observed in one-third of the 30-second observation intervals, and caregivers responded within 30 seconds to over 80% of the instances of observed infant distress. Speaking negatively or using rough physical actions with the infant was almost never observed. Attempts by the caregiver to deliberately stimulate the infant's development, however, were rare (observed in only about 6% of the intervals).

The correlation between the two composite measures of caregiving, based on the qualitative ratings and the behavior scales, was .74 (p < .001). Validation of the two ORCE measures (in-home settings) was provided by the Child Care HOME (M = 34, SD = 5.6), which was significantly correlated

TABLE 3.1. Structural and Caregivers' Characteristics of Nonmaternal Caregiving for 6-Month-Old Infants

Characteristic	n	%
Type of child care arrangement		
Father	87	15
Grandparent	98	17
In-home sitter	85	15
Child care home	201	35
Child care center	105	18
Observed group size (M = 3.3, SD = 3.2) (averaged across 2 days, .5's rounded up)		
1	219	38
2–3	168	29
4–7	119	21
8–11	46	8
> 11	24	4
Observed child–adult ratio (M = 2.1:1, SD = 1.5) (averaged across 2 days, .5's rounded up)		
1:1	244	43
2:1	146	26
3:1	93	16
4:1	39	7
5:1	23	4
≥ 6:1	21	4
Caregivers' education (M = 2.7, SD = 1.1)		
Less than high school (1)	78	14
High school diploma (2)	192	34
Some college (3)	191	34
College degree (4)	61	11
Some graduate (5)	35	6
Graduate degree (6)	8	1
Specialized training in child development (M = .9, SD = 1.3)		
None (0)	366	65
High school level (1)	24	4
Vocational certification (2)	77	14
College level courses (3)	81	14
Degree (4)	18	3
Specialized training related to infants		
No	379	71
Yes	152	29
Years of caregiving experience (M = 4.0, SD = .7)		
≤1	250	45
1–3	125	22
4–6	76	14
7–10	45	8
11–20	48	9
21–45	15	3

with both positive caregiving ratings (r = .63, p < .001) and positive caregiving frequencies (r = .40, p < .001) composites.

Structural Characteristics and Caregiver Qualifications Associated with Caregiving Behaviors

One of our major goals was to determine whether structural and caregiver characteristics were associated with the quality of caregivers' interactions with the study infant. We hypothesized that small group sizes and small child–staff ratios would be associated with infants receiving more positive caregiving. Caregivers' education and training also were expected to contribute positively to caregiving quality.

Table 3.2 shows correlations between the structural and caregivers' characteristics and the caregiving composites that were derived from the frequency counts and ratings. Higher positive caregiving ratings and frequencies were observed in child care arrangements with fewer children and with lower child–adult ratios, in settings that were assessed as safer and physically more stimulating, and in programs in which caregivers had more formal education and held more nonauthoritarian beliefs about child rearing. These significant correlations were moderate in size, ranging from .31 to .47. A statistically significant but smaller correlation (–.15) was obtained between observed caregiving and caregivers' experience, indicating that positive caregiving was more frequent among caregivers with fewer years in the field. Observed caregiving was not significantly correlated with specialized training pertaining to children.

Multiple regression analyses were conducted to determine the extent to which observed caregiving was simultaneously associated with structural and caregivers' characteristics (group size, child–adult ratio, childrearing

TABLE 3.2. Correlations between Structural and Caregivers' Characteristics and Observed Positive Caregiving

	Positive caregiving	
Characteristics	Ratings	Frequencies
Observed group size	–.36****	–.46****
Observed child–adult ratio	–.36****	–.45****
Caregivers' formal education	.11**	.03
Caregivers' specialized training in child development	–.02	–.05
Caregivers' nonauthoritarian childrearing beliefs	.14**	.09**
Caregivers' years of experience	–.07	–.15**
Physical environment (homes)	.33***	.10
Physical environment (centers)	.47***	.31**

* p < .05; ** p < .01; *** p < .001; **** p < .0001.

beliefs, experience, formal education, and specialized training). Positive caregiving frequencies (adjusted R^2 = .19, p < .0001) and positive caregiving ratings (adjusted R^2 = .27, p < .0001) were predicted by the full model including these six variables. Characteristics of the physical environment were not included in these regression analyses because different versions of the instrument were used in home-based settings and in centers.

A backward elimination procedure was then used to determine which variables in the full model could be removed without substantially reducing predictability. Group size, child–adult ratio, and nonauthoritarian child-rearing beliefs all accounted for significant variation in observed positive caregiving frequencies and ratings. Other variables included in the full model (caregivers' formal education, years of experience, and specialized training) did not significantly add to the prediction of observed positive caregiving for 6-month-olds.

Comparisons of Different Types of Care

Our second primary goal was to contrast infants' experiences in five types of arrangement. Two rival hypotheses were examined: (1) infants receive more positive caregiving in formal center-based care and (2) infants receive more positive caregiving in home-based settings. ANOVAs were used. Tukey *post hoc* comparisons indicated that child–adult ratio and group size were largest in child care centers, followed by child care homes, followed by in-home care. Not surprisingly, specialized training in child development was highest for caregivers in centers. Fathers had more formal education than did other nonmaternal caregivers, although the level of education was not higher than that of other fathers in the study. Grandparents and in-home sitters had the most authoritarian childrearing beliefs. Fathers and grandparents had the least experience providing child care, and caregivers in centers and child care homes had the most. No difference in the quality of the physical environment was found for the four home-based types of care.

Observed caregiving behaviors varied by type of care. Both composite measures of positive caregiving (ratings and frequencies) were higher for father care, grandparent care, and in-home sitter care than they were in child care homes where, in turn, they were higher than for care in centers. A significant difference also was found for the Child Care HOME scores; fathers received higher scores than other home-based caregivers.

Factors Associated with Positive Caregiving in Different Types of Care

The purpose of the fourth set of analyses was to identify the factors associated with positive caregiving in different types of care. Three types of care were examined: (1) relative home care (father and grandparents), (2) nonrelative home care (in-home caregivers and child care homes), and (3) center care. Multiple regressions were conducted within these different types of care to parallel the analyses conducted for the whole sample. Predictors were, as before, child–adult ratio, group size, caregivers' formal education, specialized training in child development, years of child care experience, and nonauthoritarian childrearing beliefs. Paralleling the analyses for the whole sample, the backward elimination procedure was used only when the full regression models were significant.

For father and grandparent care, higher ratings and frequencies of positive caregiving were associated with lower child–adult ratios and with more nonauthoritarian childrearing beliefs. Because of the high correlation between child–adult ratio and group size in these settings ($r = .99$ and $r = .87$ for fathers and grandparents, respectively), it is not surprising that only one of these variables was a significant predictor of positive caregiving. For in-home sitter care and child care homes, these two variables were not as highly correlated, and positive caregiving was associated with smaller group sizes, lower child–adult ratios, nonauthoritarian childrearing attitudes, and specialized training in child development. In center care, smaller group sizes and more formal education were associated with more frequent positive caregiving behaviors. In the within-type analyses it also was possible to include measures of the physical environment (these could not be included in the overall analyses because different instruments were used for home and for center-based care). In all three types of care, environments rated as safe, clean, and stimulating were associated with higher ratings of positive caregiving and, including the physical environment measures, significantly improved the prediction of positive caregiving ratings.

Other Factors Associated with Positive Caregiving Behaviors

For infants in centers, positive caregiving ratings and frequencies were contrasted for infants who were in classrooms consisting of infants only, infants and toddlers only, and mixed ages including preschoolers. ANOVAs were significant for frequency of positive caregiving behaviors, $F(2,100) = 4.52$, $p < .01$. Tukey *post hoc* comparisons indicated that infants in classrooms with infants only ($M = -2.1$, $n = 54$) or infant and toddler combinations ($M = -2.4$, $n = 25$) received positive caregiving less frequently than did infants in mixed-age groups ($M = -.9$, $n = 24$)—despite the fact that the groups were the same size; $Ms = 8.3$ children in infant and toddler groups versus 7.7 children in mixed-age groups; $F(1,102) = 2.2$, NS. No effect of age configuration was found for the composite ratings of positive caregiving.

In home-based settings, contrasting the positive caregiving ratings and frequencies for the study infant alone versus the study infant with any other children yielded highly significant *t*-test results: Settings where the study infant was the only child in care had significantly more positive caregiving

(M's = 16.2 for ratings, 1.6 for frequencies) than did settings with other children (M's = 14.1 for ratings, -.7 for frequencies).

DISCUSSION

Associations between Structural and Caregivers' Characteristics and Observed Caregiving

Four factors were associated with infants receiving sensitive, warm, responsive care from their caregivers. Positive caregiving, assessed in terms of frequency counts and qualitative ratings, was higher when group sizes and child–adult ratios were smaller, when caregivers had nonauthoritarian beliefs about childrearing, and when the physical environments appeared safe, clean, and stimulating.

The importance of group size and ratios for infant care is consistent with research on toddler care (Allhusen, 1992; Clarke-Stewart, Gruber, & Fitzgerald, 1994; Fosburg, 1981; Fosburg et al., 1980; Howes, 1983; Ruopp, Travers, Glantz, & Coelen, 1979; Stallings, 1980; Whitebook, Howes, & Phillips, 1990). In fact, it appears that infant child care is particularly susceptible to these structural dimensions. The closer the child–adult ratio was to 1:1, the higher was the probability of sensitive, positive caregiving. The link between the number of children and positive caregiving was moderately strong in absolute terms (r's = .36–.46); it was strong compared with associations with other structural and caregivers' dimensions and remained significant when these other dimensions were statistically controlled; and it was consistent across different types of care.

Another factor associated with observed positive caregiving in this investigation was caregivers' beliefs about childrearing. Caregivers with nonauthoritarian childrearing beliefs tended to have more positive interactions with infants than did caregivers with more authoritarian beliefs. These results are consistent with research by Arnett (1989) and McCartney (1984), which linked observed interactions with preschool-age children to caregivers' childrearing beliefs. This association was not as strong as that between the number of children and positive caregiving, however.

Our finding of a significant association between positive caregiving behaviors and characteristics of the physical environment (safe, uncluttered, age-appropriate materials) was consistent with research on somewhat older children (Dunn, 1993; Howes, 1983; Scarr, Eisenberg, & Deater-Deckard, 1994). It supports the lay views of parents and caregivers (Galinsky, Howes, Kontos, & Shinn, 1994) about the importance of the physical setting. This aspect of child care has generally been given less emphasis in the scientific community than other features such as child–adult ratios and caregivers' training. Our results suggest that the importance of the physical environment should not be underestimated.

In this investigation other factors were less clearly associated with observed positive caregiving for infants. When group size, child–adult ratio, and caregivers' childrearing beliefs were statistically controlled, experience, per se, did not affect positive caregiving. Caregivers' formal education and specialized training also did not appear to contribute substantially to the frequencies or ratings of positive caregiving, although research (McCartney, 1984; Vandell & Powers, 1983; Whitebook et al., 1990) indicates their importance with older children.

Taken together, the structural and caregivers' characteristics measured in this investigation accounted for only about one-quarter of the variance in observed positive caregiving (R^2's = .19, .27). This suggests that our conventional measures of regulable aspects of child care have a limited capacity to predict the quality of care an infant will receive. It is hoped that further research will uncover links with aspects of the child care situation as yet unrecognized as significant predictors of child care quality.

Differences Associated with Types of Care

Our second purpose was to examine variations associated with different types of care. Clear differences were documented. Group sizes and child–adult ratios were significantly larger in child care centers than in child care homes, which were significantly larger than in father, grandparent, and in-home sitter care. Caregivers in centers had more specialized training and caregiving experience than did home-based providers. Along with these descriptive differences, there were differences in observed caregiving behaviors. Sensitive, positive, and involved care was most likely in in-home arrangements, with fathers, grandparents, and sitters, somewhat less likely in child care homes, and least likely in child care centers—although there were overlapping distributions across these types of care. The most notable difference between our results and those of other researchers was that fathers and grandparents were observed to display more positive caregiving than unrelated providers in child care homes and centers.

For infants, child–adult ratio and group size were consistently associated with positive caregiving behaviors within each type of care, as they were in the whole-sample analyses. Interestingly, differences in caregivers' beliefs, which contributed significantly to the caregiving behavior of home-based providers, did not predict observed caregiving in child care centers. This lack of association may be the result of the generally large ratios and group sizes in centers, which did not allow center caregivers the opportunity to implement their beliefs as they struggled to meet the demands of caring for several babies at one time. The challenge of caring for multiple infants was further demonstrated by the age configuration analyses. In centers, caregivers responsible for groups of infants or infants and toddlers showed less positive caregiving than did caregivers with mixed-age groups.

Quality of Infant Child Care

Our third purpose was to provide a window into infant child care in the United States. The majority of infants (70–80%) observed in the NICHD study were judged to be receiving care that was moderately or highly sensitive or moderately or highly positive. Some caution should be taken in generalizing these figures to the quality of infant care in the United States. The study was not designed to be nationally representative, and our sampling plan excluded adolescent mothers, very ill newborns, and mothers who did not speak English. Infants in these families may have less access to high-quality child care than the infants of participating families. In addition, 15% of the providers who were contacted refused to participate in the study; and care in those settings may well have lowered the overall ratings. Within these constraints, observations obtained in this investigation suggest that the quality of nonmaternal infant care is not as poor as might be surmised from other investigations such as the Cost, Quality, and Child Outcomes Study (Helburn et al., 1995), the Child Care Staffing Study (Whitebook et al., 1990), and the Study of Children in Family Child Care and Relative Care (Galinsky et al., 1994), which all reported high proportions (25–40%) of inadequate care and low proportions (8–12%) of "good" care.

Many factors may have contributed to the discrepant findings. One possibility is that other studies simply used different measures to assess child care. Although the NICHD study and the other investigations assessed similar aspects of child care settings (such as caregiver sensitivity, presence of stimulating activities, and physical safety), different instruments were used, and comparisons across these instruments may not be valid.

We do not believe, however, that discrepancies are solely the result of these measurement differences, because the child care settings also differed on objective, structural characteristics. In the NICHD study the average child–adult ratio in centers was 3.2:1, whereas in the Cost and Quality study the ratio for infants and toddlers was 3.6:1, and in the Staffing study the ratio was 3.9:1. In the NICHD study 71% of centers met the 3:1 ratio recommended by the American Public Health Association and the American Academy of Pediatrics (1992); in the Staffing study, only 36% did. In the child care homes observed in the NICHD study, the average child–adult ratio was 2.7:1, whereas in the Study of Family and Relative Care, the average ratio was 3.3:1. These structural differences suggest that the NICHD study observed care in settings that had greater potential for positive caregiving.

These structural differences (and differences in observed caregiving) may partially reflect the locations in which the observations were conducted. The other large-scale studies were conducted in states such as North Carolina, Texas, and Colorado, which have minimal child care standards. Although several states in the NICHD sample overlap with those in the other investigations (California, North Carolina, and Virginia), and still other states included in the NICHD study have relatively low standards (e.g., Arkansas), the NICHD study also included states with relatively high child care standards (e.g., Washington, Kansas, and Massachusetts). The structural characteristics and observed caregiving in these states may have contributed to the overall scores that were obtained.

Another important difference between the NICHD study and the other large-scale studies was the inclusion of a broader range of care arrangements—that is, care by fathers, grandparents, and in-home sitters and care that was part time as well as full time. Almost half of the infants in the NICHD study were in such informal care arrangements. The quality of observed care in our study was, in fact, significantly higher in these arrangements than in child care homes and child care centers—the settings observed most frequently in prior studies.

4

Child Care Characteristics of Infants with and without Special Needs

Comparisons and Concerns

Cathryn L. Booth
Jean F. Kelly

Although there are no national statistics on child care usage in families with children with special needs, Landis (1992) found that mothers of children with disabilities entered the labor force at the same rate as the general population. In survey studies designed to assess the needs of parents of children with disabilities, child care issues have been among the most important problems reported (Axtell, Garwick, Patterson, Bennett, & Blum, 1995; Bailey, Blasco, & Simeonsson, 1992; Freedman, Litchfield, & Warfield, 1995; Herman & Thompson, 1995; Horner, Rawlins, & Giles, 1987; Palfrey, Walker, Butler, & Singer, 1989).

The purpose of the present report is to provide information about employment and child care characteristics, concerns, and problems in a sample of 166 families with children who had diagnosed disabilities by the age of 12 months ($n = 89$), or who had risk factors for developing disabilities ($n = 77$). These data address a primary goal of a longitudinal study that was designed to examine, within an ecological model, the influence of variations in early child care histories on the development of children with special needs. As a first step toward realizing this goal, we (1) describe the maternal

From *Early Childhood Research Quarterly*, 1998, Vol. 13, pp. 603–621. Copyright 1998 by Elsevier. Reprinted by permission.

employment patterns, child care characteristics, problems, and concerns of mothers and children with special needs and (2) compare this sample with a group of typically developing children and their families in terms of these characteristics.

The unique aspects of this investigation are as follows: First, children were studied at a relatively young age—12–15 months—and children at risk for developing disabilities, as well as those with diagnoses, were included. The rationale for including children at risk was that we expected a greater proportion of these children, compared with typically developing children, to be chronically ill, medically fragile, or more vulnerable to stress. Consequently, we expected maternal employment decisions and the timing and selection of child care to be affected in these families, as well as in families of children with diagnosed disabilities.

A second unique aspect of the study is that detailed information about child care usage, patterns, and problems was obtained from mothers, and actual observations of child care quality were conducted. These observations were the same across all types of care. Third, families were studied regardless of their child care usage and plans (including children staying at home full time with their mothers). Fourth, the sample size is substantially larger than in previous studies. Finally, we were able to compare data from the present study with similar data from a local sample of typically developing children who were participating in a national study of the effects of early child care on children's development (the National Institute of Child Health and Human Development [NICHD] Study of Early Child Care). Very few other studies have had the benefit of such a comparison sample. Thus, it has been difficult, prior to this study, to ascertain whether child care characteristics in special-needs samples are a function of the unique needs of these children and their families or whether they reflect more general patterns.

METHOD

Participants

Special-Needs Study

The participants were 166 mothers and their children, who had a diagnosed disability by the age of 12 months ($n = 89$) or who were at risk for developing a disability ($n = 77$), primarily because of peri- or postnatal biomedical factors. In general, the majority of the mothers were married/partnered (78.9%). Although educational attainment varied across the sample from less than high school graduation to advanced degrees, on average, the mothers had completed some college. The children were primarily European American, non-Hispanic (European American, non-Hispanic: 72.0%; African American, non-Hispanic: 6.7%; Hispanic: 9.2%; Asian American: 1.8%; Native American: 1.8%; other: 8.5%). More boys than girls were enrolled in the study (64% for the diagnosed group and 54.5% for the at-risk group), reflecting the tendency for boys to be overrepresented in samples of children with special needs.

Diagnoses and risk factors for the children appear in Table 4.1. The most common diagnosis was developmental delay (52%), followed by Down syndrome (29.2%). The most common risk factors were low birth weight (46.8%), severe respiratory distress syndrome (39%), abnormal neurological signs (22.1%), and maternal substance abuse (23.4%). Most of the at-risk infants had either one (45.5%) or two (41.6%) risk factors.

At 15 months of age, children with diagnoses had an adjusted (for prematurity) mean mental development score of 64.49 (+ 14.12) on the revised Bayley Scales of Infant Development (BSID-II; Bayley, 1993), and an adjusted mean motor development score of 55.08 (+ 10.92). Adjusted mental and motor scores in the at-risk group were 90.21 (+ 9.46) and 95.51 (+ 12.70). By mothers' report, 33% of the children had chronic health problems at 12 months of age, and 20% required the use of adaptive equipment.

TABLE 4.1. Children's Diagnoses and Risk Factors: Special-Needs Sample

Diagnosis or risk factor	Percentage
Children with diagnosed disabilities	
Developmentally delayed[a]	52.0%
Down syndrome	29.2%
Spina bifida	6.7%
Other	12.1%
Children at risk for developing disabilities[b]	
Birth weight < 2,000 gm	46.8%
Severe respiratory distress syndrome	39.0%
Abnormal neurological signs	22.1%
Maternal substance abuse	23.4%
Small for gestational age	9.1%
Severe chronic illness	7.8%
Neonatal seizures	6.5%
Head circumference > 97th percentile	3.9%
Ventriculoperitoneal shunt installed	2.6%
Sepsis	2.6%
Failure to thrive	2.6%
Head circumference < 3rd percentile	2.6%
Maternal mental retardation	1.3%
Maternal use of therapeutic drugs	1.3%
Blood disorder	1.3%

[a]Children with developmental delays of unknown origin—that is, they met state qualifications for special services due to a 25% or greater cognitive delay and significantly delayed adaptive functioning.
[b]Percentages are not mutually exclusive.

NICHD Study of Early Child Care

The comparison sample (n = 139) came from the Seattle site of the NICHD Study of Early Child Care. As in the special-needs sample, most of the mothers were married/partnered (82.4%). On average, they had completed some college. Approximately half of the infants were male (50.4%), and most were European American, non-Hispanic (European American, non-Hispanic: 72.7%; African American, non-Hispanic: 9.4%; Hispanic: 7.9%; Asian American: 3.6%; Native American: .7%; other: 5.7%).

Procedure and Measures—Special-Needs Study

Whenever possible, the procedures, measures, and variable-construction methods used for the special-needs sample were identical to those used in the NICHD study. However, the subject recruitment methods and ages differed according to the nature of the sample, as described in the following text and in the next section.

Recruitment

Families were recruited from 17 participating clinics or agencies providing early intervention services for infants with diagnosed disabilities, or follow-up services for infants at risk. A staff member at each agency identified infants who were the appropriate age and then gave these infants' mothers a descriptive pamphlet about the study and asked if a member of our research team could telephone them to describe the study in more detail. The names and telephone numbers of mothers who agreed to a call were forwarded to our project staff, who then contacted and recruited the families by phone. Of the 226 families contacted, 166 (73%) agreed to participate. Reasons for not participating are provided in the original version of this paper.

12-Month Home Visit

At approximately 12–13 months of age the infants and their mothers were visited at home. Mothers were interviewed to obtain information about demographics, child care usage/plans, and child care concerns and problems. The BSID-II (Bayley, 1993) was also administered to the study children, yielding the Mental Development Index (MDI).

Mothers also gave their consent for their children's medical records to be obtained. Information about risk factors or disabilities were obtained from these records. Some of the data collected at the 12-month visit pertained to employment and child care concerns related to the children's special needs. Mothers were asked about the extent to which their child's special needs affected their work plans; their satisfaction with child care in the areas of location, cost, and quality; and the severity of their problems with child care in the areas of finding good-quality care, confidence in the staff, transportation, integrating child care with other services, cost of child care, special equipment or medications needed, and distance to child care.

14-Month Phone Call

When their child was approximately 14 months of age, mothers were called to obtain updated child care information. The following child care variables were summarized from the 14-month phone call: (1) primary type of care (mother, father, relative, nonrelative in home, child care home, and child care center); (2) age of entry into any amount of regular nonmaternal child care; (3) average weekly hours in care during any months that the child was in care; and (4) simultaneous number of arrangements in which the child spent time.

15-Month Child Care Visits

For those children spending at least 10 hours per week in a regular nonmaternal child care arrangement, two child care visits, approximately 1 week apart, occurred at 15 months of age. For children with more than one child care arrangement, observations took place in the setting in which the child spent the most time. If the child spent equal time in two arrangements, the more "formal" or institutional arrangement was observed. Observation and data collection procedures were identical regardless of the type of care (e.g., grandparent and center care) being observed. Of the observable arrangements, 9.2% were not observed for various reasons (e.g., scheduling difficulties and caregiver refusal).

For six children receiving combined early intervention and child care, observations were conducted during regular child care rather than during intervention. Note that "father care" of at least 10 hours per week, while the mother was employed or in school, was considered to be a regular child care arrangement for the purposes of this study (and the NICHD study).

The primary measure of the quality of observed care was the Observational Record of the Caregiving Environment (ORCE; see Chapters 1–3). In addition to the ORCE, two other observational instruments were used. The Home Observation for Measurement of the Environment (HOME) Inventory (Caldwell & Bradley, 1984), with some of the wording modified by Caldwell and Bradley to make the items more appropriate for child care situations, was completed in all home settings. The Child Care HOME uses an interview and observation format to assess caregivers' responsivity, acceptance, and involvement with the child, the organization of learning materials, and the variety of experiences offered the child. The 45 items, scored yes or no, had a Cronbach's alpha of .79. In child care centers, the Assessment Profile for Early Childhood Programs (Profile; Abbott-Shim & Sibley, 1987) was also used (see Chapter 3 for further details). Child care visitors were trained on the observational measures by one of the observers from the NICHD study.

Procedure and Measures: NICHD Study

Recruitment

Subjects were recruited from four hospitals in the Seattle area. During selected 24-hour sampling periods, 886 women who gave birth were visited in the hospital. Of these, 563 met the eligibility criteria for the study and agreed to be contacted after their return home from the hospital. From these, 139 families (58% of those contacted) were recruited for the study from the Seattle site.

Sources of Comparison Data

The procedures and methods used in the NICHD study are described in detail in Chapter 1. In terms of comparison with the special-needs sample, demographic variables that would not change over time (such as child sex and ethnicity) were obtained from data collected during a 1-month home visit. Additional demographic and descriptive data (such as child's health rating and mother's partner status) were obtained from an update phone call to the mother at 12 months. The BSID was administered at 15 months rather than at 12 months, and the original (Bayley, 1969) rather than the revised version was used. Finally, as noted later, the child care observations differed slightly in the two studies. However, all variables derived from the child care visits and all the other variables described for the special-needs sample were identical to those generated for the NICHD sample.

15-Month Child Care Visits

Children spending at least 10 hours per week in a nonmaternal child care arrangement were observed on two occasions at 15 months, using the same rules for selection of arrangement to be observed, and so forth, as described previously. Of the observable arrangements, 10.9% were not visited. The Profile, the Child Care HOME, and the ORCE were used to obtain indicators of the quality of the caregiving environment.

In terms of the ORCE, the differences between the two studies were that in the NICHD study (1) the observation cycles were slightly longer (44 minutes vs. 38 minutes), (2) the final ratings for a given cycle were based on four 10-minute observation periods rather than three, and (3) during the 10-minute observation periods, frequencies of specific behaviors were recorded to yield an additional index of quality (positive caregiving frequencies). Note that the additional 10-minute observation period and longer total observation time in the NICHD study were needed to ensure that adequate time was available for making qualitative ratings, apart from the time allocated for recording behavioral frequencies. The behavioral frequencies were not used in the special-needs study because in the NICHD study, the frequency index proved to be highly correlated ($r = .72$) with the positive caregiving ratings. Therefore, the additional training and reliability efforts required to add the frequency index were not warranted.

RESULTS

Demographic Differences

The NICHD, at-risk, and diagnosed samples were compared in terms of demographic characteristics, to select variables to act as covariates in the substantive analyses. Based on these comparisons, four covariates were selected for use in the substantive analyses: mothers' education, income-to-needs ratio, child ethnicity (minority, nonminority), and birth order.

Maternal Employment Patterns

Across groups, the majority of mothers (78.7%) were employed or in school part time (17.4%) or full time (61.3%) prior to the study child's birth, with average weekly hours of 38.62 ($\pm$ 14.94) among those who were working or attending school. Comparisons of the groups indicated that they did not differ significantly in terms of prebirth hours. A chi-square analysis, including all the subjects, also indicated that the groups did not differ significantly in terms of distribution by categorical hours (i.e., full time [> 30 hours], part time [10–30 hours], or less).

At 1 year of age, across groups, only 48.9% of the mothers were employed or in school part time (20.0%) or full time (28.9%). The majority of the mothers in the special-needs groups were employed or in school less than 10 hours per week, but the mothers in the NICHD group were distributed more evenly across categories. Among the mothers who were employed or in school, the NICHD group tended to have more hours than the mothers in the at-risk group, $F(2, 158) = 2.72$, $p = .07$. This trend remained the same when the mothers' prebirth employment/school hours were used as an additional covariate, $F(2, 147) = 2.56$, $p = .08$. Also, the groups differed in their distribution of hours, $\chi^2(4, N = 305) = 10.70$, $p < .05$. In the special-needs groups, fewer mothers were employed or in school full time, and more mothers were spending less than 10 hours per week in school or at work, compared with the NICHD group.

Child Care Patterns

Data about child care patterns appear in Table 4.2. On average, children entered child care relatively early in the first year of life ($M = 5.12 \pm 3.98$ months). However, an analysis of covariance (ANCOVA) by group revealed that the children with special needs entered care significantly later than the children in the NICHD sample, $F(2, 212) = 10.25$, $p < .001$. Among children who had entered care prior to 15 months, the mean weekly hours in care

TABLE 4.2. Child Care Characteristics by Group at 15 Months

Variable	NICHD (n = 139)	At risk (n = 77)	Diagnosed (n = 89)
Age of entry (months)	3.92(.37)	6.21(.54)	6.49(.51)
Hours in care (weekly)[a]	30.92(1.52)	29.84(2.23)	24.17(2.10)
Number of arrangements	1.43(.06)	1.18(.08)	1.26(.07)
Observed child–adult ratio	2.78(.23)	2.39(.30)	2.42(.31)
Positive caregiving ratings	14.97(.39)	15.74(.50)	16.08(.52)
Child care HOME	37.69(.72)	38.06(.81)	37.61(.97)
Profile–centers	12.74(.58)	13.48(1.19)	14.52(.78)
Type of care			
Mother (no child care)	29.8%	41.6%	41.6%
Father/partner	12.1%	13.0%	14.6%
Relative	10.5%	19.5%	20.2%
Nonrelative, in home	7.3%	6.5%	5.6%
Child care home	23.4%	9.1%	7.9%
Child care center	16.9%	10.4%	10.1%

Table entries (except for type of care) are means, adjusted for covariates, and standard error in parentheses. For all variables except age of entry and hours in care, 14- or 15-month data were used.
[a]Average weekly hours in care for the months that child was actually in care.

was 28.88 ($\pm$ 16.02). The groups differed significantly on this variable, with the diagnosed group spending fewer hours in care than the NICHD group, $F(2,212) = 3.40$, $p < .05$. At 14 months of age, children were spending time, on average, in more than one child care arrangement ($M = 1.32 \pm .53$), but the at-risk children had fewer arrangements than did the NICHD children, $F(2,177) = 3.09$, $p < .05$.

In terms of the primary type of care arrangement at 14 months, 36.6% were cared for by their mothers (i.e., they were not in child care), 13.1% by their fathers, 15.9% by another relative, 6.6% by a nonrelative in the child's home, 14.8% in a child care home, and 13.1% in a child care center. A chi-square analysis revealed a significant difference by group, $\chi^2(10, n = 290) = 20.44$, $p < .05$, with more of the special-needs children being cared for by their mothers or another relative and fewer being cared for in a child care home or center. Although the observed child–adult ratio was smaller in the special-needs groups than in the NICHD sample, a significant difference was not obtained.

The measures of quality of child care indicated that, on average, the children were receiving relatively high-quality care. The mean score was 15.46 ($\pm$ 2.90) out of a possible 20 points on the ORCE positive caregiving ratings; 37.79 ($\pm$ 4.58) out of a possible 45 points on the Child Care HOME; and 13.39 ($\pm$ 2.37) out of a possible 17 points on the Profile for child care centers. ANCOVAs on these quality measures indicated that the groups did not differ significantly on any of them.

To determine whether quality differed by group within type of care, a Type × Group ANCOVA was performed on the ORCE composite. To maximize the n per cell, and to form logical groupings, the types used were (1) father/partner or relative, (2) child care home, and (3) child care center. The analysis yielded a significant effect of Type, $F(2,102) = 17.92$, $p < .001$. Follow-up pairwise comparisons revealed that the (adjusted) scores for father/partner or relative ($M = 17.04$, $SE = .35$) were higher than the scores for child care homes ($M = 15.02$, $SE = .55$), which were higher than the scores for child care centers ($M = 13.37$, $SE = .51$). As expected, the Group effect was not significant. The Type × Group interaction term was also not significant, indicating that quality did not differ by group within each type.

DISCUSSION

One of the strengths of the present study, compared with previous research on child care for children with special needs (e.g., Landis, 1992; Warfield & Hauser-Cram, 1996), is that a comparison sample of typically developing children was included. Thus, employment and child care patterns in the special-needs group can be interpreted within the context of what is known about the "usual" child care patterns and characteristics in the same geographic area. Despite some demographic differences between the samples, when these variables were controlled statistically, comparisons of the groups revealed significant effects. Specifically, although the mothers' prebirth employment (and school) patterns were comparable in the two groups, the mothers of children with special needs did not return to the workforce by the time their child was 1 year of age at a rate comparable to that of the mothers of typically developing children. Similarly, the children with special needs entered child care at an older age, and for fewer hours per week (for those with diagnoses). The children's special needs were an important issue in making employment decisions and in finding child care for about one-third of the sample.

When these children did enter child care, they were more likely to be cared for by a relative and less likely to be enrolled in a child care home or center. Care by relatives, across all groups of children, was generally of higher quality than other types of care. Thus, we would expect the children with special needs to have higher average scores for the quality of care. In fact, scores on the ORCE ratings were higher in the special-needs groups than in the NICHD group, but these differences did not reach statistical significance. The groups also did not differ in terms of the quality of the physical environment in which the care was taking place.

It is important to note that care by relatives, though of higher quality than other types of care in both the special-needs and NICHD studies

(NICHD Early Child Care Research Network, 1996) was not found to be as positive in the Study of Children in Family Child Care and Relative Care (Galinsky, Howes, Kontos, & Shinn, 1994), an investigation involving 226 providers in three communities. In the latter study, two crucial factors were that the majority of relatives were living in stressful poverty conditions and were providing child care as a way to help the mother, rather than because they wanted to care for children. Thus, in any individual care situation (including exclusive maternal care), the quality of care cannot be assumed on the basis of the type of caregiver alone.

In addition to comparing children with and without special needs in this chapter, it is also instructive to compare the results of this study with previous investigations of child care for children with special needs. Regarding postbirth maternal employment, about 22% of the mothers in the present study were employed full time at 12 months, compared with 33% in the Landis (1992) study, and 36% in the Warfield and Hauser-Cram (1996) study. These differences may be a function of the older ages of the children in these published reports (0–3 years and 5 years, respectively), because we would expect maternal employment to increase as children age. Despite these apparent differences in hours of employment, children in the Warfield and Hauser-Cram study were spending an average of 22.2 hours per week in child care, compared with 26.3 hours in the present study.

An additional concern is that there were a significant number of mothers who were employed (or in school) prenatally but who did not return to work during their child's first year. Although 70% of the women who were not employed at 1 year indicated that this was what they had planned, 30% of the women cited their child's special needs as an important concern in making this decision. It is possible that many of the mothers in the latter group could afford to stay home without adverse economic consequences. However, for others, the lack of income resulting from this decision could severely affect the family's living conditions. For these families, either the lack of available and affordable child care and/or their belief that their infant's needs are best met at home could lead to a decision resulting in economic hardship and possible dependence on welfare. Several recent studies report that low-income families are more likely to turn to welfare when they cannot get child care (Ebb, 1994; Siegel & Loman, 1991) and underscore the importance of affordable child care for the working poor. On the other hand, the family's decision for the mother to stay at home because of the infant's special needs suggests the importance of strengthening family-leave policies to include more low-income families that might benefit from job-protected leave under the provisions of the Family and Medical Leave Act (FMLA).

In a recent survey of early childhood child care providers, lack of knowledge regarding care requirements of young children with special needs was cited most often as a barrier to including them in child care arrangements (Dinnebeil, McInerney, Fox, & Juchartz-Pendry, 1998). Therefore, it seems likely that one way to increase inclusive child care options is to provide special training for caregivers so that more settings are available for these families. From a policy perspective, such training can be addressed most easily in licensed or more formal child care arrangements (e.g., Demchak, Kontos, & Neisworth, 1992). However, most of the families of children with special needs in this study opted to use less formal arrangements. It is not clear whether this decision reflects a genuine desire to have the child cared for by a relative or in a one-to-one situation or indicates a lack of other child care choices. It could be that the child care issues reported in the literature, such as lack of staff training (NICHD Early Child Care Network, 1996), high staff turnover (Helburn, 1995; Whitebook, Howes, & Phillips, 1990;), and low staff wages and benefits (Helburn, 1995; Whitebook et al., 1990) combine to make appropriate center care for children with special needs especially difficult to locate.

One of the limitations of this study is that about 10% of the child care arrangements were not observed, and nonobserved situations typically are of lower quality. Thus, the results pertaining to quality of child care could look more positive than they actually are. However, this is a problem in any study of child care, including the NICHD study.

A second limitation is that the methods and procedures for the NICHD study and the special-needs study were different in some ways and could have accounted for some of the results. However, the fact that the special-needs sample differed from the NICHD sample on some child care variables but were comparable to other special-needs samples on these variables leads us to believe that these small differences in methods were not of consequence. Nonetheless, it would be ideal to conduct a study in which all the children with and without special needs were recruited and studied at the same time.

A third limitation is that both the special-needs and NICHD samples had higher income and educational levels than did national norms, reflecting a general trend in the Puget Sound area. Thus, the generalizability of these data is limited.

Despite these limitations, the results indicate some ways in which child care for children with special needs is different and some ways in which it is similar to child care for typically developing children. As these children mature, we will evaluate child care characteristics further and will be using a longitudinal ecological model to address the effects of child care, in interaction with child characteristics, family characteristics, home characteristics, and the early-intervention environment, on child cognitive, language, and social–emotional outcomes.

5

A New Guide for Evaluating Child Care Quality

NICHD EARLY CHILD CARE RESEARCH NETWORK

The words "quality care" are frequently heard on the lips of teachers and administrators, parents and reporters, researchers, and policymakers. All these concerned adults want to be sure that children receive "quality care." But what is quality care? According to child care expert Sandra Scarr (1998), "There is an extraordinary international consensus among child care researchers and practitioners about what quality child care is: It is warm, supportive interactions with adults in a safe, healthy, and stimulating environment, where early education and trusting relationships combine to support individual children's physical, emotional, social, and intellectual development" (p. 100). But can anyone walk into a center or a child care home and know at a glance if it meets these criteria for good quality care? If the person is a trained observer—an NAEYC (National Association for the Education of Young Children) accreditor perhaps—he or she can make an objective and educated evaluation. But what about a new teacher or child care provider, a parent, a teacher-to-be, or an inexperienced director whose experience is primarily administration? How can they recognize quality care?

From *Zero to Three*, 2001, Vol. 21, pp. 40–47. Copyright 2001 by Zero to Three: National Center for Infants, Toddlers, and Families. Reprinted by permission.

WAYS OF EVALUATING THE QUALITY OF CARE

There are, of course, many different ways to evaluate the quality of a child care program, and these vary with the goals of the evaluation. If the purpose of the evaluation is professional accreditation, all aspects of the arrangement must be probed in great depth. The NAEYC accreditation involves assessing the qualifications of the staff, the behavior of the teachers, and the physical environment of the center (Bredekamp & Glowacki, 1996). If the purpose of the evaluation is licensing, the evaluator must establish that the caregiver is an adult who has some training and passes a criminal background check, that there are not more children than the county allows, that the setting complies with minimum space requirements, that equipment is easily accessible to the children, that vehicles are equipped with age-appropriate safety carriers, that cleaning materials are not accessible to children, and that there are periodic health appraisals of the staff. Determining quality, in this case, requires a trained evaluator with a detailed checklist and a nose for infractions. If the purpose of the evaluation is program improvement, the assessment of quality might be based on ratings of the overall quality of the program. One of the assessments most commonly used for this purpose is the Early Childhood Environment Rating Scale (ECERS; Harms & Clifford, 1980). Although the ECERS is useful to program developers, it is not so useful for inexperienced observers such as parents, new teachers, or directors. Using the ECERS requires an observer who has been thoroughly trained to use this instrument and has observed the quality of care in a large number of programs (Helburn, 1995).

So what can parents, teachers, or administrators do to decide whether a program is of "good quality"? Their purpose is not to license or accredit the program. What they want to know is whether the program is excellent, good, fair, or poor. Teachers-to-be are interested in seeing what high-quality care looks like. New teachers want to know whether it is a place they would like to work. Lead teachers may want to know how a particular child in the class is faring. Administrators want to know whether a particular teacher or classroom is meeting their expectations. Parents simply want to know if they have found the best program for their child. These individuals typically do not have training in making detailed evaluations. How can they evaluate quality?

HOW CAN A NOVICE OBSERVER
EVALUATE THE QUALITY OF CARE?

One predictor of high quality care is the number of children for whom the caregiver is responsible (NAEYC, Zero to Three, or the American Public Health Association and the American Academy of Pediatrics, 1992). Another predictor of high-quality care is the caregiver's level of training. But research shows that the best evaluation of the quality of care comes from observing the child's actual experiences in the care arrangement (Clarke-Stewart, Vandell, Burchinal, O'Brien, & McCartney, 2002; McCartney, Scarr, Phillips, Grajek, & Schwartz, 1982).

HELP FROM A NATIONAL STUDY OF CHILD CARE

As researchers in the National Institute of Child Health and Human Development (NICHD) Study of Early Child Care, we have developed a way of evaluating child care that is better than guessing—a simple checklist that can be used to observe children's experiences in care. We have devised a tool that we believe can be used by relatively inexperienced observers to estimate the quality of a program in a center or home in a brief period. This tool is based on 3,477 observations of diverse child care settings, and we believe it is a practical and useful instrument which, in combination with other sources of information, can help observers evaluate the quality of child care programs.

In the NICHD Study of Early Child Care, we followed more than 1,000 children who were selected for the study soon after birth. Mothers of newborn infants were approached in hospital in 10 locations around the country. When the children were 6 months old, and then, again, when they were 15, 24, 36, and 54 months old, their mothers were called and asked about the child's care. The care provider in any care arrangement that the children were in for at least 10 hours a week was then contacted and asked if the researchers could schedule a visit to observe the child. If the child was in more than one care arrangement, the observers visited the setting in which the child spent the most time. Observations were conducted on two different days at each age.

At each visit, observers used an instrument especially designed to assess the quality of care that the child experienced, the Observational Record of the Caregiving Environment (ORCE): The first part is a checklist on which the observers record the occurrence of specific caregiver and child behaviors in half-minute intervals (Figure 5.1); the second part is a set of rating scales, which the observers use for coding the nature and manner of the caregiver's behavior. The rating scales were selected by study investigators to represent what child development researchers and child care professionals believe reflects good-quality care for infants and young children.

After the data were collected, these specific ratings for each child were combined to create an overall rating of good-quality caregiving at each age observed. These ratings were then analyzed to see if they were related to measures of how well the children were developing. Children who were in child care settings that received higher overall ratings for quality of caregiving had fewer behavior problems on a standardized checklist at 24 and 36 months (NICHD Early Child Care Research Network, 1998a). Their interactions with other children were more positive at 24 months (NICHD Early Child Care Research Network, 2001c). They also did better on tests of cognitive and language development at 24 and 36 months (NICHD Early Child Care Research Network, 2000b) and 4½ years (NICHD Early Child Care Research Network, 2002a).

A SIMPLER SOLUTION: THE NICHD CAREGIVER LANGUAGE CHECKLIST

The next step was to relate these overall ratings to some simpler and more specific measures of the child's experience in care that could be used by less experienced observers. The combined rating of overall quality of caregiving was divided into four levels: poor, fair, good, and excellent. In "poor" programs, sensitivity, responsiveness, and stimulation were not at all characteristic of the caregivers, and detachment and intrusiveness were very characteristic; in excellent programs, sensitivity, responsiveness, and stimulation were highly characteristic of the caregivers, and detachment and intrusiveness were not at all characteristic. These levels of quality were then related to the following specific behaviors, which the observers had recorded in the half-minute intervals in the first part of the ORCE: The caregiver (1) responds to the child's vocalization, (2) reads aloud to the child, (3) asks the child a question, (4) praises or speaks affectionately to the child, (5) teaches the child, (6) directs other positive talk to the child, (7) has close physical contact with the child; and the child (8) is unoccupied or (9) is watching TV.

Data analyses showed that these specific behaviors were significantly related to the overall rating of the quality of care (tables containing details on the statistical relations between the specific behaviors and the ratings of quality are available from the authors). In general, in programs that were rated highest for overall quality, caregivers responded to children's vocalizations more often, read to them more, asked them more questions, praised them more, instructed them more, talked to them more in other positive ways, and had more close physical contact with them; the children spent less time doing nothing or watching TV.

The strongest and most consistent predictors of overall child care quality involved the kinds of language caregivers directed to the children: responding to vocalizations, asking questions, praising, teaching, and talking to the children in other positive ways. The NICHD Caregiver Language Checklist includes just these behaviors. It is this checklist that a novice observer could use to evaluate the quality of a program or a particular child's experience.

Definitions

Caregiver responds to the child's vocalization

Responds verbally to what the child is saying or trying to say, repeats the child's words, comments on what the child has said, or answers the child's question.

Caregiver asks the child a question

Examples: "Are you hungry?" "Who is that?" "You're sleepy, aren't you?" "You like green ones?"

Caregiver praises, says something affectionate to child

Examples: "I love you." "You're a cutie." "You did it!"

Caregiver teaches the child

Caregiver instructs the child: "This is a ball." "Say 'ball.'" "That's a ball." For children aged 2 years and older, teaching should involve an academic skill, that is, the three R's—counting, naming shapes, saying the ABCs, pointing out letters or words in a book, teaching the meaning of a new word, labeling alphabet blocks, showing how to put together a puzzle, correcting the child's language, comparing objects of different sizes, suggesting the child work on academic materials.

Caregiver directs other positive talk to the child

Describes an object or event, comforts or entertains the child, sings a song, tells a story. Examples: "We're going outside." "The bottle is empty." "I'm going to put your bib on." A single sentence will do. **Does not include** negative talk (insults, criticizes, rejects, reprimands, teases, yells) or directive talk (giving orders).

Record Form

Caregiver language	30-second observation intervals															
	1	2	3	4	5	6	7	8	9	10	11	12	13	14	15	Subtotal
Responds to child's vocalization[1]																
Asks child a question																
Praises, says something affectionate[2]																
Teaches child																
Directs other positive talk to child																

	16	17	18	19	20	21	22	23	24	25	26	27	28	29	30	Subtotal
Responds to child's vocalization[1]																
Asks child a question																
Praises, says something affectionate[2]																
Teaches child																
Directs other positive talk to child																
	31	32	33	34	35	36	37	38	39	40	41	42	43	44	45	Subtotal
Responds to child's vocalization[1]																
Asks child a question																
Praises, says something affectionate[2]																
Teaches child																
Directs other positive talk to child																
	46	47	48	49	50	51	52	53	54	55	56	57	58	59	60	Subtotal	Total
Responds to child's vocalization[1]																	
Asks child a question																	
Praises, says something affectionate[2]																	
Teaches child																	
Directs other positive talk to child																	

[1]Do not code at 54 months.
[2]Do not code at 6 months.

FIGURE 5.1. NICHD Caregiver Language Checklist.

83

A USER'S GUIDE:
HOW TO OBSERVE CAREGIVERS' BEHAVIOR

Users of the NICHD Caregiver Language Checklist record and tally the language directed by caregivers to children in the child care program. They pick out a child at the beginning of the observation and focus their attention on that child for a period of 1 hour. The child might be a child selected by chance or a child in whom they were interested for some particular reason. If the observers are parents, it would make sense to focus on a child that reminded them of their own. To find out about the overall quality of the program, it would be best to observe several children, in turn, each for 1 hour, or to observe the same child for 1 hour on several different days. The observer then observes and records the language of any caregiver who interacts with the particular child being watched during the observation period. The child may be alone or part of a group; there may be one caregiver or more than one who interacts with the child during the observation; what is important is that the observer notes all the caregivers' language that the child hears during the period of the observation.

Observers use a watch with a second hand or a timer that beeps every half minute to divide their observations into alternating half-minute "observe" and "record" intervals. During "observe" intervals, the observer watches the child, keeping track of what happens to him or her, specifically, what language a caregiver directs to him or her or to the group to which he or she belongs. Then, during the next half-minute interval, the "record" interval, the observer scans the checklist and marks off all the different types of caregiver language he or she has observed. For example, if a caregiver asks the child one or more questions, the observer puts a checkmark in the box beside "Asks question"; if a caregiver compliments the child, the observer puts a checkmark in the box beside "Praises." A maximum of five check-marks can thus be given in any observation interval.

After an hour, the observer has a total of 60 intervals recorded on the checklist. (If the observation has to be interrupted for some reason, the observer can continue it later, until a full hour observation is made for the particular child.) Observers then total up the number of intervals in which each type of language was observed and compare those numbers to the NICHD Quality Guidelines graph for the age closest to the age of the child they have observed. These quality guideline graphs (shown at the end of this chapter) tell the observer how the observed program lines up with the programs observed in the NICHD study and what quality rating was given to programs similar to the one just observed. To get the best snapshot of quality, the observer should choose to observe on a typical day for the children, at a time when there are different activities going on—not just lunch or nap time.

HOW TO USE THE QUALITY GUIDELINE GRAPHS

The NICHD Quality Guidelines show how caregiver behaviors mapped onto the four levels of quality at each age in the NICHD study. For each level of quality—poor, fair, good, excellent—the center of the bar indicates how often the observed behavior occurred on average, and the two ends of the bar indicate a "standard deviation" above and below the average. What this means is that just over two-thirds of the caregivers with that quality designation received behavior scores that fell between the ends of the bars.

To use the graphs, first, select the graph that applies to the age of the child who has been observed. Second, mark on the graph the scores for each of the observed behaviors. Third, determine whether each of these scores reflects poor, fair, good, or excellent quality. Fourth, assign an estimate of overall program quality by seeing which rating is marked most often. If the scores are totally inconsistent from behavior to behavior (for instance, if the caregiver does a lot of teaching and is in the "excellent" range for this behavior but never praises the child or says anything nice, scoring "poor" for this behavior), the observer might conclude that the quality is "mixed" and decide to observe for another hour on a different day.

For example, when the child observed is an 8-month-old infant: The observer totals up the caregivers' behaviors; she finds that a caregiver responded to the child's vocalizations in 10 of the 60 half-minute observation intervals, asked a question in 23 intervals, instructed the child in 7 intervals, and talked to the child in another positive way in 40 intervals. The observer looks at the graph for "Quality at 6 Months" and discovers that each of these behaviors is as frequent as the caregivers given "excellent" ratings in the NICHD study (see "Example of Excellent Quality at 6 Months"). She concludes that the quality of care in the observed program is excellent. If, on the other hand, a caregiver responded to the child's vocalizations in only 3 intervals, asked a question in 5 intervals, instructed the child in 3 intervals, and talked to the child in another positive way in 16 intervals, the observer would conclude that the quality of care was "fair" (see "Example of Fair Quality at 6 Months").

ARE THERE DIFFERENT PROFILES
FOR DIFFERENT TYPES OF CARE?

It is possible that evaluating the quality of care depends on the care setting—that is, whether the care is being provided in a home or center setting. There are differences in children's experiences depending on whether they are in a home care setting or a center—because there are usually fewer children in home settings and a more educational agenda in centers. In the NICHD study, these differences were reflected in the fact that children in home care, especially in their own home with a relative or nanny, had more conversations with their caregivers than did children in centers (they were asked more questions and received more frequent responses to their vocalizations), and, at the older ages (36 and 54 months), children in centers received more instruction from their caregivers than did children with relatives or nannies. There were no differences in how much caregivers read to, praised, or had close physical contact with the children.

What are the implications of these differences for an observer evaluating a new program? Is there a difference in what the observer should look for in centers and in home care? The findings and graphs we have discussed apply to child care of all types—a relative in the child's home, a nanny, a child care home, or a center. In both homes and centers, the overall quality of care was related to these caregiver behaviors. Thus, basically, observers can look for the same set of characteristics in different settings. However, if they want to compare the quality of care across different types of settings (i.e., in homes and centers), because home caregivers converse more and center caregivers teach more (with older children), they might want to hold home caregivers to a higher standard for the frequency of conversations and center caregivers to a higher standard for the frequency of instruction.

WHAT SHOULD OBSERVERS DO
WITH THEIR EVALUATION?

The guidelines we have presented for evaluating whether a program offers poor, fair, good, or excellent quality care are just that–guidelines. They are not guarantees. Observing that a program meets the criteria to receive an excellent rating does not confer a seal of approval. These guidelines should not be used to give a program a grade that can be posted on the front door. They should not be used as the basis for granting or withdrawing a license or awarding or denying accreditation. They are intended to help parents, teachers, and administrators make informed judgments about the quality of care in particular programs and help them decide whether a more detailed, in-depth evaluation is warranted.

NICHD QUALITY GUILDELINES

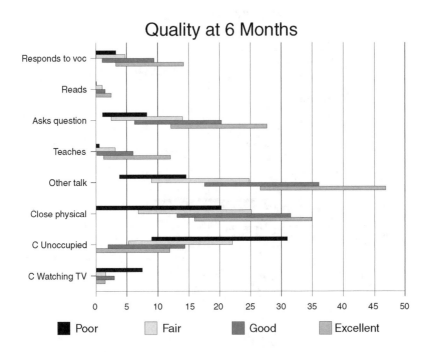

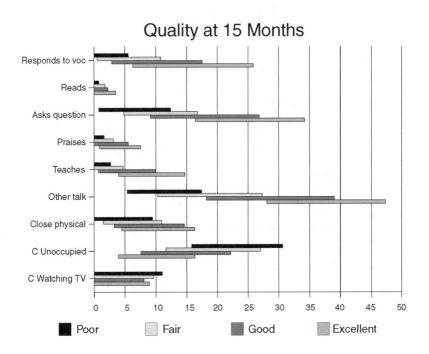

Quality at 24 Months

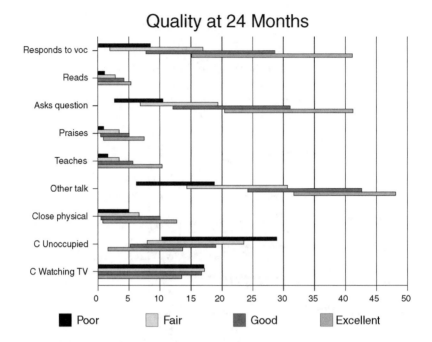

Quality at 36 Months

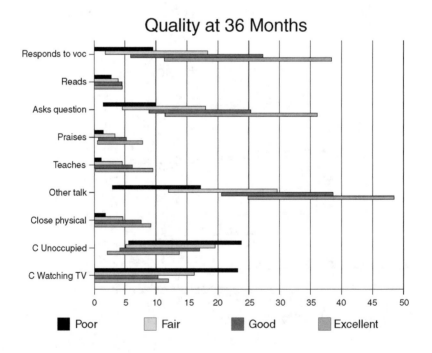

Quality at 54 Months

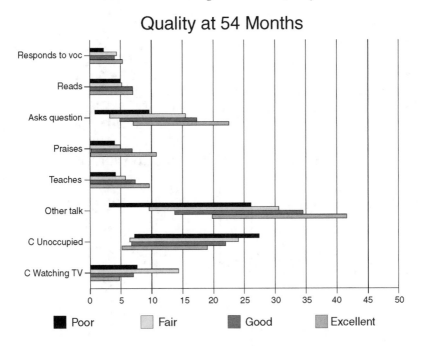

Poor   Fair   Good   Excellent

Example of Excellent Quality at 6 Months

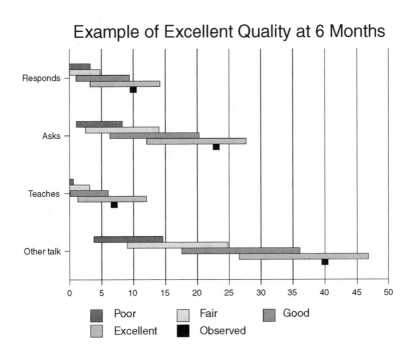

Poor   Fair   Good

Excellent   Observed

Behavior	Count	Rating
Responds to vocalization	10	Excellent
Asks question	23	Excellent
Teaches	7	Excellent
Other talk	40	Excellent
Most common rating		Excellent

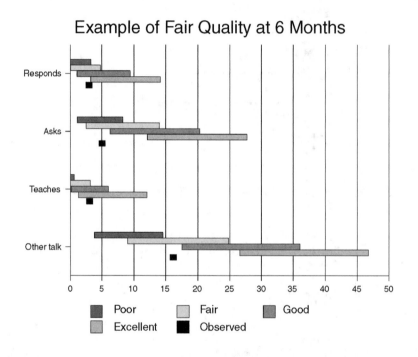

Behavior	Count	Rating
Responds to vocalization	3	Fair
Asks question	5	Poor
Teaches	3	Good
Other talk	16	Fair
Most common rating		Fair

6

Characteristics and Quality of Child Care for Toddlers and Preschoolers

NICHD Early Child Care Research Network

As the 21st century dawns, child care is a fact of life for the majority of young children in the United States who spend at least some time in nonmaternal care before they embark on kindergarten or enter first grade. Concerns have been raised about the quality of these child care arrangements—about what kind of care children are receiving, how it varies in different types of care with different caregivers, and what structural (i.e., child–adult ratio, group size, physical characteristics of the child care setting) and caregiver characteristics (i.e., education, specialized training, experience, childrearing beliefs) are linked to the quality of care. These are important issues for parents, policymakers, and, of course, children. They are also relevant for researchers. It would be useful for us, as well, to know which observable characteristics of the care arrangement predict higher-quality care. It also would be valuable to have an indication of the quality of child care in the United States today, taking into account different types of care, ages of children, and family circumstances. Child care in America does not have a good reputation (Greenspan, 1997); we should know whether its negative reputation is deserved.

It was our goal in this study to investigate each of these issues. First, we examined the relation between structural and caregiver characteristics and observed caregiver behavior to see which factors predicted more positive

From *Applied Developmental Science*, 2000, Vol. 4, pp. 116–135. Copyright 2000 by Lawrence Erlbaum Associates. Reprinted by permission.

caregiving. Second, we analyzed differences in levels of positive caregiving associated with the type of child care centers, child care homes, in-home sitters, grandparents, and fathers—at three different child ages. Third, we used our observations of positive caregiving, stratified by type of care, child age, and maternal education, in conjunction with the 1995 National Household Education Survey (Hofferth, Shauman, Henke, & West, 1998), a nationally representative survey of child care usage, to extrapolate from our sample to the nation, by adjusting for bias in our estimate along these three dimensions relative to the population of 1- to 3-year-olds in the United States. To investigate these issues, we used the data from the National Institute of Child Health and Human Development (NICHD) Study of Early Child Care (NICHD Early Child Care Research Network, 1996, 1997c, 1998b, 1999b).

METHOD

Procedure

At 15 months of age, 612 children who were in care for 10 hours or more per week were observed in their care setting; at 24 months of age, 630 children in care were observed in their care setting; and at 36 months of age, 674 children were observed in their care setting. Of those who were in child care 10 hours or more per week, 127 children at 15 months of age, 137 children at 24 months of age, and 128 children at 36 months of age were not observed in care because of caregiver or parent refusal or because the child care visits could not be scheduled within the 2-month assessment window. Participation rates were highest for in-home caregivers (92%) and centers (91%), somewhat lower for fathers (83%) and grandparents (79%), and lowest for child care homes (75%).

Demographic characteristics of the total sample at recruitment and of the observed and unobserved samples at 15, 24, and 36 months of age show that, at 15 and 24 months, African American children were less likely than other children to be observed, $\chi^2(3; n = 801, n = 814) = 9.50, p < .02, 18.83, p < .001$, respectively. At all three ages, mothers in the observed sample had higher levels of education, $\chi^2(4; n = 801, n = 814, n = 849) = 11.66, p < .02, 17.66, p < .001, 12.79, p < .01$, respectively.

Two half-day visits to the children's primary care arrangement were conducted at 15, 24, and 36 months of age (a total of six visits) to observe and assess children's experiences. At the first visit, observers completed two observation cycles and then filled out the physical environment checklist. At the second visit, two additional observation cycles were completed and then interviews and questionnaires were administered to the caregiver or caregivers. An observational instrument, the Observational Record of the Caregiving Environment (ORCE), which could be used in all types of child care settings, was designed for this study. Observers using this instrument focus on caregivers' behavior with a specific child (in this case, the study child) rather than on what happens in the setting at large. They record frequencies of specific behaviors and make qualitative ratings of caregivers' behavior. We included both behavior frequencies and qualitative ratings in this instrument so that we might estimate both the quantity or amount of positive caregiving experienced by each child and the quality or nature of that positive caregiving. Chapters 3 and 5 provide further details about the ORCE.

At 15 months of age, *positive caregiving frequency* was defined as the sum of 14 categories of behavior that had been individually standardized. These behaviors, all directed to or involving the study child, included the following: The caregiver expresses positive affect, has positive physical contact, speaks positively, asks questions, responds to the child's vocalization, reads, initiates other talk to the child, stimulates the child's cognitive development, stimulates the child's social development, facilitates behavior, restricts activity, speaks negatively, exhibits negative physical actions, and does not interact with the child (the child is unoccupied). The last four behavior categories were reverse coded before being included in the composite variable (Cronbach's alpha = .78).

At 24 months of age, the composite measure of positive caregiving frequency consisted of the sum of the following 12 individually standardized categories of behavior with the child: The caregiver has positive physical contact, talks, speaks positively, responds to child's talk, asks questions, teaches academic skill, has mutual exchange with child, exhibits negative-restrictive actions, speaks negatively, and does not interact with child (the child watches, is unoccupied, or makes transition). The last three behavior categories were reverse-coded (Cronbach's alpha = .78).

At 36 months of age, the composite consisted of the sum of 10 individually standardized variables: The caregiver has positive physical contact with child, talks, speaks positively, responds to talk, asks questions, teaches academic skill, has mutual exchange with child, exhibits negative-restrictive actions, speaks negatively, and does not interact with child (the child watches, is unoccupied, or makes transition). The last three behavior categories were reverse coded (Cronbach's alpha = .76).

The coherence of these *a priori* composite measures of the frequency of caregivers' behavior, based on types of behavior that the investigators believed best reflected positive caregiving for toddlers and preschoolers, was supported by confirmatory factor analyses.

Qualitative ratings of positive caregiving were made as part of the ORCE method. At 15 and 24 months of age, the composite rating of positive caregiving quality was the mean of five ratings of the caregiver's behavior: sensitivity to child's nondistress signals, stimulation of child's development, positive regard toward child, detachment, and flatness of affect. The last two scales were reverse coded before being included in the composite variable (Cronbach's alphas = .88 at 15 months and .87 at 24 months). The coherence of this *a priori* composite was confirmed by principal component factor analysis. At 36 months of age, the composite qualitative rating for positive caregiving quality was the mean of seven variables: sensitivity to the child's nondistress signals, stimulation of child's development, positive regard toward child, fosters child's exploration, detachment, flatness of affect, intrusiveness; the last three scales were reverse coded (Cronbach's alpha = .83). The qualitative composite measure was available for 907 caregivers and 612 children at 15 months, 976 caregivers and 630 children at 24 months, and 1,109 caregivers and 674 children at 36 months. The qualitative ratings used in this chapter were for a single caregiver for each child at each age; for children interacting with more than one caregiver during the observation, the caregiver selected was the one for whom the most information was available, that is, the one who received qualitative ratings for more observation cycles.

At the beginning and end of each ORCE cycle (there was a maximum of four cycles), observers recorded the composition of the group of adults and children in the care setting. Variables derived from these records included the following: *group size* (average across ORCE cycles of the number of children under 13 years of age observed in the child's room or defined space) and *child–adult ratio* (average across the ORCE cycles of the number of awake children observed per caregiver).

Global rating of care. At the end of each visit, observers gave an overall evaluation of the quality of the care in the setting from 1 (terrible), 2 (poor), 3 (fair), 4 (good), to 5 (excellent). They were not specifically trained to make this global rating, and its points were not defined beyond these labels. This "commonsense" rating was highly correlated with ratings of positive caregiving, r's = .75, .68, .72, p's < .0001, at 15, 24, and 36 months, but it was based on a wider range of observations. It included all the dimensions observable in the setting—the quality of the physical environment, the curriculum, and peer interactions as well as the behavior of caregiver or caregivers.

Structured interviews and questionnaires were administered at the end of the second child care visit at each age. Caregivers' education was scored as 1 (less than high school graduation), 2 (high school diploma or GED), 3 (some college), 4 (bachelor's degree), 5 (some graduate work, including master's degree), or 6 (EdD, PhD, or other post–master's degree). Specialized training in child development or early education was scored from 0 (none) to 1 (high school or vocational level courses) to 2 (college-level courses). Caregiver experience was calculated as the number of years of providing child care or working in a child care or early childhood center.

Caregivers' beliefs about childrearing were assessed with a 30-item questionnaire (Schaefer & Edgerton, 1985). A principal component factor analysis yielded a single dimension of child-centered (nontraditional and nonauthoritarian) beliefs about childrearing. The 30 responses were summed with a range of possible scores between 30 and 150 with higher scores reflecting more child-centered beliefs. Cronbach's alphas were .90 at 15 months, .89 at 24 months, and .89 at 36 months.

Assessment of *the physical-learning environment* was based on the Assessment Profile for Early Childhood Programs (Abbott-Shim & Sibley, 1987) and was used at 15, 24, and 36 months in both center care and child care home settings. Three additional items from Wachs (1991) were added to assess quiet, crowding, and clutter. Higher scores reflected environments that were cleaner and safer, were less crowded and cluttered, and offered more numerous and varied developmentally appropriate toys and learning materials. Details about the items selected are available in the full article (NICHD Early Child Care Research Network, 2000a). Cronbach's alphas ranged from .48 to .76.

As we have described previously (NICHD Early Child Care Research Network, 1996), observers at the 10 sites were trained to a high level of *interobserver agreement* before data collection began and checks were maintained throughout data collection.

RESULTS

Three sets of analyses were conducted. Their purpose was to (1) determine univariate and multivariate relations between structural and caregiver characteristics and positive caregiving at the three ages (15, 24, and 36 months); (2) compare different types of care at the three ages in terms of their structural features, caregiver characteristics, and positive caregiving; and (3) estimate the quality of observed and unobserved care in the NICHD sample and use these figures to extrapolate to the quality of care in the United States by weighting them based on a nationally representative data set. Table 6.1 presents mean levels and descriptive statistics for all dependent and independent variables at each age.

Associations between Structural and Caregiver Characteristics and Observed Positive Caregiving Ratings

Pearson correlations (see Table 6.2) between the structural and caregiver characteristics and observed positive caregiving ratings revealed that positive caregiving was higher when child–adult ratios were lower and group sizes were smaller and when caregivers had higher levels of education and held more child-centered beliefs, at all three ages (all p's < .01). Caregivers' child care experience and specialized training were not correlated with positive caregiving ratings at any of the ages assessed.

Differences in the magnitudes of the significant correlations at the three ages were tested using a multivariate regression technique in a Seemingly Unrelated Regression Equation (Zellner, 1962). (The Seemingly Unrelated Regression Equation technique takes into account the fact that the same participants were studied over time and that the obtained correlation

TABLE 6.1. Descriptive Statistics for Structural and Caregiver Characteristics and Observed Positive Caregiving

	Age								
	15 months			24 months			36 months		
Child care variable	n	$M(\%)$	SD	n	$M(\%)$	SD	n	$M(\%)$	SD
Child–adult ratio	612	2.6	1.7	630	3.3	2.2	674	4.6	3.0
Group size	612	3.8	3.3	630	5.1	4.5	674	7.3	6.0
Caregiver education	607	2.7	1.1	585	2.7	1.0	636	2.9	1.1
Caregiver beliefs	556	101.9	18.9	610	103.6	18.0	665	104.8	17.9
Caregiver experience	603	4.0	5.9	585	4.6	6.3	633	5.4	6.2
Caregiver specialized training	612	0.6	0.8	587	0.7	0.8	636	0.8	0.9
Physical-learning environment[a]									
Child care homes	183	19.9	4.1	209	18.9	4.6	–	–	–
Centers	120	12.3	2.6	172	12.8	2.3	269	26.2	1.6
Type of care (%)									
Father	107	17.5	–	89	14.1	–	83	12.3	–
Grandparent	80	13.1	–	67	10.6	–	62	9.1	–
In-home	97	15.8	–	79	12.5	–	67	9.9	–
Child care home	200	32.6	–	211	33.5	–	168	24.9	–
Center	128	20.9	–	184	29.2	–	294	43.6	–
Positive caregiving frequency (whole sample)	612	0[b]	7.1	630	0[b]	5.8	674	0[b]	5.7
Positive caregiving rating (whole sample)	612	2.93	0.57	630	2.81	0.56	674	2.80	0.46
Positive caregiving rating (nonparental sample)	518	2.89	0.57	553	2.79	0.55	595	2.79	0.46
Positive caregiving rating (imputed for whole sample)[c]	764	2.87	0.60	784	2.78	0.55	819	2.79	0.45
Positive caregiving rating (imputed for nonparental sample)[c]	638	2.84	0.60	677	2.76	0.55	712	2.77	0.44
Positive caregiving rating (extrapolated for U.S.)	–	2.81	–	–	2.71	–	–	2.76	–

[a]Physical-teaming environment measures are not on the same scale across assessments.
[b]Standard scores.
[c]Correcting for sample selection and attrition; n's include children who had observable care that was not observed but not children who dropped out of the sample; means are adjusted for dropouts based on demographic characteristics.

TABLE 6.2. Pearson Correlations between Structural and Caregiver Characteristics of Care and Observed Positive Caregiving

	Age							
	6 months[a]		15 months		24 months		36 months	
Child care variable	Rating	Frequency	Rating	Frequency	Rating	Frequency	Rating	Frequency
Child–adult ratio	-.36*****	-.45*****	-.33****	-.41****	-.34****	-.49****	-.14*****	-.41****
Group size	-.36*****	-.46*****	-.34****	-.35****	-.33****	-.43****	-.11****	-.37****
Caregiver education	.11***	.03	.11***	.14***	.14***	.10***	.19*****	.06
Caregiver beliefs	.14***	.09**	.13***	.10***	.11***	.06	.22*****	.04
Caregiver experience	-.07	-.15**	-.08	-.07	.02	-.06	.06	-.07
Caregiver specialized training	-.02	-.05	.02	.03	.02	-.06	.05	-.04
Physical-learning environment								
Child care homes	.33*****	.10	.34****	.25****	.30****	.06		
Centers	.47*****	.31***	.49****	.42****	.15**	.15**	.20*****	.11*

[a]Figures for 6 months of age are from NICHD Early Child Care Research Network (1996, p. 290).
*p < .05; **p < .01; ***p < .001; ****p < .0001.

coefficients themselves were correlated.) Although they were statistically significant at all three ages, the correlations between positive caregiving ratings and observed ratios and group sizes were significantly smaller at 36 months than at either 15 or 24 months (p's < .001). Correlations between positive caregiving ratings and caregivers' education and beliefs increased in size as children got older, but the differences across age were not significant.

In the regression analyses, ratings of positive caregiving were significantly associated with the set of independent variables at all three ages, adjusted R^2's ranging from .12 to .21, p's < .001. Positive caregiving ratings were significantly higher when caregivers had more child-centered beliefs (at all three ages); higher levels of education and more experience providing child care (at 24 and 36 months); more specialized training (at 15 months); and when there were fewer children per adult and fewer children in the group (at 15 and 24 months).

To determine whether caregiver and structural characteristics contributed to positive caregiving in the same ways in different types of care, the homogeneity of the regressions across the five types of care was tested. Significant interactions between care type and other predictors were found for positive caregiving ratings at 36 months, $F(42, 516) = 1.56$, $p < .02$. Lower child–adult ratios were more strongly predictive of positive caregiving for fathers, grandparents, and in-home caregivers than for caregivers in centers or child care homes, $F(3, 516) = 3.12$, $p < .03$.

To determine whether the quality of the physical-learning environment was associated with observed positive caregiving, multiple regressions were recomputed, adding the physical-learning environment score in a second step. The addition of the physical-learning environment measure significantly improved the prediction of positive caregiving ratings, over and above the other structural and caregiver characteristics, in all these analyses.

Associations between Structural and Caregiver Characteristics and Observed Positive Caregiving Frequencies

Although there was a high degree of overlap in the patterns of association between structural and caregiver characteristics and positive caregiving ratings and frequencies, there were some differences. Frequencies of positive caregiving were more strongly related to child–adult ratio and group size than ratings were, significantly so at 36 months, r's in Table 2 = –.41 versus –.14 for ratio, –.37 versus –.11 for group size, p for differences < .01; regression weights for ratio and group size were significant for caregiving frequencies but not for ratings. On the other hand, ratings of positive caregiving were more strongly related to caregivers' education than frequencies were, particularly at 36 months, r's in Table 6.2 = .19 versus .06; regression weights for caregiver education were significant for caregiving ratings but not for frequencies. Ratings were also more consistently related to the quality of the physical-learning environment than were frequencies; all five associations between ratings and the physical-learning environment were significant, but only those at 15 months were significant for frequencies.

Characteristics of Care and Positive Caregiving in Different Types of Care at Different Ages

Mixed-model, repeated-measures analyses were used to test effects of type of care (father, grandparent, in-home, child care home, and center) and age (15, 24, and 36 months) and the interactions between type of care and age on structural and caregiver characteristics and positive caregiving ratings and frequencies. Consistent main effects associated with type of care were evident for child–adult ratio, $F(4, 811) = 19.83$, $p < .001$, and group size, $F(4, 811) = 581.15$, $p < .001$. Child–adult ratios were larger in child care centers ($M = 5.5$) than in child care homes ($M = 3.5$), which were larger than ratios with in-home caregivers ($M = 1.6$), grandparents ($M = 1.4$), and fathers ($M = 1.6$), $F(4, 811) = 19.83$, $p < .001$. Group sizes were largest in centers ($M = 10.5$), followed by child care homes ($M = 4.3$). Group sizes with fathers, grandparents, and in-home caregivers did not differ (M's = 1.7, 1.7, and 1.8, respectively).

Caregivers' education, beliefs, experience, and specialized training also differed by type of care, $F(4, 796) = 18.14$, $F(4, 777) = 18.81$, $F(4, 794) = 15.40$, $F(4, 801) = 30.57$, respectively, all p's < .001. Center caregivers ($M = 3.0$) and fathers ($M = 3.0$) had higher levels of education than did in-home caregivers ($M = 2.3$) and grandparents ($M = 2.2$; $p < .001$); the level of child care home providers' education was in between. Center caregivers had the highest level of specialized training in child development ($M = 1.0$), and fathers ($M = 0.3$) and grandparents ($M = 0.3$) had the lowest level. Center caregivers had the most child-centered beliefs about childrearing ($M = 108.1$), followed by caregivers in child care homes ($M = 104.5$), and fathers ($M = 103.7$). Grandparents ($M = 93.9$) and in-home caregivers ($M = 95.1$) had the least child-centered (most traditional or authoritarian) beliefs. Caregivers in child care homes and centers had the most experience providing child care (M's = 6.3 and 6.1 years, respectively), and fathers had the least experience ($M = 0.3$ years).

Significant linear trends for child age were found for caregiver experience, child–adult ratio, and group size. All three increased as children got older from 15 to 36 months $F(1, 794) = 11.91$, $F(1, 812) = 97.33$, $F(1, 812) = 46.31$, respectively, all p's < .001. For group size and child–adult ratio, increases with age were modified by interactions with type of care, $F(8, 812) = 16.62$; $F(8, 812) = 31.97$, p's < .001. The largest increases in group size and child–adult ratio occurred for children in centers (group size increased from 8.4 to 12.8; ratio increased from 4.0 to 7.3).

Accompanying these differences in structural and caregiver characteristics were differences in observed positive caregiving. Fathers, grandparents, and in-home caregivers were rated as providing more positive caregiving than child care home caregivers (M's for fathers, grandparents, and in-home caregivers = 3.0 vs. 2.8 for child care home providers), who received higher ratings than center caregivers (M = 2.7), F(4, 811) = 19.83, p < .001. The same pattern was found for the frequency of positive caregiving behaviors. Children received the greatest number of positive caregiving behaviors from fathers (M = 2.1), grandparents (M = 2.4), and in-home caregivers (M = 2.9), and less frequent positive caregiving from child care home caregivers (M = −0.5), and even less frequent positive caregiving from center caregivers (M = −2.9), F(4, 812) = 38.06, p < .001.

Positive caregiving ratings decreased as children got older (M's = 3.0, 2.9, and 2.8 at 15, 24, and 36 months, respectively, overall). This decrease was evident in all care types except centers (M's = 2.6, 2.6, 2.7 for centers), type of care × age interaction, F(8, 811) = 3.25, p < .001.

Quality of Caregiving

The final issue examined in this study was an estimation of the quality of care within the NICHD sample and an extrapolation from that estimate to the quality of care nationally. As a first step, mean scores for the qualitative ratings of positive caregiving at each age were converted to categories. Settings in which the caregiver's behavior was "not at all characteristic" of positive caregiving were rare (6.3% of the observed caregivers at 15 months, 8.1% at 24 months, and 4.1% at 36 months). Settings in which caregivers offered care that was "highly characteristic" of positive caregiving were also quite uncommon (17.8% at 15 months, 13.0% at 24 months, and 5.8% at 36 months). About 30% of the children across ages and types of care received care in which positive caregiving was "somewhat characteristic." The most common category at all three ages was "somewhat uncharacteristic" of positive caregiving (42.1% at 15 months, 50.1% at 24 months, and 57.6% at 36 months).

On the global ratings observers completed at the end of each visit, combining observations across the three ages, 11% of the care observed was judged to be of terrible or poor quality (ratings 1 to < 2.5), 31% was fair (ratings 2.5 to < 3.5), 41% was good (ratings 3.5 to < 4.5), and 17% was excellent (ratings 4.5 or higher). These observed percentages did not reflect caregiving quality for children whose child care setting could not be observed, nor does it reflect care used by families that had dropped out of this study. Thus, these percentages may provide a biased estimate for the entire sample. To remedy this problem, we imputed missing data using multiple imputation and propensity scores (Little & Rubin, 1987)—imputation methods widely accepted among statisticians. The imputed values for the sample tend to be only slightly lower than the values based on observed, uncorrected data.

Extrapolated positive caregiving ratings for the nation. We then used the imputed figures to provide our best guess as to the quality of child care in the United States. This "best guess" was created by using the imputed means and proportions from the NICHD sample for nonparental care and weighting those values with the estimated number of children in various types of care nationally as reported in the National Household Education Survey (NHES; Hofferth et al., 1998). The NHES included questions about amount and type of child care and demographic characteristics for a nationally representative sample. We categorized the data in the NHES data set based on the child's age, type of care, and maternal education. These strata were selected because, as documented in this chapter, differences in positive caregiving in child care are related to both type of care and child's age. In other analyses (NICHD Early Child Care Research Network, 1997c), we identified maternal education to be a family factor that also is consistently related to positive caregiving. Children's ages were classified as infants (0–11 months old), 1-year-olds (12–23 months of age), 2-year-olds (24–35 months of age), and 3-year-olds (36–47 months of age). Type of care was coded as center, child care home, sitter in own home, and relative care. Care by fathers was excluded because relative care in the NHES did not include paternal care. Maternal education was coded as less than high school, high school, some post–high school training or college, BA or BS degree, or graduate training. A national extrapolation was created by using the numbers of children in each stratum in the NHES data as a weight when combining strata means and proportions on positive caregiving from the (imputed) NICHD sample. The extrapolated figures for positive caregiving quality were slightly lower than the observed and imputed NICHD sample means and proportions. These values suggest that positive caregiving is "very uncharacteristic" for 8.1% of children in the United States ages 1 to 3 years, "somewhat uncharacteristic" for 53.2% of the children, "somewhat characteristic" for 29.6% of the children, and "highly characteristic" for 9% of the children.

Discussion

The results of the NICHD Study of Early Child Care presented in this chapter, obtained when the children in the study were 15–36 months old, extend those reported earlier when the children were 6-month-old infants. Continuities appeared in all three areas examined: (1) relations between structural and caregiver characteristics and observed positive caregiving, (2) differences in structural and caregiver characteristics and observed positive caregiving associated with type of care, and (3) overall quality of care.

Predicting Positive Caregiving

As had been found at 6 months of age, caregivers' observed behavior was significantly related to a set of structural characteristics, which consisted of child–adult ratio, group size, and characteristics of the physical-learning environment, and to caregiver characteristics, which included education, specialized training, experience, and beliefs. Approximately 25% of the variance in observed caregiving was accounted for by ratio, group size, and caregiver characteristics.

What was surprising was the finding that caregivers' specialized training in child care and child development was not strongly and consistently related to observed caregiving. Perhaps this lack of a strong and consistent association reflects a need for a more differentiated measure of caregiver specialized training. Researchers using more fine-grained assessments of caregiver specialized training have reported significant predictability from this variable (e.g., Howes, 1997).

Differences between frequencies and ratings of positive caregiving. Although there was a high degree of overlap in the predictions of positive caregiving frequencies and ratings when the children were 15 and 24 months old, the patterns diverged at 36 months of age. The findings suggest that the amount of attention a child receives is more strictly determined by the number of children (ratio, group size) than is the quality of that attention, at least by the time the child is 3 years old.

Changes in prediction of positive caregiving with age. At the three younger ages in the NICHD study (6, 15, and 24 months), ratings of positive caregiving were strongly related to the number of children and less strongly related to caregiver characteristics, but by 36 months the association with the number of children was significantly weaker and caregivers' characteristics had become relatively more important predictors of positive caregiving. This change with age had been predicted on the basis of earlier studies and the rationale that, as children become preschoolers, caregivers' educational backgrounds should play a more important part in determining whether they act in ways that are sensitive to children's signals and stimulate their development.

Links between positive caregiving and the physical-learning environment. Replicating the findings of the study at 6 months, a measure of the safety, stimulation, and order in the physical-learning environment was related to ratings of caregivers' positive caregiving, above and beyond the contributions made by other structural and caregiver characteristics. Perhaps the most important message from these associations is that safety, stimulation, and order evident in the physical setting can be used as one clue for parents and others seeking to evaluate caregiving quality.

Differences Associated with Type of Care

As we had observed at 6 months, compared with other types of care, centers had the largest groups, the highest child–adult ratios, and the most highly trained and experienced caregivers. Despite their higher levels of education, specialized training, experience, and child-centered beliefs, caregivers in centers offered children the lowest levels of positive caregiving (in terms of both ratings and frequencies of behavior), whereas in-home caregivers, including fathers and grandparents, offered the highest levels. Although positive caregiving was lowest in centers overall, it is worth noting that ratings of positive caregiving for center providers followed an upward trajectory from 15 to 36 months, whereas ratings of fathers, grandparents, and other home-based caregivers were decreasing. By the time the children were 36 months old, discrepancies in the ratings of positive caregiving in different types of care had diminished.

Quality of Care

The profile of care quality presented in this study is better than that reported in other large studies. It is difficult to make comparisons across studies because different researchers have used different rating scales and labeled them in different ways, but in all such comparisons the care observed in the NICHD study appears to be of higher quality than that in other research. In the three studies with which our results can be compared (Galinsky, Howes, Kontos, & Shinn, 1994; Helburn, 1990; Whitebook, Howes, & Phillips, 1990), researchers used a 7-point rating scale, whereas in the NICHD study we used a 4-point scale. To create a common metric, we converted their scores and ours to a 10-point scale. In Helburn's (1990) and Whitebook and colleagues' (1990) studies of child care centers, the average rating of quality observed in preschool classrooms (on the Early Childhood Environment Rating Scale) using the 10-point scale was 5.7, compared with our rating of positive caregiving in centers, which was 6.6. For toddlers, their average ratings were 4.9 and 5.4 compared with our rating of 6.5 for 15- and 24-month-olds. In Galinsky and colleagues' (1994) study of home-based care, the average rating of quality was 4.9, compared with our rating of positive caregiving, which was 7.1. Similar differences appear when we compare proportions of child care settings given ratings of good or excellent. It is difficult to say whether these differences reflect real, objective differences in quality of care or differences in the eyes of the beholders. Comparing the objective standard of child–adult ratio across the three studies of centers is inconclusive. Child–teacher ratios in the NICHD study were better than the ratios observed in the Whitebook and colleagues study (3.2 vs. 3.9 for infants, 4.8 vs. 5.6 for toddlers, and 7.3 vs. 8.4 for preschoolers, although note that our preschoolers were younger than theirs), but they were not as good as those in the Helburn study (4.4 vs. 3.6 for infant-toddler classes and 7.3 vs. 6.3 for preschool classes).

There is more agreement between our study and these others in the proportion of settings rated as poor: 10% of the preschool classes in Helburn's (1990) and Whitebook and colleagues' (1990) investigations and 12% in the NICHD study were given ratings of poor or worse, and 35% of the homes observed by Galinsky and colleagues (1994) and 41% in the NICHD study were observed to be inadequate (Galinsky et al., 1994) or poor or fair (NICHD).

As we have already indicated, none of these studies offers a comprehensive and representative picture of the quality of care throughout the United States, and all have sampling and measurement limitations. Using sampling plans that over sampled for low-income families or states that had only minimal child care standards, other studies may have underestimated the quality of care throughout the United States. Efforts were not made in these studies to correct for these biases. The sampling plan used in the NICHD study, in contrast, may have overestimated the quality of available care because it excluded adolescent, non-English-speaking mothers with childbirth complications, living in unsafe neighborhoods. However, we tried to alleviate this problem by imputing values to compensate for sample selection and attrition. Extrapolating from these corrected results to child care in the United States, by using known statistics describing child care users, suggests that the quality of care nationally is just slightly worse than observed in this study. Until a nationally representative observational study of child care in the United States can be done, we believe that this extrapolation of quality based on data from nine states may serve as a best guess for overall caregiving quality in the United States.

In terms of objective criteria of child care quality, our results are consistent with the results of the most representative estimate of child care demographics available: the Profile of Child Care Settings study (Profile; Kisker, Hofferth, Phillips, & Farquhar, 1991), a national telephone survey of center directors and child care home providers. The average group size for 2-year-olds in the Profile study was 12; the average child–adult ratio was 7.3. These statistics are quite similar to the average group size of 12 and child–adult ratio of 6.6 for 24- and 36-month-olds in centers in the NICHD study Kisker and colleagues (1991) concluded that the average quality of care in centers in the United States is adequate but does not meet the strictest professional recommendations (e.g., having ratios not exceeding 6:1 for 2-year-olds). Our results, too, suggest that most young children in this country receive child care that is "adequate"—neither outstanding nor terrible but leaving plenty of room for improvement. Our findings also suggest that it might be possible to improve the quality of care young children receive by lowering child–caregiver ratios and group sizes, boosting caregivers' levels of education, and increasing the safety and stimulation of child care environments. Until and unless such efforts are made, to maximize the likelihood of obtaining high-quality care, parents would be well advised to select care arrangements that are characterized by a low child–adult ratio, a clean and orderly physical environment, a variety of toys and learning materials, and a caregiver with a college education.

III

Why Consider Family Effects in a Study of Child Care?

One of the strengths of the National Institute of Child Health and Human Development (NICHD) Study of Early Child Care is the inclusion of information about families in addition to their socioeconomic status. Researchers in this study collected demographic information (e.g., income and number of individuals in the household), data about family and maternal characteristics (e.g., parents' education level and attitudes about raising children), and information about the quality of the home environment (e.g., warmth of relations and availability of cognitively stimulating materials and practices). Throughout, the qualitative features assessed in the home and child care environments were similar, and data were collected in these two contexts during the same time frame (when the children were 6, 15, 24, 36, and 54 months of age).

In this section, two chapters illustrate the ways in which family characteristics influence the child care experiences provided to young children, including the type, quality, and amount of care. Other chapters indicate the ways in which family characteristics, sometimes in conjunction with child care, affect early cognitive and social development although more information of this kind can be found in Part VII in this book. One major achievement of the reports grouped in Part III is that they identify those family characteristics that need to be statistically controlled in evaluating the relations of child care to children's development. For example, if analytic methods aimed at showing the link between child care and developmental outcomes do not statistically control for relevant family variables, the findings about child care may not be valid. Instead, they could be telling us about family effects masquerading as child care effects.

In Chapter 7, the investigators examine the family, economic, and psychosocial factors that account for the age of initiation, amount, type, and quality of nonmaternal infant care. Although economic factors were most consistently associated with the amount and nature of nonmaternal care received, maternal personality and beliefs about maternal employment were also important. Relations varied depending on whether type, amount, and quality of child care was the focus of analysis. While both maternal and family income affected every aspect of child care experience, other conditions including maternal personality and beliefs, as well as ethnicity, family size, and maternal education, were also relevant.

Chapter 8 describes the early life histories of a large sample of 3-year-old children from three family income levels—in poverty, near poverty, and above poverty. Developmental characteristics of children in the three groups were studied and related to other family characteristics and to experiences in child care. On most of the cognitive and social measures, the income groups differed significantly, such that functioning generally ranged downward from above poverty to poverty. However, the considerable variability found on all measures is striking—a pattern that is not usually stressed but that has major implications for planning in programs such as Head Start.

In Chapter 9, the investigators report how changes in families' income-to-needs during the first 3 years of the child's life were related to child outcomes (e.g., language, school readiness, social competence, and behavior problems). Although changes in family income were not important for the development of children from relatively affluent families, they did matter for children initially living in poverty. Decreases in family financial resources were associated with worse outcomes, while increases were associated with better outcomes. The findings have obvious importance to social planners as well as to students of family and child care in relation to child development.

According to Chapter 10, mothers who were chronically depressed during the child's first 3 years were least sensitive in interacting with their children across this time span. Their children performed less well cognitively and behaviorally than did children of nondepressed mothers. The findings were strongest for mothers living in poverty and least strong for affluent women.

In Chapter 11, three clusters of family risk factors (psychosocial, socioeconomic, and sociocultural), child care quality and hours in child care, and the interactions among these variables were examined as predictors of behavior problems, prosocial behavior, and language skills between 24 and 36 months. Family risk factors were the strongest predictors of outcome. Child care factors, while related to outcome, were considerably less strong, and moderation effects were not generally evident.

Taken together, this selection of chapters demonstrates that a number of demographic and psychological family variables predict families' selection of child care for their children and the child outcomes that are believed to be linked to child care. Many of the findings reinforce the importance of statistically controlling for these factors in examining the net effect of child care and thus influence the analytic strategies used elsewhere in this book. Altogether, this collection of chapters provides straightforward answers to the question posed by the title of this section: Why consider family effects in a study of child care?

7

Familial Factors Associated with the Characteristics of Nonmaternal Care for Infants

NICHD Early Child Care Research Network

As a result of the increasing number of mothers with young children in the workforce (U.S. Bureau of the Census, 1992) and the consequent increase in the number of children cared for by someone other than their mother for varying periods of time, researchers have turned their attention to examining the effects of nonmaternal care on children's development (Belsky, 1988; Caughy, DiPietro, & Strobino, 1994; Clarke-Stewart, 1988, 1993; Field, 1991; Howes, 1990). Understanding the effects of early care is complicated for several reasons. One problem is that family decisions concerning nonmaternal care may be affected by maternal, child, and familial characteristics already in place before care begins. Information about these preexisting conditions is required before the effects of nonmaternal care on children's development can be fully understood. A second problem is that most previous researchers have focused on organized child care that is provided in centers or by home day-care providers, but a substantial amount of the nonmaternal care that young children receive is informal and much is family based, where parents share childrearing or a grandmother or other relative is the caregiver. The extent to which early nonmaternal care presents risks or benefits to infants cannot be fully understood until all types of care provided in the mother's absence are examined.

From *Journal of Marriage and the Family*, 1997, Vol. 59, pp. 389–408. Copyright 1997 by the National Council of Family Relations, 3889 Central Ave. NE, Suite 660, Minneapolis, MN 55421. Reprinted by permission.

We examine how four aspects of nonmaternal infant child care—age of entry, amount, type, and quality—are affected by preexisting family characteristics, economics, and psychosocial factors. Our findings help set the stage for subsequent research that appreciates the ecological complexities of children's experiences in child care.

FACTORS ASSOCIATED WITH AGE OF ENTRY AND AMOUNT OF CARE THAT CHILDREN RECEIVE

A major factor in the selection of child care is the earning power of the mother. Mothers who can earn more are likely to have children who receive nonmaternal care earlier and in greater quantity (Leibowitz, Klerman, & Waite, 1992; Symons & McLeod, 1993). A mother's employment during pregnancy and her level of education, job status, hourly wage, and proportionate contribution to family income predict how early she returns to paid employment and whether she works full time or part time (e.g., Fuller, Holloway, & Liang, 1995; Volling & Belsky, 1993). In contrast, total family income shows little relation to the amount of nonmaternal care that children receive. Beyond economics, survey results show more use of nonmaternal care by African American families than European Americans, more by single mothers than two-parent families, and more by small rather than large families (Hofferth, Brayfield, Deich, & Holcomb, 1991).

Mothers who have high levels of work commitment tend to return to employment after childbirth more quickly than those who are less committed (Symons & McLeod, 1994; Volling & Belsky, 1993). Mothers who report relatively high levels of separation anxiety (the desire of the mother to provide care for her child herself, accompanied by the belief that there will be negative results if someone else provides care) are likely to stay home full time with their children (Hock, DeMeis, & McBride, 1988; McBride & Belsky, 1988).

Less certain is our understanding of the effects of maternal mental health and personality on child care (Belsky & Rovine, 1988; Owen & Cox, 1988; Weinraub & Jaeger, 1990). Factors such as depression and extraversion may influence mothers' decisions about employment and subsequent child care arrangements. In addition, individual differences in infant health and temperament may affect the age at which children begin nonmaternal care and the amount of care they experience.

FACTORS ASSOCIATED WITH PARENTAL SELECTION OF TYPE AND QUALITY OF CARE

Type of Care

Because some types of child care are expensive and because desirable child care arrangements are not always available (e.g., Chilman, 1993;

Phillips, 1995), parents do not always select the child care that they consider ideal. Many mothers, particularly those living in poverty, report that they would change their arrangements if they could (e.g., Hofferth, 1995; Meyers & van Leuwen, 1992). Furthermore, although many parents of infants state a preference for care by a relative (Sonenstein & Wolf, 1991), not all parents are able to share child care with each other or have a relative nearby.

Families with very low incomes tend to choose center care more frequently than other forms of care (Fuller et al., 1995; Hofferth et al., 1991). Mothers with higher levels of education and income choose in-home care for their infants (Erdwins & Buffardi, 1994) but center care for their preschoolers (e.g., Becerra & Chi, 1992; Fuller et al., 1995). Children living in rural areas are more likely to be cared for by relatives and less likely to receive any kind of organized care (Atkinson, 1994; Lehrer, 1983). In the southeastern United States, where more center-based care is available, more children are placed in centers than is true in other regions of the country (Hofferth et al., 1991; Hofferth & Wissoker, 1992).

Families under stress are more likely to use informal care by relatives or friends, multiple care arrangements, and lower-quality care (e.g., Eichman & Hofferth, 1993; Hofferth & Wissoker, 1992). Among poverty-level mothers, those who fear strangers are likely to select care by relatives (Meyers & van Leuwen, 1992). Mothers with middle to upper-middle incomes believe exposure to other adults and children is beneficial, and they are more likely to choose center care (Erdwins & Buffardi, 1994). Mothers who report high levels of separation anxiety tend not to use center-based care (Hock et al., 1988).

Quality of Care

A nationwide survey of child care centers found no difference in quality among infant classrooms in centers serving low-, middle-, or upper-income families (Phillips, Voran, Kisker, Howes, & Whitebook, 1994). By contrast, a study of infants and toddlers receiving home-based care showed clear associations between family income and the quality of care observed (Galinsky, Howes, Kontos, & Shinn, 1994). Some research suggests that the relation between income and quality is curvilinear; children from high- and low-income families receive higher-quality care than those from families with moderate incomes (Phillips et al., 1994; Waite, Leibowitz, & Witsberger, 1991).

Howes (1990) reported that mothers with less education were more likely to have children in lower-quality care, and she also found that boys receive lower-quality care than girls. Other studies have found no significant effects for demographic variables other than income (McCartney, 1984; Waite et al., 1991).

Parental attitudes and values regarding childrearing also influence the quality of care that children receive. In a Bermuda sample, parents who valued social skills were more likely to place their children in high-quality care than were parents who valued conformity (McCartney, 1984), and U.S. parents with authoritarian attitudes have been found to choose lower-quality child care arrangements (Bolger & Scarr, 1995).

Covariation in home and child care environments has been well documented (e.g., Phillips, McCartney, & Scarr, 1987; Vandell & Corasaniti, 1990). Parents who provide a sensitive, stimulating home environment are likely to select an arrangement with these same characteristics.

RESEARCH QUESTIONS

As this chapter indicates, a number of factors are thought to be associated with the use of nonmaternal care, but few studies have examined this question in a comprehensive manner. No prospective, longitudinal study has considered demographic and psychosocial factors simultaneously, examined informal as well as formal nonmaternal care arrangements, included observational measures of the quality of care, or focused specifically on infant care.

We address the following questions relating to use of nonmaternal care:

- *Question 1:* What is the relation between family demographic factors (e.g., ethnicity, number of children, and mother's education) and the infant's age at the initiation of nonmaternal care, the hours in care, the type of care selected, and the quality of that care?
- *Question 2:* What is the relation between economic factors (both maternal and nonmaternal income) and the amount, type, and quality of nonmaternal care?
- *Question 3:* To what extent are mothers' childrearing values, beliefs about the benefits and risks of employment, and separation anxiety associated with the timing, amount, type, and quality of the nonmaternal care their infants receive?

METHOD

Participants

Information about the research participants is provided in Chapter 1. Analyses presented in this report are based on the 1,281 children (52% male) who participated in the study through age 15 months. (The attrition rate from 1 month to 15 months was 6%.) Demographic characteristics of the families used for these analyses are provided in Tables 7.1 and 7.2. There were no significant differences between these families and the sample initially enrolled.

TABLE 7.1. Characteristics of Participating Families When Infants Were 15 Months Old

	n	%
Child's ethnicity		
White, nonHispanic	985	76.9
Black, nonHispanic	158	12.3
Hispanic	51	4.0
Other	87	6.8
Number of children in family		
1	522	40.7
2 or 3	677	52.8
4 or more	82	6.4
Maternal education		
< 12th grade	122	9.5
High school graduate or GED	267	20.8
Some college	430	33.6
Bachelor's degree	272	21.2
Postgraduate work	190	14.8
Husband or partner at home	1,100	85.9
Other relatives in household	176	13.7
Hours of maternal employment at 6 months		
0 hours	459	36.7
1–19 hours	136	11.6
20–39 hours	255	15.4
40 or more hours	400	32.0
Hours of maternal employment at 15 months		
None	435	35.0
1–19 hours	124	10.0
20–39 hours	251	20.2
40 or more hours	422	34.7

Note. n = 1,281.

TABLE 7.2. Incomes of Participating Families When Infants Were 15 Months Old

	n	M	SD
Maternal income from earnings (for all mothers)	1,278	$17,000	$16,310
Maternal income from earnings (for mothers with some income)	1,112	$19,530	$16,000
Nonmaternal income	1,278	$34,870	$31,150
income-to-needs ratio	1,278	3.24	2.83

Data Collection Procedures

Mothers and infants were visited at home when the children were 1, 6, and 15 months old. Phone contacts were made at 3, 9, and 12 months. At each home visit, mothers completed questionnaires and responded to a standardized demographic interview. Observers measured the quality of the home environment when the children were 6 and 15 months old. Children receiving 10 or more hours per week of regular, nonmaternal care at 6 and 15 months of age also were observed in the child care setting in which they spent the most time.

Design

We examined three sets of variables for their association with characteristics of nonmaternal care: (1) family characteristics—ethnicity, education, and family structure; (2) economic circumstances, including maternal and nonmaternal sources of income; and (3) psychosocial characteristics describing mother and child and the home environment. Multivariate analyses were used to examine the extent to which each of these three sets of variables was related to the four characteristics of nonmaternal care: age of initiation, amount, type, and quality.

Measures

Family Characteristics

The ethnicity of the child (based on the mother's report) was classified as African American (not Hispanic), European American (not Hispanic), Hispanic (any race), and all others.

The sex of the child was recorded from the mother's report at 1 month.

For analyses with age of entry, amount, and type of care, we measured the number of children in the family at 15 months. For analyses with quality measures at 6 and 15 months, we used the number of children at 6 and 15 months, respectively.

Maternal education was measured when the child was 1 month old and scored as a five-level variable (less than a high school education, high school graduate, some post–high school, college graduate, some post-college).

Partner presence or absence from the home was assessed at each contact (1, 3, 6, 9, 12, and 15 months). For most analyses, partner presence at 1 month was used as a predictor variable; for analyses predicting the number of hours of nonmaternal care, the percentage of occasions (out of six) when a partner was present also was included.

We coded the presence of other relatives in the home as "yes" if one or more adult relatives lived in the home when the child was 1 month old.

Economic Characteristics

We collected three measures of family income (see Table 7.2) during interviews of the mothers when the child was 1, 6, and 15 months old: (1) Maternal income from earnings was the mother's average income across all postbirth occasions when her income was greater than zero, (2) nonmaternal income was all household income other than the mother's at 6 or 15 months, and (3) income-to-needs ratio was measured as the total family income (from earnings and investments in that year) divided by the poverty threshold (U.S. Bureau of the Census, 1992) for each family size. Another variable—maternal work hours or the total number of hours that mothers worked for pay at all jobs—was also included.

Psychosocial Characteristics

Five sets of psychosocial characteristics were measured: maternal well-being and personality, social support and stress, maternal attitudes, child health and temperament, and the quality of the child's home environment.

For maternal well-being and personality, four measures indicated the mother's overall emotional health and personality. Depression was measured at 1 month using the Center for Epidemiological Studies—Depression (CES-D) scale (Radloff, 1977), and we used scores from the extraversion, agreeableness, and neuroticism scales of the Neuroticism Extraversion Openness (NEO) Personality Inventory (Costa & McCrea, 1985) that was administered at 6 months.

We measured social support at 1 month with the Relationships with Other People Scale (Marshall & Barnett, 1993). We measured parenting stress at 1 month using 25 items from the Abidin Parenting Stress Index (Abidin, 1983). We measured financial stress at 1 month by summing answers to three questions:

1. How satisfied are you with your financial situation?
2. How often do you worry about financial matters (reflected score)?
3. How predictable is your income from month to month?

Principal components analysis of the three items indicated a single component accounted for 61% of the total item variance.

Maternal attitudes toward separation were measured at 1 month using the 21 items from subscale I, maternal separation anxiety, of the Separation Anxiety Scale (Hock, Gnezda, & McBride, 1983). Two scales were taken from the Attitudes toward Maternal Employment Questionnaire (Greenberger, Goldberg, Crawford, & Granger, 1988) and were administered at 1 month. Nonauthoritarian beliefs about childrearing were assessed at 1 month using a questionnaire that discriminates between "modern" and "traditional" childrearing beliefs (Schaefer & Edgerton, 1985).

To measure child health when the child was 1 month old, the mother rated the child's health on a 4-point scale from poor to excellent. Child temperament was measured using 14 items from three subscales (intensity, mood, and adaptability) of the Early Infant Temperament Questionnaire (Medoff-Cooper, Carey, & McDevitt, 1993) completed at 1 month.

To measure the quality of the infant's experiences at home, trained observers administered the Home Observation for Measurement of the Environment (HOME) Inventory (Caldwell & Bradley, 1984) during home visits when the child was 6 and 15 months old. Interobserver reliability on the HOME is reported in Chapter 3.

With the exception of two measures, Cronbach's alpha ranged from .74 (for agreeableness on NEO) to .92 (for separation anxiety). For nonauthoritarian childrearing beliefs, the Cronbach's alpha was .60, and for temperament, the Cronbach's alpha was .67.

Characteristics of Child Care

To measure the age at which nonmaternal care was begun, children were categorized into five groups, depending on the age (in months) at which, on a regular basis, they began 10 or more hours per week of nonmaternal care: 0–2 months, 3–5 months, 6–11 months, 12–15 months, and no regular care by 15 months.

To measure hours in care at 6 and 15 months, the mother reported the number of hours per week that her child was cared for on a regular basis by someone other than herself.

To indicate the type of care, we grouped nonmaternal care arrangements into five categories: coparental, grandparent (in the child's home or in the grandparent's home), in-home (care in the child's own home by anyone other than a parent or grandparent), child care home (care in someone else's home by someone other than a parent or grandparent), or child care center. We defined coparental care as the mother's report that the child's father assumed full care for the child for at least 10 hours per week on a regular, prearranged basis.

The quality of the child's primary nonmaternal child care setting was assessed at 6 and 15 months; observations were conducted on two half-day visits scheduled within a 2-week interval. Visits were conducted within 2 weeks of the child's 6-month birthday and within 4 weeks of the child's 15-month birthday. Observers scored four measures designed to assess both the individual child's experience and the degree to which the child care setting met standards considered to index quality in child care environments. These standards focus on the degree to which individuals providing care are attentive and appropriately responsive, express positive affect and affection, are not excessively restrictive or intrusive, and offer activities likely to promote the infant's cognitive and social development. Previous research (Clarke-Stewart, 1993; Scarr & Eisenberg, 1993) has demonstrated that these characteristics are associated with children's development.

Two of these measures were obtained using the Observational Record of the Caregiving Environment (ORCE). We calculated a composite variable, positive caregiving frequency and a second composite variable, positive caregiving ratings. Further details about the ORCE and these two composite measures is available in Chapters 3 and 5 of this volume. Reliability estimates (Pearson correlations) at 6 and 15 months, respectively, for positive caregiving frequency were .98 and .91 (videotapes) and .86 and .97 (live). For positive caregiving ratings, reliability estimates were .94 and .86 (videotapes) and .90 and .89 (live).

For all home-care arrangements, the quality of child care also was measured using a HOME Inventory (Caldwell & Bradley, 1984) modified by Caldwell and Bradley to fit child care situations. The total score of the Child Care HOME was used.

An abbreviated form of the Assessment Profile for Early Childhood Programs (Profile; Abbott-Shim & Sibley, 1987) was collected in both child care homes and centers but not in settings in which the relative or another parent cared for the child. For child care homes, the Profile consisted of items selected from two scales: safety and health and learning environment (play materials and spaces). In child care centers, the Profile included these scales plus individualizing (having spaces and plans for each child), adult needs (providing opportunities for staff development and communication with parents), and physical environment (organization and adequacy of space). We added three items to assess quiet, crowding, and clutter in the environment (from Wachs, 1991).

Descriptions of these measures of child care quality, their intercorrelations, and relationships to other measures are reported in the National Institute of Child Health and Human Development (NICHD) Early Child Care Research Network (1996).

Overall Analytic Approach

We used regression analyses to evaluate the extent to which each of the three sets of family factors, entered individually and in combination with the other sets, was associated with characteristics of nonmaternal care. Generalized logit analysis was used for the categorical dependent variables of age of initiation and type of care. Ordinary least-squares regressions (OLS) were used to examine the continuous variables of hours in care and quality of care.

We used a hierarchical approach to determine the contribution made by demographic, economic, and psychosocial factors to the selection of child care. In each regression model tested, family characteristics were entered first. In models that included economic factors, these variables were entered second. Psychosocial variables were entered last, one set at a time. Fewer variables were used in the analyses predicting the quality of care because these had to be run separately within each type of care, thus restricting the number of subjects in each analysis.

Because we anticipated that sites might differ, we controlled site differences whenever possible. For regressions, as the first step we entered sites as a dummy factor. Because including sites in the logit analyses would have reduced the degrees of freedom more than the model could bear, we tested interactions between site and age of entry and between site and type of care. For age of entry, these interactions were negligible, but they were large and significant for the type of care, suggesting that some of the reported differences among types of care may reflect characteristics on which sites differed.

RESULTS

Child's Age When Nonmaternal Care Began

In the first model we analyzed family characteristics. On the whole, children in larger families began nonmaternal care later than did those in smaller families. However, children entering care between 3 and 5 months of age came from smaller families than those who began nonmaternal care earlier. Children beginning nonmaternal care between 3 and 5 months were also the most likely of any group to have highly educated mothers, mothers with higher incomes, and mothers who scored highest on extraversion and agreeableness. Families with children beginning nonmaternal care between 3 and 5 months had the second highest nonmaternal income, just under the average nonmaternal income for families of children not yet in any nonmaternal care.

Economic factors were added in the second model. We performed parallel analyses using an income-to-needs ratio and the proportion of family income from maternal earnings. The results were quite similar to those reported here. The highest overall family incomes (maternal plus nonmaternal income) were reported for children beginning care between 3 and 5 months. Mothers of these children earned more than other mothers, and nonmaternal income was also relatively high. The children beginning care earliest (0–2 months) had families with low nonmaternal incomes; these families were more dependent than other families on the mother's earnings. Children who were not in nonmaternal care by age 15 months came from families with relatively high nonmaternal incomes. With income included in the model, the effect of the mother's education on age when nonmaternal care began was reduced considerably, and the number of children in the family became nonsignificant.

Two sets of psychosocial variables were significantly related to age of entry into care (Models 3 and 4). Maternal well-being and personality were important predictors. Even with demographic and income variables included in the model, extraversion and agreeableness were highest for mothers whose infants entered care between 3 and 5 months. Mothers' attitudes about the benefits associated with their employment also showed a strong relation to the child's age of entry into nonmaternal care (Model 4). The greater the perceived benefits, the earlier the child entered care. However, with the effects of these psychosocial factors in the model, the effect of the mother's education was no longer significant.

Hours in Care

The children included in the analyses of the number of hours in care were those who received any nonmaternal care (i.e., children not in child care were excluded).

Analysis of family characteristics (Model 1) showed that they accounted for relatively little (about 3%) of the variance. Children from African American or other ethnic backgrounds spent more hours in nonmaternal care than did Hispanic or European American children. Compared with those from smaller families, children with more siblings spent less time being cared for on a regular basis by someone other than the mother. Low maternal education was associated with relatively long hours in nonmaternal care, particularly when the mother's income and work hours were included in the model.

Because we expected mother's work hours to predict how many hours the child was in nonmaternal care, we ran regressions for demographic and income effects first without work hours in the predictor set (Model 2). Then we entered work hours alone (Model 3), and finally we included work hours as part of the set of economic variables (Model 4). Family income variables were potent predictors of the time infants spent in nonmaternal care and accounted for an additional 20% of the variance over family characteristic variables. The two sources of family income had opposite relations to children's hours in nonmaternal care. The higher the mother's earnings, the more time children spent in nonmaternal care, whereas the higher the nonmaternal income, the less time children spent in nonmaternal care. Mother's work hours were the best predictor of the child's hours in nonmaternal care. However, a mother's income made an independent contribution. That is, for mothers who worked a comparable number of hours, those with higher earnings had children who spent more time in nonmaternal care.

We entered each set of psychosocial variables into the analyses after the demographic set alone (e.g., Model 5) and after both the demographic and economic (excluding work hours) sets of variables (e.g., Model 6). Only maternal beliefs and attitudes accounted for significant amounts of variance in these analyses. Mothers who believed in the benefits of maternal employment had children with more nonmaternal care, whereas those who thought its risks were high had children with fewer hours of nonmaternal care. Mothers with more traditional attitudes about rearing children were also likely to have children with fewer hours of nonmaternal care than those with more progressive attitudes. These patterns appeared both with and without controlling income.

Because we were concerned that including coparental care may have distorted the effects of predicting nonparental care, we also ran the regression analyses with hours in coparental care deleted. At 6 and 15 months, the results of these analyses were essentially the same. Only one item at 15 months showed differences in the two sets of analyses. With hours of coparental care included in the amount of child care, the amount of variance added to the model when work hours were added to family demographic variables was 16%. When we omitted hours in coparental care from analyses, maternal work hours added 37% of the variance to the prediction of child care.

Type of Care

The significant demographic variables associated with the type of care (Model 1) were the number of children in the home, the mother's education, the presence of a partner in the home, and the presence of a relative in the home. Children with in-home caregivers and those receiving coparental care came from families with more children than those in other types of care. Mothers' education was lowest for families using shared parental care or grandparent care and highest for families using in-home caregivers who were not relatives.

The addition of economic variables (Model 2) showed that families using in-home care had the highest incomes, both maternal and non-maternal. Most striking, families using care with an unrelated in-home caregiver had average nonmaternal incomes that were $20,000 a year higher than those of families using any other type of care.

Mothers' concern about the risks associated with maternal employment was the only psychosocial variable predicting the type of care used (Model 3). Mothers who thought employment had high risks were more likely than others to use shared parental or grandparent care; those who thought employment had relatively low risks were more likely to use formal care in child care homes or centers.

Quality of Care

Because the structural arrangements of the caregiving setting and the relationships between family and nonmaternal caregivers varied so much across the five types of nonmaternal care, analyses combining children in all types of care were difficult to interpret. Factors associated with quality were, therefore, analyzed separately for each type of care using OLS regressions. The number of cases in each analysis was limited. Thus, a reduced set of predictor variables (omitting family structure, social support and stress, and maternal attitudes about the risks and benefits of work) was chosen on the basis of previous research that has linked these variables to quality. In addition, we categorized ethnicity as minority versus white, non-Hispanic. We expected the major relation between income and quality to result from the family's overall ability to purchase the care of their choice. Therefore, we used a single index of income. Similarly, we did not expect the presence or absence of a partner or other adult relative to affect quality within the type of care, so these variables were omitted from the analyses.

In general, family characteristics and economics were more highly related to scores on the Child Care HOME and the Profile than to observed frequency and ratings of positive caregiving, and associations were stronger at 15 months than at 6 months.

In all care settings that were not child care centers, at both 6 and 15 months Child Care HOME and Profile scores were higher for white, non-Hispanic children than for children from other groups, but these differences did not appear on measures of observed caregiving. Thus, except perhaps for center-based care, children from all ethnic groups received equally sensitive and positive care, but the physical environment of care was different for children from ethnic minority groups.

Across all types of care, there were no consistent sex differences in the quality of care at 6 months. At 15 months in group situations (in child care homes and, to a smaller extent, in centers), caregivers of girls scored higher on measures of positive caregiving than did caregivers of boys. There were similar tendencies, though nonsignificant, in all other types of care. The child care homes where girls were cared for also received higher scores on the Child Care HOME and Profile than did child care homes of boys.

The number of children in the family was negatively related to several indices of quality in coparental care at 6 and 15 months and in grandparent care at 15 months. Because most of this care was provided only for the study child and his or her siblings, more siblings generally meant an equivalent decrease in the adult–child ratio, which would be expected to decrease positive caregiving. There was no effect of family size on quality of care in day care homes or centers. The linear effect of the income-to-needs ratio was tested both with and without demographic predictors in the models. At neither age was the income-to-needs ratio strongly associated with the quality of care provided by fathers and grandparents. With one exception, the income-to-needs ratio did not account for a significant amount of additional variance above family characteristics. For in-home care, the income-to-needs ratio was significantly associated with the frequency of positive caregiving and the Child Care HOME when children were 15 months old. In child care homes, however, the income-to-needs ratio was associated with high scores on the Child Care HOME and the Profile at both 6 and 15 months. In addition, at 15 months, children from higher-income families received more frequent and more highly rated positive caregiving than did those from lower-income homes. In child care centers, by contrast, there was little indication of a linear relation of income to any quality indicator.

Because earlier research on child care centers serving preschoolers suggests a nonlinear relation of income to the quality of care, with children at the low and high ends of the income continuum receiving higher-quality care than those in near-poor and moderate-income families, all of the above analyses were repeated with income dummy-coded into five levels: income-to-needs ratio < 1.0 (below poverty threshold), 1.0–1.99 (near poor), 2.0–2.99, 3.0–3.99, > 3.99. The near-poor group was the excluded one, against which the others were compared. A nonlinear pattern was evident only for child care centers. In general, the quality of center care was lowest for children in families just above the poverty level. At both 6 and 15 months, the near-poor children in families with income-to-needs ratios ranging from 1 to 3 received less positive caregiving and attended centers scoring lower on the Profile than did children either from families at the poverty level or from more affluent families. At 15 months, caregivers of poverty-level children were also rated significantly higher on positive caregiving than caregivers serving children from families just above the poverty threshold.

Childrearing attitudes were the only psychosocial variables showing any association with the quality of care. At 6 months, mothers' non-authoritarian, less traditional attitudes about childrearing predicted relatively high ratings of positive caregiving from in-home caregivers (beta = –.055, SE = .025, p < .05); and high scores on the Child Care HOME in grandparent care (beta = –.077, SE = .035, p < .05) and child care homes (beta = –.081, SE = .038, p < .05). At 15 months, more nontraditional childrearing attitudes were associated with higher scores on the Child Care HOME (beta = –.112, SE = .027, p < .001), and the Profile (beta = –.100, SE = .0305, p < .001) in child care homes.

The quality of the infants' experiences at home (measured by the HOME) was directly related to the quality of the child care homes in which 6-month-olds received care, indexed by positive caregiving ratings (beta = .176, SE = .055, p < .01) the Child Care HOME (beta = .500, SE = .123, p < .001); and the Profile (beta = .408, SE = .093, p < .001). By age 15 months, the quality of the child's experiences at home was related to all quality measures in child care homes: positive caregiving frequency (beta = .183, SE = .056, p < .01); positive caregiving ratings (beta = .241, SE = .056, p < .001); Child Care HOME (beta = .485, SE = .101, p < .001); and Profile (beta = .324, SE = .1125, p < .001). Home environment did not predict any aspects of the quality of center care.

Table 7.3 presents a summary of family characteristics, economic factors, and psychosocial factors associated with the four child care variables when all predictor variables were considered simultaneously.

DISCUSSION

This chapter focuses on factors that predict a number of characteristics of nonmaternal infant care. The results indicate that, overall, family economics, rather than other demographic characteristics, account for both the

TABLE 7.3. **Factors Associated with Use of Nonmaternal Care, Controlling for All Other Variables**

	Age of entry	Hours in care	Type of care	Quality of care
Family characteristics				
Child ethnicity		*		*1
Child's sex				*1
Family size		−	*	−
Maternal education		−	*	
Partner in home			*	NA
Economic factors				
Maternal income	*	+	*	NA
Nonmaternal income	*	−	*	NA
Income/needs	NA	NA	NA	+1
Maternal work hours	NA	+	NA	NA
Psychosocial factors				
Maternal well-being and personality	*			
Social support and stress				NA
Maternal attitudes and beliefs				
Separation anxiety				
Benefits of work	−	+		NA
Risks of work		−	*	NA
Nonauthoritarian childrearing beliefs		+		+1
Child's health and temperament				
Quality of infant's experiences at home	NA	NA	NA	+1

Note. + indicates a positive relationship, − indicates an inverse relationship, * indicates that effects were not linear, and 1 indicates the relationship in some types of care only. NA indicates that the variable or set was not analyzed.

amount and kind of nonmaternal care that infants receive. Family and mother's income affect every aspect of children's experiences in nonmaternal care. But the picture that emerges from these results is complex. The age at which infants begin nonmaternal care is affected not only by economic variables but also by their mothers' personalities and beliefs concerning the benefits of employment. Furthermore, once infants begin regular nonmaternal care, a number of family characteristics affect how much nonmaternal care the infant receives. The number of hours an infant is in care is affected not only by the mother's work schedule, her earning power, and the family's total income but also by individual differences in ethnicity, family size, and the mother's education. Mothers' beliefs and attitudes about childrearing also affect how much nonmaternal care infants receive.

What kind of nonmaternal care children receive is affected by family size, maternal education, household composition, and economics and by mothers' beliefs about the risks associated with maternal employment. Children whose primary form of nonmaternal care is coparental—about one-quarter of our sample in nonmaternal care—tended to have less well educated mothers and mothers who earned lower incomes than those in other forms of nonmaternal care. Nonmaternal income was also lower for families using coparental care and the care of grandparents than for families using other types of care. Coparental care tended to be used by mothers who were very concerned about the risks of maternal employment. Sharing care with their husbands may have been the only way these mothers were willing to return to employment. Compared with other highly involved fathers, fathers who take primary responsibility for their children's care in the mother's absence may be unique. Subsequent reports from this project will address the characteristics of fathers that may have influenced families' selection of coparental care.

The quality of care that infants experience is related to a wide range of family, economic, and child characteristics, depending on the type of care. Because demographic, economic, and attitudinal factors were included in the same analyses, these findings add depth to previously reported results and define factors that must be considered when studying the effects of nonmaternal care. Of particular importance for child care policy is the finding that in child care centers serving infants, family income had a curvilinear relation to quality. Children at the lowest and highest income levels receive higher-quality care than do those in the middle. This pattern is consistent with earlier findings for centers serving preschool children (Phillips et al., 1994; Waite et al., 1991). One reason for this pattern may be the distribution of federal subsidies. The care provided for children from families with very low incomes is often directly subsidized, and families with higher incomes receive an indirect subsidy in the form of the child care tax credit. Those in the middle are less likely to receive any federal benefit (Phillips & Bridgman, 1995).

The results also indicate that nonmaternal family income and mothers' income had opposite effects on the amount of nonmaternal care that children received. Nonmaternal income tended to be negatively related to the hours per week that children were in child care, whereas mothers' income was positively related to the hours that children were in child care. That maternal and nonmaternal income operate in contrary directions to influence the amount of care that children receive demonstrates the importance of considering the mother's income separately from nonmaternal income whenever possible. It appears that families are more likely to use more nonmaternal care when mothers are able to earn more in the labor force but less likely to do so when there are adequate sources of nonmaternal income.

Demographic variables other than income predicted only 3% of the variance in the amount of nonmaternal care that children experienced at 6 and 15 months of age. No single demographic factor was consistently significant.

Child ethnicity was significantly related to the quality of nonmaternal care, measured by the Child Care HOME, in all settings except centers. This finding was robust and held even when family income and mother's education were controlled statistically. However, observed, positive caregiving did not differ by ethnicity.

A startling finding with regard to the quality of nonmaternal care was that at 15 months boys received less responsive care than girls in both child care homes and centers. That such differences were observed with unrelated caregivers but not relatives suggests that fathers and grandparents may be responding more sensitively to the unique characteristics of the children in their care, but care providers who are not relatives may be responding more stereotypically to the boys and girls in their care.

Mothers' beliefs about the effects of maternal employment predicted both the age at which infants entered nonmaternal care and the type of child care setting selected, even after controlling for demographic and economic variables. Mothers' beliefs in the benefits of their employment were associated with beginning nonmaternal care earlier. Mothers' concerns about the risks of employment, on the other hand, predicted fewer hours of care and the use of more informal types of arrangements. Mothers who were least concerned about the risks associated with their employment were more likely to have their infants in child care centers, whereas those who were most concerned tended to leave their infants in the care of grandparents or to share care with their husbands.

Unlike previous studies, this study found that mothers' separation anxiety did not appear to predict any aspect of the nonmaternal care selected for their infants. This discrepancy may be due to the fact that other attitudinal measures, such as mothers' beliefs about childrearing and the effects of the mother's employment on children's development, were found to be both correlated with separation anxiety and more strongly related to the timing, amount, and nature of care.

Our findings extend previous research in a number of ways. The sample used was large, with adequate minority representation, and the children and their families were followed prospectively from birth to 15 months. The nonmaternal care settings included coparental care, grandparent care, and informal family-based care, as well as day care homes and centers. We investigated a wide range of measures of family characteristics, economics, and psychosocial factors simultaneously, so that we could explore the effects of each of these sets of variables, controlling for the others.

Two weaknesses of measurement within this study limit the generalizations that can be drawn. First, our measure of mothers' earnings was based on the amount of mothers' income averaged across the first 15 months of their child's life. This measure of income is not unrelated to work hours, and, therefore, covariation may have inflated the relationships we observed. We attempted to circumvent this problem by including maternal work hours as well as income in the regression equations predicting hours in care. Nevertheless, this study did not include an assessment of mothers' potential earnings, independent of actual earnings.

Second, the availability of child care in the community in which each family lived was not measured. The focus of this study has been on the characteristics of the care that children receive, rather than on parental choice.

The results inform the child care research community of the factors correlated with nonmaternal care that must be considered when analyzing for the effects of early child care experiences on child outcomes. Future studies will need to take into the consideration the effects of mothers' income, family income, ethnicity, maternal attitudes toward employment, and the quality of the child's experience at home, at the very least, when evaluating the effects of early child care on children's development.

From a policy standpoint, the results of this study demonstrate the importance of economic factors and parental values in some aspects of decision making about child care. Parents are placing their young infants in nonmaternal care early and for long hours for two kinds of reasons: because the family needs the income that the mother earns at her jobs and because mothers want to continue working. In either case, child care makes employment possible. These decisions about child care are congruent with mothers' belief systems already in place. Moreover, families may be choosing the types of care they do largely for economic reasons. Shared parental care or low-cost care provided by relatives or in subsidized centers is not available to all families, and in-home care is prohibitively expensive for many parents. When families choose day-care homes, they tend to select settings similar in quality to their own home environment.

8

Before Head Start

Income and Ethnicity, Family Characteristics, Child Care Experiences, and Child Development

NICHD EARLY CHILD CARE RESEARCH NETWORK

Since the launching of Head Start in 1965 as an enrichment program for poor children prior to formal school entry, a wealth of data has been collected on participants, their families, and the communities in which the programs operate. As the result, a great deal is now known about the participants (children and parents) at the point of exit from the program, at school entry, or beyond. However, surprisingly little effort has been devoted to the task of carefully describing the children and the constellation of life experiences in which their development is embedded at the time of entry into the preschool program (i.e., age 3). Such information is needed to provide an appropriate match between entry characteristics and program design.

Extensive assessment of behavioral competencies of the children at the time of enrollment is generally not feasible in individual Head Start centers across the country. One way to accomplish the equivalent of entry assessment is to examine existing data bases dealing with a broad array of family and child characteristics during this very early time of life. The National Institute of Child Health and Human Development (NICHD) Study of Early Child Care (NICHD Early Child Care Research Network, 1994) has such a data set collected from 10 different cities across the country. It provides

From *Early Education and Development*, 2001, Vol. 12, No. 4, pp. 545–576. Copyright 2001 by *Early Education and Development*. Reprinted by permission of Wide Range, Inc.

empirical data about the early life histories of children from different economic backgrounds from birth until 3 years, the earliest age at which, until the recent launching of Early Head Start, children from poor families could enter Head Start.

SCOPE OF THE ANALYSIS

This chapter provides both a within-group description of children in poverty families and a relational picture that also encompasses two nonpoverty groups—near poverty and above poverty. The main questions that guided the study were:

- How do children in the three income groups—poverty, near poverty, and above poverty—differ in family backgrounds, child growth, health, developmental characteristics, and child care experiences up to age 3 years?
- Are there interactions between poverty and ethnicity in the observed patterns?
- Is experience in child care associated with different patterns of child development in the different income groups?

For all family and child care measures collected at more than one time point, longitudinal information was utilized, thus allowing cumulative influences to be represented. For the associated child variables, a cross-sectional slice of data at age 3 was taken, representing essentially a frozen section of the gestalt of these influences.

METHOD

Data for this chapter came from a large-scale, prospective, longitudinal study—the NICHD Study of Early Child Care.

Study Participants

As this chapter was designed to describe characteristics of Head Start children and their families at the point in time at which the children were eligible to enter the program, the participants were those children and families still in the study when the children were 3 years of age. In the original sample of 1,364 children, there were 66 children whose ethnicity was described by their mothers as Asian, Native American, or Other. These were excluded because the small numbers of individuals in each group precluded any assumption of cultural homogeneity. Family income data were missing on 9 children. This left a total of 1,289 children and families (1,034 European American, 173 African American, and 82 Hispanic). Of this total, 133 had been lost to the study at some time point between 1 and 36 months of age. The remaining 1,156 participants comprised the sample for most of the data analyses reported in this chapter.

When the 1,156 families were compared with the 133 families for whom we had incomplete data, it was found that the families lost to attrition were disproportionately more likely to be poor (45% vs. 15%), $\chi^2(2, n = 1,289) = 80.3$, p < .001, African American (26% vs. 12%), $\chi^2(2, n = 1,289) = 24.5$, p < .001, and include a single mother (26% vs. 13%), $\chi^2(1, n = 1,289) = 15.2$, $p < .001$ with less education ($M = 13.3$ vs. 14.3), $t(1,286) = 5.4, p < .001$. Of this remaining sample, 683 children (59%) were in at least 10 hours per week of nonmaternal child care at age 36 months, and 592 (87%) of these children were observed in their primary child care arrangement.

Income Group Membership

The designation of income groups used for the present analysis was the income-to-needs ratio. This measure is considered to be a reliable indicator of economic ease or hardship faced by a family (Bradley & Whiteside-Mansell, 1997). The ratio is obtained by dividing the total family income (without income transfers) by the federal poverty threshold, which is determined by family size and number of children under 18. For this study we used three ratio cuts to define our groups: *poverty* (ratio ≤1), *near poverty* (ratios > 1 and ≤ 1.8), and *above poverty* (ratios > 1.8). These cutting points are consistent with those generally used to characterize family economic security (Brooks-Gunn, Duncan, & Maritato, 1997) and mirror those used for eligibility for some federal and state support programs. For example, families above poverty but earning less than the 1.8 income-to-needs ratio sometimes qualify for WIC (Women's, Infants' and Children), Medicaid, and some states' child care assistance programs. The group designated by these ratios as near poverty could be thought of as a proxy for families currently trying to move from welfare to work. Applying these ratios to our participants produced a sample of 235 poverty, 180 near-poverty, and 874 above-poverty families, for a total of 1,289.

Family Context Measures

Family Demographics

At the 1-month visit, the mothers reported their child's *ethnicity*. Then at each subsequent assessment they provided information about other family demographics. These included *family income* (which provided the information necessary to establish the *income-to-needs ratios* and to calculate *duration of poverty* on the basis of the percent of occasions when family income was below the poverty level); *family composition* (percent of assessment occasions when the parent was a single caregiver, i.e., not living with a partner/spouse or extended family); *maternal education* (years of school completed at child's birth); and *average hours per week that the mother was employed or attended school.*

Maternal Characteristics

This category included five measures of maternal and parenting characteristics. These were:

1. *Maternal depression,* measured by the Center for Epidemiologic Studies–Depression (CES-D) scale (Radloff, 1977), administered to the mothers at each assessment period and averaged for these analyses. A score of 16 or greater on this scale is considered indicative of clinical depression.

2. *Benefits of work,* a score obtained from the Attitudes toward Maternal Employment scale (Greenberger, Goldberg, Crawford, & Granger, 1988), which gives an indication of the extent to which mothers perceive employment as beneficial (higher scores) or harmful to children. Mothers completed this questionnaire when their infants were 1 month of age.

3. The *Home Observation for Measurement of the Environment (HOME) Inventory* (Caldwell & Bradley, 1984) assessed the level of support for development available in the home at 6, 15, and 36 months. The HOME is based on both observation and interview and summarizes behaviors that describe the stimulation and responsiveness of the mothers, their involvement with their children, availability of play and learning materials, organization and variety of the physical environment, and acceptance of the child's behavior. The HOME is often used as a marker for socioeconomic status. Although it serves this purpose to some extent in the NICHD study, it was used in this analysis because of the picture it provides of nurturant maternal care within the child's home. The proportion of positive scores from each assessment period was averaged to create a summary score.

4. *Maternal sensitivity* was measured by an adaptation of the three-boxes procedure of Vandell (1979). Mothers interacted with their young children in a semistructured play session at 6, 15, 25, and 36 months. Three sets of appealing toys were assembled, and the mothers were asked to play with their children sequentially with the three sets in any way they chose. The 15-minute sessions were videotaped at the 10 data collection sites and coded at a central site by carefully trained coders blind to family and child care histories of the children. Intercoder reliability ranged from .83 to .87. A composite sensitivity measure derived from each play session was based on maternal supportive presence, absence of intrusiveness, and absence of hostility (see NICHD Early Child Care Research Network, 1997c, for details). These composite measures were averaged across the four data collection points to yield an overall sensitivity measure for the first 3 years.

5. *Maternal health* was a rating by mothers of their own health at the 36-month interview on a 4-point scale—poor, fair, good, or excellent—with a higher score indicating better health.

Child Care Measures

For any child who had experienced at least 10 hours per week of routine nonmaternal care at one or more of the assessment occasions, several child care measures were obtained. If a child was in more than one care environment, the primary arrangement (the one in which the most time was spent) was observed. Some of the information came from maternal interview, some from caregiver interview, and some from direct observation.

The amount and stability of care were measured by *number of hours per week* averaged over all assessment occasions in which the child was in nonmaternal care, child's *age at entry* into 10 or more hours per week, and *number of starts* in different care settings. These data on amount and stability of care covered all of the child's first 3 years of life. The remaining child care measures pertained to the actual care the children were receiving at 36 months.

Information about the structural aspects of care received at 36 months was obtained from the child care provider. *Type of care* was coded into a five-category classification: (1) care by the father or partner, (2) care by a relative in the child's or relative's home, (3) in-home care by a nonrelative, (4) child care home (family day care), or (5) child care center. The provider also reported information about structural characteristics such as *group size, caregiver's education*, and amount of *caregiver's formal training* in child development or early childhood education.

The caregiving environment was also assessed by direct observation. The *ratio of children to adults* was noted by the observer at each visit. The overall quality of the environment was assessed using a coding procedure developed specifically for the NICHD study—the Observational Record of the Caregiving Environment (ORCE). (For details about the observation procedure, see NICHD Early Child Care Research Network, 1996.)

Child Development Measures

When the study children were 36 months of age, cognitive and socio-emotional functioning, physical growth, and health were assessed. The cognitive domain was covered by two published and carefully standardized instruments. The first was the Reynell Developmental Language Scales (Reynell & Gruber, 1977), which measure *expressive language* and *verbal comprehension*. Scores were standardized with a mean of 100. The second measure consisted of five subtests of the Bracken Basic Concept Scale (Bracken, 1984)—colors, letter identification, numbers/counting, comparisons, and shapes. These subscales yield an estimate of *preschool readiness*. Scores on the Bracken could range from 1 to 19, with a standardized mean score of 10.

Two composite behavioral scores were created. Children's *cooperation and social competence* at 36 months was measured by having the mothers complete the Express and Comply subscales of the Adaptive Social Behavior Inventory (ASBI) developed by Hogan, Scott, and Bauer (1992). Scores were standardized and assigned a mean of 0 and a standard deviation of 1, with higher scores indicating more prosocial and adaptive behavior. *Incidence of problem behavior* consisted of the Externalizing, Internalizing, Sleep Problems, and Somatic Problems scores from the Child Behavior Check List (CBCL; Achenbach & Edelbrock, 1991) and the Disruptive subscale of the ASBI, both completed by the mother. Scores were standardized and assigned a mean of 0 and a standard deviation of 1, with higher scores indicating more behavior problems.

Children's Growth and Health

Three measures of children's health at 36 months were available: *overall health of child* as rated by the mothers on a 4-point scale—poor, fair, good, or excellent—and the measured *height* in centimeters and *weight* in kilograms of the children.

Analytic Plan

To answer the research question about differences among the three income groups and to control for multiple tests of significance, multivariate analyses of variance (MANOVAs) were performed for the following groups of variables: family demographic characteristics, maternal and parenting characteristics, child development measures, child growth and health, and child care experiences. When the multivariate F for a group of variables was significant, individual analyses of variance (ANOVAs) testing single variables and pairwise comparisons between the income, ethnic, and child care groups were conducted. Chi square was used for nonlinear measures. When appropriate, the total sample was used for the analyses; for analyses dealing with child care variables, only the subsample of children (and their families) in care for more than 10 hours a week at 36 months of age was used.

RESULTS

(Note: In this abridged version of this chapter, most of the text description of the findings has been retained, but further information may be gleaned from the figures and tables provided in the full version of this chapter.)

Income and Ethnicity

The income-to-needs ratios at the five assessment points were averaged to represent an aggregate income status over the child's first 3 years of life. This average is used in all statistical analyses relating to family income.

In the total sample, 18% of the families were in poverty during the first 3 years of the child's life, whereas this characterized only 10% of the child care subgroup. This obviously reflects the fact that use of child care generally occurs as a result of maternal employment and that such employment helps to keep families out of poverty.

In the total sample, only 11% of European Americans were in poverty, with 76% above poverty. Among African Americans, 57% were in poverty and only 25% above poverty. Half of the Hispanics lived above poverty, with the remainder divided equally between the poverty and near-poverty groups. Ethnicity and income status were significantly related, $\chi^2(4, N = 1{,}289) = 245.6$, $p < .001$. Ethnicity and income status were also significantly related in the child care subsample, $\chi^2(4, N = 683)=145.6$, $p < .001$, with African Americans and Hispanics overrepresented in the low-income groups.

Family composition also differed as a function of ethnicity. Two-parent families were far more common in European American and Hispanic than in African American families, with extended families and single-parent families accounting for slightly more than half of the African American sample ($\chi^2 = 123.294$, $p = .001$).

Family Context Variables

All analyses conducted on the family context variables used the entire available sample regardless of prior child care experience. The first MANOVA dealt with the demographic variables. The demographic variables differed significantly by income, $F(8, 1180) = 259.11$, $p = <.0001$, and ethnicity, $F(8,1180) = 12.9$, $p < .0001$, with no significant interaction between income and ethnicity. Lower income was related to a longer duration of poverty, more time spent as a single parent, lower maternal education, and fewer hours of employment or school. The pairwise comparisons showed almost identical patterns within each ethnic group. The one exception was that for Hispanic mothers, the near-poverty and above-poverty groups were not significantly different in percent of time spent as a single parent, whereas for European American and African American mothers, above-poverty mothers spent significantly less time single than did near-poverty mothers. For all ethnic groups, the above-poverty and near-poverty groups did not differ in maternal educational level or in number of hours per week that the mothers were at work or in school, but both groups were employed significantly more hours and had higher education than poverty mothers. Thus poverty mothers stand out as a distinct group in these highly significant areas of social competence.

The MANOVA on maternal and parenting characteristics revealed significant income, $F(10, 2286) = 16.41$, $p < .0001$, and ethnicity differences, $F(10, 2286) = 13.01$, $p < .0001$, and a significant interaction, $F = 2.08$, $p < .01$. The univariate F's for income on each constituent variable were also significantly different. Many of the pairwise comparisons of the income groups within ethnic groups were statistically significant, although the pattern was not as similar across ethnic groups as it was for demographic characteristics because of the interaction. Maternal depression was highest in the poverty group and lowest in the above-poverty group across ethnicities, although only for European Americans was the near-poverty group significantly different from the poverty or above-poverty group. Although the univariate F for the benefits of work measure was statistically significant, none of the pairwise comparisons was significant, indicating that the significant group differences arose from ethnicity differences. Sensitivity, whether measured by the mother–child play observations or the more naturalistic HOME Inventory, was always lowest in the poverty group and highest in the above-poverty group, with almost the same pattern across all three ethnicities. For mothers' health status, the above-poverty group had the highest rating among Hispanics and European Americans, but there was no income group difference for African Americans.

Child Care Measures

The analyses presented thus far dealt with all the children in the project who were still participating in the NICHD study at 36 months. Child care measures could obviously be made on only those children in care. It was not possible to visit all the child care settings or to get every item of information in all those where visits were made. Accordingly, N's will vary in the different analyses.

As indicated earlier, fewer of these families lived in poverty (10%) than was the case for the total sample (18%). Ethnic distributions were very similar in the two samples, with African American and Hispanic families accounting for 19% of the total group and 17% of the child care subsample.

Type of Care

A major area of interest about child care experiences of children from all economic backgrounds pertains to the type of care used. For children in nonmaternal care more than 10 hours per week, type of care as a function of income group and ethnicity was examined by means of chi square. Type of care used by the three income groups at 36 months differed significantly, $\chi^2(8, N = 592) = 35.887, p < .001$. Center care was the most common type of care in all three groups, accounting for 37–44% of the arrangements across groups. A child care home was the next largest category for above-poverty families, but the third most used care arrangement for poverty and near-poverty families. The near-poverty group used father or partner care twice as often (23%) as the poverty (12%) or above-poverty (11%) groups. The poverty sample used other relative care (30%) more than either the near-poverty (18%) or the above-poverty (11%) group. The only group that used in-home nonrelative care to any extent was the above-poverty group (11%).

Type of child care for children in care more than 10 hours a week also differed by ethnic group, $\chi^2(8, N = 654) = 26.15$, $p < .001$. As was true for all income groups, the most common care arrangement for all ethnic groups at 36 months was center care, ranging from a low of 40% in the Hispanic group to 46% in the African American group. About two-thirds of the care used by European Americans was in centers or child care homes. Hispanics used father/partner care more than the other two groups, and both Hispanics and African Americans used other relatives to a considerable extent (19% and 26%, respectively). Neither Hispanics nor African Americans had a single instance of in-home care by a nonrelative.

Amount and Stability of Care

Table 8.1 presents results from the MANOVA covering a child care composite embracing amount and stability of care, structural aspects of care, and observed measures of quality for the child care subsample.

Child Development Variables

Cognitive and Socioemotional Functioning

Three measures of cognitive development and two measures of socioemotional functioning were used as the dependent variable set in a MANOVA with family income and ethnicity as the independent variables. There was a main effect for income, $F(10, 2076) = 8.06$, $p < .0001$, and for ethnicity, $F(10, 2076) = 8.61$, $p < .0001$, but no interaction between income and ethnicity. The pattern of significant pairwise comparisons was similar across ethnic groups, with the poverty group scoring lowest on every measure, the above-poverty group highest, and the near-poverty group about halfway between the extremes. However, although the near-poverty group scored between the other two income groups, the relevant pairwise comparisons were not consistently significant in any of the ethnic groups. On the cognitive measures (Reynell and Bracken) the children from poverty families were, on the average, about two-thirds of a standard deviation below the above-poverty children, the near-poverty children about one-third below. On the socioemotional measures, the magnitude of the differences, although statistically significant, was not as great. There was considerable variability on all the measures.

Children's Growth and Health

Results from the MANOVA that included child's height and weight and mother's rating of child's general health as dependent variables, with income and ethnicity as independent variables show that the multivariate F for income was statistically significant, $F(6, 2054) = 2.18$, p .05, but not for

TABLE 8.1. Child Care Experiences by Income and Ethnicity Status: Child Care Sample

	Poverty (n = 61)			Near poverty (n = 76)			Above poverty (n = 455)			Group differences (n = 592)		Significant pairwise comparisons[a]		
	EA (n = 27) M (SD)	AA (n = 28) M (SD)	HP (n = 6) M (SD)	EA (n = 49) M (SD)	AA (n = 12) M (SD)	HP (n = 15) M (SD)	EA (n = 413) M (SD)	AA (n = 23) M (SD)	HP (n = 19) M (SD)	F	p	EA	AA	HP
Amount and stability														
Mean hr in care	18.92 (10.72)	24.24 (13.44)	27.15 (-10.88)	27.20 (14.03)	30.24 (11.57)	31.11 (11.80)	30.37 (13.07)	35.10 (10.23)	34.90 (11.65)	4.33	.0001	P < N,A	P < A	
Age onset (mo)	10.63 (10.42)	7.21 (9.48)	4.17 (3.92)	5.29 (6.87)	2.83 (1.75)	4.33 (4.67)	4.76 (5.99)	3.61 (3.65)	5.10 (5.02)	3.51	.0006	A,N < P		
Total no. starts	5.63 (3.00)	6.43 (2.81)	6.33 (3.33)	6 (3.18)	5.92 (2.23)	6.87 (1.88)	5.52 (2.82)	5.61 (2.61)	5.84 (2.99)	0.88	.5303			
Structural quality														
Obs. group size	8.68 (6.53)	7.2 (6.54)	4.94 (4.46)	4.82 (4.41)	5.22 (4.90)	7.95 (7.06)	7.68 (6.32)	8.58 (4.83)	7.6 (5.81)	1.78	.0773	N < P,A		
Obs. ratio	4.91 (3.21)	4.17 (3.31)	2.8 (1.10)	3.56 (2.87)	3.64 (2.72)	4.84 (3.74)	4.71 (3.13)	5.77 (3.01)	4.41 (2.82)	1.68	.1000	N < A	N < A	
Crgv. educ. (1-6 scale)	2.82 (1.14)	2.87 (1.01)	3 (1.55)	2.61 (1.02)	2.92 (1.08)	2.53 (0.92)	2.96 (1.05)	2.7 (1.15)	2.84 (1.07)	2.14	.0307	N < A		
Crgv. formal training	1.52 (1.42)	1.36 (1.54)	1.67 (1.86)	0.74 (1.22)	0.75 (1.14)	1.07 (1.28)	1.48 (1.45)	1.26 (1.57)	1.95 (1.35)	2.35	.0174	N < P,A		
Observed quality														
ORCE Qual. Comp.	19.16 (2.83)	17.46 (3.30)	20.29 (1.60)	19.82 (3.46)	18.42 (3.28)	18.21 (3.08)	19.94 (3.21)	17.31 (3.25)	20.7 (2.89)	4.58	.0001			N < A
ORCE Positive Int.	-1.59 (5.56)	-2.65 (4.00)	1.65 (5.87)	1.48 (5.88)	-0.44 (5.45)	-3.28 (5.87)	0.45 (5.82)	-2.88 (4.30)	0.87 (5.50)	3.26	.0012	P < N		N < A
MANOVA														
Income										2.0767	.0052			
Ethnicity										1.6702	.0386			
Income × ethnicity										0.7970	.8003			

Note. EA, European Americans; AA, African Americans; HP, Hispanics.
[a]The pairwise comparisons are between poverty groups within ethnic groups.

ethnicity. None of the univariate tests was significant. On the general health rating, the means for all three groups indicated that they were in "good" health. Children in the three income groups did not differ significantly from one another on height or weight or general health.

Child Development and Child Care Experiences

The foregoing analyses show clearly that the cognitive and socioemotional development of the children bore a strong relation to poverty and its co-factors. They also show that alternative care patterns are often different in the various income and ethnic groups. A major question for both theory and policy is whether extrafamily experiences during the first 3 years of life can interrupt some of the associations between early poverty and subsequent developmental difficulties.

This chapter examined the question in two ways. First, amount of child care exposure was introduced as an additional independent variable along with income and ethnicity in an examination of the child development outcomes (cognitive, socioemotional, and health) in children from all three income groups. Second, an observational index of quality was related to the same child development measures.

The first analysis used the entire sample, segmenting child care usage into three categories: less than 10 hours per week of nonmaternal care, between 10 and 30 hours per week, and more than 30 hours per week. With regard to income and child development, this analysis confirmed the existence of a strong association between income and cognitive and social outcomes ($F = 16.65$, $p < .001$). The poor children scored lowest and the above-poverty children highest, with the working-poor children scoring in between. There was also a significant association between ethnicity and cognitive and social outcomes ($F = 10.67$, $p < .001$). However, once income and ethnicity were taken into account, the relationship between amount of care and the cognitive and socioemotional outcomes was not statistically significant ($F = .81$, $p = $ NS). Although the middle group (10–30 hours) appears to have a slight edge in the child development measures, variability in all groups was great and the differences were not significant. Amount of care was, however, related to the health measures, $F (6, 2058) = 2.98$, $p = .007$. Mothers rated their children as slightly less healthy if they were in part-time or full-time care than if they were in little or no child care.

Although no association could be established between sheer amount of child care attendance per week and the child development variables, that finding does not address the issue of quality of the child care experience. To determine whether quality of care made a difference, we used the positive caregiving rating of child care quality based on direct observations in the child care settings and the cognitive and social outcomes (Reynell, Bracken, cooperation, and problem behavior). Structural indices of quality, such as child–adult ratios and group size, are confounded with type of care and were therefore not used in this analysis. And, as a major objective of this study was to determine whether and how child care experiences had an impact on children likely to be eligible for Head Start, we included in this analysis only those children in the poverty and near-poverty groups who spent at least 20 hours a week in either a child care home or a center. This restriction reduced the size of the sample to 79 children. Results of a linear regression using income and quality as independent variables and the cognitive and social measures as dependent variables showed no effect of income when the above-poverty group was excluded from the analysis. Quality was not related to the two measures of social functioning but was related to children's overall cognitive and language functioning at 3 years of age, $F(73,3) = 4.30$, $p = .008$, with better scores found for poor and near-poor children participating in programs of higher quality. On the individual measures, total quality was predictive of the Reynell expressive language standard score ($F = 4.73$, $p = .03$) and the Bracken school readiness standard score ($F = 10.92$, $p = .002$).

DISCUSSION

This study was undertaken to explore early life experiences of children eligible for federally subsidized preschool programs, such as Head Start. It has been exhaustively documented in landmark historical studies (Deutsch, 1967; Klaus & Gray, 1968; Lazar & Darlington, 1982; Weikart, Deloria, Lawser, & Wiegerink, 1970) and in research exclusively concerned with Head Start (Administration on Children, Youth and Families, 1996; McKey et al., 1985) that children from poverty backgrounds enter kindergarten and first grade significantly behind their more economically privileged agemates on a host of developmental measures. Furthermore, there is an impressive literature on family functioning during early childhood (Beckwith, 1990; Bradley & Caldwell, 1984), which shows that these delays are associated with family environments providing reduced stimulation and support. Less is known about children's experiences outside the family—especially those in the first 3 years of life—and how these experiences, interacting with conditions and experiences within the family, affect development. In this chapter we have attempted to add to the knowledge base in this area by examining family characteristics, child care experiences, child health, and child development characteristics of children living in poverty and contrasting them with samples just above the poverty line and substantially above poverty. Then, recognizing the influence of various co-factors of poverty, we have included ethnicity in our analyses.

An oversimplified summary of our findings would be that, on most of the family background variables and in the cognitive and social child outcomes, the income groups differ significantly, with the levels of reported and observed functioning generally ranging downward from above poverty to poverty. The near-poverty group sometimes looked more like the above-poverty group and at other times more like the poverty group but generally fell somewhere between the two extreme groups. Exceptions to this pattern occurred (e.g., health measures), but they were too infrequent to invalidate the generalization.

In some respects the data from this study, dealing with only the first 3 years of life, echo the findings of previous research: The developmental achievements of poor children lag behind those of children from families that have more wealth. However, in all the measured attributes, there is considerable variability. This mandates an early education curriculum adapted to a wide range of abilities and experiences. The observed variability does not, however, eradicate the need that many poor and near-poor children have for additional support during the first 3 years of life both within and outside their families. The fact that some of the children who grow up in poverty arrive at the preschool door with a full complement of cognitive and social skills cannot mask the evidence that many of them will need intervention services to enable them to realize their full developmental potential. And such services are most likely to be effective only if of high quality. It is by highlighting both the variability and the predominant patterns of functioning shown by families and children in poverty that our data can be of greatest benefit to the planners and operators of Head Start and other early education programs.

9

Change in Family Income-to-Needs Matters More for Children with Less

ERIC DEARING
KATHLEEN MCCARTNEY
BECK A. TAYLOR

One of the most consistent findings in the developmental literature concerns the association between childhood poverty and negative developmental outcomes (Duncan & Brooks-Gunn, 2000; Duncan, Yeung, Brooks-Gunn, & Smith, 1998; Huston, McLoyd, & Garcia Coll, 1994; McLoyd, 1998). Researchers and policymakers alike have used these collective findings to argue that redistributions of wealth, such as income transfers, will improve the life chances of children in poverty (e.g., Duncan & Brooks-Gunn, 2000). That is, change in family economics is assumed to lead to change in child outcomes, albeit indirectly. Causal inferences, however, have been limited by methodological concerns, including a lack of research modeling change in economic resources for individual families, which is the focus here.

We examined changes in family income-to-needs using data from 1 to 36 months from the National Institute of Child Health and Human Development (NICHD) Study of Early Child Care. The advantage of this data set over others lies in the richness of the data, which include observational assessments of the family context as well as child outcomes. Using these data, we modeled patterns of change for individual families, as well as associations between these patterns and child outcomes. Thus, this chapter

From *Child Development*, 2001, Vol. 72, pp. 1779–1793. Reprinted with permission of the Society for Research in Child Development.

study extends the poverty literature in at least three ways. First, because family economics are dynamic and vary within families, modeling change at the level of the individual family should provide a more accurate account of the association between economic well-being and child outcomes than static or categorical approaches have provided. Second, as Duncan and colleagues (1998) have suggested, patterns of change are relevant for discussions of causality in nonexperimental research. Third, change is particularly relevant for this topic of study; policymakers want to know whether increases in family economic resources lead to improvements in child outcomes.

Growth curve analysis is now recognized as a preferred method for studying patterns of change over time for both groups and individuals within those groups (Bryk & Raudenbush, 1992; Rogosa, 1995; Willett, Singer, & Martin, 1998), yet no studies of income dynamics have used this approach to date. Growth curve analysis is conducted with statistical methods that have been referred to using a number of different titles (e.g., hierarchical linear models, Bryk & Raudenbush, 1992; mixed-effects or random-effects models, Laird & Ware, 1982) and is available in a number of different statistical packages (e.g., hierarchical linear modeling [HLM], Bryk & Raudenbush, 1992; LISREL, Rovine & Molenaar, 1998; and SAS PROC MIXED, Singer, 1998). The method is an extension of repeated-measures analysis of variance with the advantage that change at the level of the individual is measured directly rather than via the interaction of time by subject.

In this study, growth curves were used to model family economics over time. More specifically, HLM (Bryk & Raudenbush, 1992) was used to estimate initial status (i.e., 1 month) and change for family income-to-needs through 36 months. Associations between change and child, mother, and family characteristics were then examined in an attempt to identify potential sources of bias. Based on a large body of demographic research (e.g., Corcoran & Chaudry, 1997; Hanson, Heims, Julian, & Sussman, 1995), we hypothesized that maternal education and changes in family structure would be associated with change in income-to-needs.

A series of regression analyses was used to investigate associations between change in income-to-needs and 36-month child cognitive, language, and behavioral outcomes. The first set of regressions included an interaction term of income-to-needs by nonpoverty status. We hypothesized that associations would be stronger for families living in poverty, for whom changes would be more salient. A change model was used in the second set of regressions by adding a 15-month measure of children's intelligence as a predictor for the cognitive and language outcomes. That is, change in family income-to-needs was used to predict change in children's cognitive outcomes. We hypothesized that these associations would be significant.

Finally, we investigated whether the quality of the home environment mediated associations between change in family income-to-needs and child outcomes. Based on the results of studies that have investigated the home environment as a mediator of static measures of income (for a review, see Duncan & Brooks-Gunn, 2000), we hypothesized that the home environment would explain approximately half of the variance between change in income-to-needs and the child outcomes.

METHOD

Participants

A total of 1,364 families enrolled in the study, 89% (1,216) of which continued to participate through 36 months. (A detailed description of the study participants is provided in Chapter 1 of this volume.) There were some demographic differences between families that dropped out and those that continued to participate. Specifically, mothers in families that dropped out were less likely than the other mothers to be partnered (75% vs. 87%, $\chi^2 = 13.55$, $p < .001$) and had fewer years of education (13.38 vs. 14.34, $t = -4.362$, $p < .001$). In addition, children in families that dropped out were more likely than the other children to be African American (23% vs. 11%, $\chi^2 = 17.83$, $p < .001$).

Measures

Demographics

Mother's education was assessed when the children were 1 month of age and was coded as number of years of schooling. Child ethnicity was divided into two dummy variables representing African American versus other and Latino American versus other. For family structure, three variables representing whether the mother was partnered during all assessments, single during all assessments, or changed from partnered to single status were created using effect coding; that is, the excluded group (family structures that changed from single to partnered status) was coded as –1 for each of the three variables. Thus, the family structure variables represented the "effects" of always-partnered status, always-single status, and partnered-to-single status (i.e., the group mean minus the grand mean).

Family Income-to-Needs

At 1, 6, 15, 24, and 36 months, the ratio of family income to needs was computed by dividing total family income by the poverty threshold for the appropriate family size (U.S. Bureau of the Census, 1999b). In addition, a categorical variable (i.e., nonpoverty status) was created for which families were coded as having an income-to-needs ratio of greater than or equal to 1 during all assessments versus having an income-to-needs ratio of less than 1 (i.e., poor) at any time between 1 and 36 months. Effect coding was used such that nonpoor families were coded as 1 and poor families were coded as −1.

Home Environment

The quality of the home environment was assessed at 36 months using the Home Observation for Measurement of the Environment (HOME; Caldwell & Bradley, 1984). The measure has demonstrated excellent reliability (e.g., alpha = .93, Caldwell & Bradley, 1984). For the NICHD Study of Early Child Care sample, the internal consistency for the measure was excellent (alpha = .87). (See Chapter 1 for details.)

Cognitive and Language Outcomes

During the 15-month home visit, children's cognitive development was assessed using the Mental Development Index (MDI) from the Revised Bayley Scales of Infant Development (BSID-II; Bayley, 1993). The MDI has been validated via strong correlations with other measures of children's intelligence such as the Stanford–Binet (Bayley, 1993). The measure is also highly reliable; in the standardization sample, the split-half reliability for the MDI was .80 (Bayley, 1993).

Children's cognitive development was also assessed during the 36-month home visit using the school readiness composite from the Bracken Basic Concept Scale (Bracken, 1984). The 51-item measure assesses children's abilities in the areas of color recognition, letter identification, number/counting skills, comparisons, and shape recognition. The school readiness composite has demonstrated excellent validity via strong correlations with intelligence measures and academic performance in kindergarten (Laughlin, 1995; Zucker & Riordan, 1987). In the present sample, the internal consistency of the measure was excellent (alpha = .93).

During the laboratory visit at 36 months, children's language performance was assessed using the Reynell Developmental Language Scale (Reynell, 1991). The 67-item scale is divided into two subscales: receptive language and expressive language (see previous chapters). In the NICHD sample, both scales were internally consistent (alpha = .93 for the receptive scale and .86 for the expressive scale).

Behavioral Outcomes

During the laboratory visit at 36 months, child behavior was assessed via maternal report. Specifically, mothers completed both the Child Behavior Checklist (CBCL; Achenbach, Edelbrock, & Howell, 1987) and the Adaptive Social Behavior Inventory (ASBI; Hogan, Scott, & Bauer, 1992, as mentioned in Chapters 1 and 8).

Based on factor analysis (for a detailed description, see NICHD Early Child Care Research Network, 1999b), child behavior composites representing behavior problems and positive social behavior were formed by summing results from multiple subscales of the CBCL and ASBI. Specifically, the behavior problems composite consisted of the Externalizing (i.e., aggressive and destructive problem behaviors), Internalizing (i.e., social withdrawal and depression related behaviors), Sleep Problems, and Somatic Problems subscales from the CBCL, as well as the Disrupt (i.e., resistant and agonistic behavior) subscale from the ASBI. In the present sample, the Cronbach's alpha for these subscales ranged from .60 to .89 and correlations among the scales ranged in size from .40 to .70. The positive social behavior composite consisted of the Express (i.e., sociable and empathic behaviors) and the Comply (i.e., cooperative and prosocial behaviors) subscales of the ASBI. In the present sample, the Cronbach's alpha for these two subscales was .76 and .82, respectively; the correlation between the two was .49. The behavior problems and positive social behavior composites were validated via correlations with a variety of family, maternal, and child characteristics including maternal psychological functioning and child temperament (NICHD Early Child Care Research Network, 1998a).

RESULTS

Initial Status and Change in Family Income-to-Needs

Two-level HLM (Bryk & Raudenbush, 1992) was used to estimate initial status (intercept) and linear change (slope) from 1 to 36 months for family income-to-needs, as well as to test associations between these estimates and characteristics of children and families. In the first level of HLM, ordinary least-squares (OLS) estimates of initial status and change are computed for the population (i.e., fixed effects) as well as for each individual (i.e., random effects). Initial status and change were weakly associated, tan = .15, such that families that started with lower income-to-needs ratios were somewhat less likely to experience positive change in income-to-needs.

The mean value for the OLS estimates of initial status was 3.07; note that an income-to-needs ratio of about 3 is indicative of middle-class families (see Conger, Conger, & Elder, 1997). There was, however, significant variability in initial status. In fact, 24% of the sample was in poverty at 1 month, as defined by an income-to-needs ratio of less than 1. The mean value for the OLS estimates of change was .02; note that this represents the amount of change per month. Thus, on average, families experienced a positive change of .70 in income-to-needs between 1 and 36 months. There was also significant variability across families. In fact, nearly 30% of the sample experienced losses in income-to-needs between 1 and 36 months. Empirical Bayes (EB) estimates of initial status and change are also computed in the first level of HLM. In our data, the mean value of the EB estimates for initial status was 3.08, $SD = 2.44$, and for change was .014, $SD = .013$.

HLM Estimates and Characteristics of Children and Families

In the second level of HLM, the EB estimates of initial status and change are analyzed as outcomes of a specified set of fixed-effect predictors. To identify child and family characteristics associated with income-to-needs, measured both statically at 1 month and dynamically through 36 months, we specified a set of standard child and family predictors. The child characteristics included sex, two ethnicity dummy variables for African American and Latino American status, and birthweight. The family characteristics included maternal education, three dummy variables for partner status, and a dummy variable that represents nonpoverty status. There is modest covariation among predictors with one exception—nonpoverty status was strongly related to both maternal education and always-partnered status.

The HLM analyses showed that for initial status, at 1 month, income-to-needs was negatively associated with being African American, positively associated with maternal education, and associated with all three indices of partner status. Change in income-to-needs was positively associated with maternal education and negatively associated with change in partner status from partnered to single.

Regression Models Predicting 36-Month Child Outcomes

Standard regression analyses were used to model 36-month child outcomes. Although there were no problems of multicollinearity, we report tolerance values for each variable so that intervariable dependency can be interpreted.

Each of the five outcomes was regressed separately on the predictors (see Tables 9.1 and 9.2). Note that the tables include three separate standardized regression coefficients for the effect of change in income-to-needs. Specifically, coefficients representing the average effect of change for children from nonpoor and poor families, the effect of change for children from nonpoor families, and the effect of change for children from poor families are reported in the tables. Also note that the interaction of change by nonpoverty status tests whether these latter two coefficients significantly differ from one another. In other words, is the effect of change in income-to-needs qualitatively different for children from nonpoor and poor families?

Table 9.1 presents results for the three cognitive and language outcomes. Initial status was positively associated with school readiness and receptive language. That is, children whose families started with higher income-to-needs ratios scored higher on these two measures than other children. Furthermore, the average effect of change in income-to-needs and nonpoverty status were positively associated with all three outcomes such that children whose families experienced positive change in income-to-needs and were not in poverty scored higher than other children. However,

TABLE 9.1. Regression Models Predicting School Readiness, Receptive Language, and Expressive Language

Predictor	School readiness[a]			Receptive language[b]			Expressive language[c]		
	r	β	Tolerance	r	β	Tolerance	r	β	Tolerance
Child characteristics									
Gender	-.16***	-.15***	.98	-.20***	-.18***	.98	-.16***	-.15***	.98
African American	-.32***	-.21***	.78	-.35***	-.24***	.78	-.19***	-.08*	.79
Latino American	-.07*	-.04	.96	-.12***	-.09***	.96	-.09***	-.05	.96
Birthweight	.08**	.04	.96	.06*	.03	.96	.09***	.07*	.96
Family characteristics									
Maternal education	.43***	.26***	.65	.44***	.27***	.65	.31***	.19***	.64
Always partnered	.23***	-.01	.72	.26***	.02	.72	.18***	.04	.73
Always single	-.11**	.00	.84	-.12**	-.03	.84	-.08**	-.04	.83
Partnered to single	-.01	-.01	.85	.06	.06*	.85	-.05	.05	.84
Income-to-needs									
Initial status	.40***	.15***	.55	.40***	.12***	.55	.27***	.06	.55
Change[a]	.22***	.13** (.01) [.25**]	.44	.20***	.12** (.02) [.21**]	.44	.12**	.09* (-.05) [.23**]	.44
Nonpoverty status	.35***	.11*	.34	.36***	.10*	.34	.27***	.15**	.34
Change × Nonpoverty	-.12*	-.12*	.27		-.10*	.27		-.14**	.27

The top coefficients represent the average effect of change in income-to-needs for children from nonpoor and poor families. The coefficients in parentheses represent the effect of change in income-to-needs for children from nonpoor families and the coefficients in brackets represent the effect of changes in income-to-needs for children from poor families.

*p < .05; **p < .01; ***p < .001.
[a]R^2 = .30***; n = 1,149.
[b]R^2 = .34***; n = 1,148.
[c]R^2 = .16***; n = 1,121.

the regression coefficients for change in income-to-needs were substantially different for children from poor versus nonpoor families.

Consider the effect of change for school readiness. For children in poor families, the standardized coefficient for change in income-to-needs was .25, but for children in nonpoor families this coefficient was only .01. In fact, the interaction of change and nonpoverty status was significant for each of the cognitive and language outcomes, showing that change in income-to-needs had little impact on children from nonpoor families but great impact on children from poor families.

Table 9.2 presents results for the two behavior outcomes. The average effect of change in income-to-needs and nonpoverty status was positively associated with positive social behavior. As with the cognitive and language outcomes, however, the effect of change for positive social behavior was markedly different for children from poor and nonpoor families (i.e., .23 and −.05, respectively). The interaction of change and nonpoverty status was, in fact, significant for this outcome. Change in income-to-needs had lit-

TABLE 9.2. Regression Models Predicting Positive Social Behavior and Behavior Problems

Predictor	Positive social behavior[a]			Behavior problems[b]		
	r	β	Tolerance	r	β	Tolerance
Child characteristics						
Gender	−.09***	−.08**	.98	−.02	−.03	.98
African American	−.22***	−.16***	.80	.08**	.00	.80
Latino American	−.04	−.02	.96	−.01	−.04	.96
Birthweight	.02	−.01	.96	.03	.00	.96
Family characteristics						
Maternal education	.24***	.15***	.64	−.22***	−.17***	.64
Always partnered	.14***	.00	.73	−.15***	−.08*	.73
Always single	−.09**	−.03	.83	.07*	.02	.83
Partnered to single	.03	.03	.85	.02	.02	.85
Income–to–needs						
Initial status	.20***	.03	.54	−.08**	−.01	.54
Change[a]	.09**	.09*	.46	−.16***	−.04	.46
		(−.05)			(.02)	
		[.23**]			[−.11]	
Nonpoverty status	.22***	.14**	.35	−.17***	−.08	.35
Change × Nonpoverty		−.14**	.28		.07	.28

The top coefficients represent the average effect of change in income-to-needs for children from nonpoor and poor families. The coefficients in parentheses represent the effect of change in income-to-needs for children from nonpoor families and the coefficients in brackets represent the effect of changes in income-to-needs for children from poor families.
[a]R^2 = .11*** (n = 1,167)
[b]R^2 = .06*** (n = 1,167).
*p < .05; **p < .01; ***p < .001.

tle influence on the positive social behavior of children in nonpoor families but had great influence on the positive social behavior of children in poor families. Again, these maternal ratings were similar for children from poor and nonpoor families when they experienced increases in income-to-needs that were approximately one standard deviation above the mean for poor families.

A Change Model

We reestimated the regression models for school readiness and the Reynell language scales, including the Bayley MDI, assessed at 15 months. Conceptually, the MDI measure is an appropriate control for early cognitive and language ability; it was, in fact, the strongest predictor in the model for Reynell receptive language, beta = .31, $p < .001$, and expressive language, beta = .20, $p < .001$, and it was second to maternal education as a predictor of school readiness, beta = .18, $p < .001$. The significant main effects and interactions for income-to-needs in models that did not include the MDI (see Table 9.1) were again evident in these change models. Among non-experimental designs, change models, like this one, provide better support for causal argument than models that do not account for change, because modeling change controls for unobserved influences associated with both the outcome and predictor.

Quality of the Home Environment as a Mediator

We used Baron and Kenny's (1986) two-stage regression strategy in order to test whether the home environment served as a mediator between change in family income-to-needs and child outcomes. For children in poverty, including the HOME in the regression analyses slightly decreased the size of the standardized coefficients for change in income-to-needs from .25 to .20 for school readiness, .21 to .16 for receptive language, .23 to .18 for expressive language, and .23 to .19 for positive social behavior.

The Practical Importance of Change in Income-to-Needs for Families in Poverty

To evaluate the practical importance of change in income-to-needs, we decided to compare its effects with those of maternal education, which is not only a well-established influence on child development but also the largest predictor in our analyses other than the MDI in the simple change models (see McCartney & Rosenthal, 2000, for a discussion of evaluating practical importance). We reestimated our regressions for the 373 children from families that had lived in poverty at some time between 1 and 36.

Table 9.3 contains the effect size estimates (i.e., partial correlations) for initial status and change in income-to-needs as well as for maternal educa-

TABLE 9.3. Partial Correlations from Regression Models for Families in Poverty

Predictor	School readiness	Receptive language	Expressive language	Positive social behavior
Income-to-needs initial status	.15	.15	.13	.03
Income-to-needs slope	.10	.12	.10	.10
Maternal education	.21	.17	.12	.18

tion. Note that the effect sizes for initial status in income-to-needs were similar to those for change. Although they might be considered small by some standards (e.g., Cohen & Cohen, 1983), they are not much smaller than those for maternal education. In fact, if we compute an average effect size across outcomes, the effects for initial status in income-to-needs, $M = .12$, and change in income-to-needs, $M = .11$, are each approximately two-thirds the size of that for maternal education, $M = .17$.

DISCUSSION

Using data from the NICHD Study of Early Child Care, the sequelae of changes in income-to-needs for a variety of 36-month child outcomes were identified. For four of the five child outcomes, there was an interaction between nonpoverty status and change in income-to-needs. Change in income-to-needs was of little importance for children from nonpoor families but of great importance for children from poor families. In other words, change in family income-to-needs mattered more for children with less.

These results are consistent with past research documenting nonlinear effects for static measures of income-to-needs (e.g., average family income-to-needs); that is, differences between children that are associated with family income-to-needs are often greatest at the low end of the income distribution (see Duncan & Brooks-Gunn, 1997; Duncan et al., 1998). Surprisingly, however, we found that children in poor families that experienced gains in income-to-needs scored similarly as those from nonpoor families. Thus, a positive change in income-to-needs was a powerful protective factor for children from poor families. Our results are also consistent with research estimating the effects of economic loss on children and adolescents (Flanagan & Eccles, 1993; Elder, Van Nguyen, & Caspi, 1985; Galambos & Silbereisen, 1987; McLoyd, Jayaratne, Ceballo, & Borquez, 1994).

Nearly 17% of children in the United States live in poverty (U.S. Bureau of the Census, 1999a); thus, the importance of these findings, especially with respect to risk and prevention, is great from an incidence validity perspective (see Fabes, Martin, Hanesh, & Updegraff, 2000). From these find-ings, we know that naturally occurring decreases in family income-to-needs were associated with worse developmental outcomes for children from poor families. Conversely, we know that naturally occurring increases in family income-to-needs were associated with better developmental outcomes for children from poor families. In fact, a change in income-to-needs one stan-dard deviation above the mean for poor families was associated with compa-rable performance for children from poor and nonpoor families. Even more modest increases over time in income-to-needs, however, led to improvements in children's performance, *even as early as 3 years of age.*

10

—

Chronicity of Maternal Depressive Symptoms, Maternal Sensitivity, and Child Functioning at 36 Months

NICHD Early Child Care Research Network

Maternal depression, whether defined in terms of self-reported symptoms or clinically diagnosed disorder, is considered a risk factor for children's socioemotional and cognitive development (Beardslee, Bemporad, Keller, & Klerman, 1983; Field, 1992; Gelfand & Teti, 1990; Zahn-Waxler, Iannotti, Cummings, & Denham, 1990). The effects of maternal depression may be especially evident when children are very young because they are more dependent on nurturance, stimulation, and support from primary caregivers (Beardslee et al., 1983; Cummings & Cicchetti, 1990).

Clinically significant depression is characterized by sadness, fatigue, irritability, and emotional withdrawal (American Psychiatric Association, 1994), symptoms that are likely to foster less sensitive and engaged maternal care as well as more maternal negativity (Beardslee et al., 1983; Cohn, Campbell, Matias, & Hopkins, 1990; Cummings & Davies, 1994; DeMulder & Radke-Yarrow, 1991). In turn, emotional unavailability, lack of responsiveness, and negativity from primary caregivers may place young children at risk for an array of developmental problems, as reflected, for example, in poorer regulation of negative affect, less reciprocity and shared positive affect, less compliance, and less interest in mastering the world of

From *Developmental Psychology*, 1999, Vol. 35, pp. 1297–1310. Copyright 1999 by the American Psychological Association. Reprinted by permission.

objects (e.g., Cohn & Campbell, 1992; Field, 1992; Murray, 1992; Radke-Yarrow, Cummings, Kuczynski, & Chapman, 1985; Tronick, 1989). Although biological/genetic mechanisms may play a role in the link between maternal depression and problematic infant/toddler development, proximal mechanisms such as the quality of mothering and mother–child interaction also are important factors to consider (Cohn & Campbell, 1992; Cummings & Davies, 1994; Field, 1992; Radke-Yarrow et al., 1985).

For this report we examine the link between maternal depression and mother–child interaction and their relations with children's functioning at 36 months. Specifically, we test a model that includes the chronicity of maternal depressive symptoms assessed from the birth of the study child to 36 months, and common co-occurring risk/protective factors such as household income, education, partner presence, and social support. We hypothesize that mothers who report more chronic symptoms of depression across this 3-year period will be less sensitive and responsive to their infants during play, and that the effects of the chronicity of depressive symptoms on mother–child interaction will be moderated by other risk/protective factors. Thus, women with chronic depressive symptoms who also have substantial resources and few psychosocial risks will be more sensitive with their babies than women who report chronic symptoms but also have few resources and little support from others. We also test the hypothesis that children whose mothers report chronic symptoms of depression will display more negative and less positive mood during play. Finally, our longitudinal data permit us to explore whether sensitive and responsive mother–child interaction changes over the first 36 months of life as a function of the chronicity of symptoms and other risk factors.

The second part of the model focuses on the predictors of child outcomes at 36 months, specifically behavior problems, cooperation and compliance, self-control, and cognitive–linguistic development. Children's outcomes are examined first as a function of maternal reports of chronic depressive symptoms and second as a *joint* function of maternal depressive symptoms and maternal sensitivity over the first 36 months of life. We expect that maternal sensitivity will partially mediate the effect of depressive symptoms on child outcomes. Finally we examine the moderating effects of maternal sensitivity on children's outcomes within the depressed groups.

METHOD

Participants

Data for this report are based on 1,215 families (89% of the initial National Institute of Child Health and Human Development [NICHD] sample) with questionnaire and observational data on mother–child interaction through 36 months. These 1,215 families were more advantaged on several measures than those not included in these analyses because of missing data. Based on data collected during a home visit at 1 month (see next paragraph), the women included in this report were more educated (M = 14.4 vs. 13.2 years of education, t = 5.17, p < .001), had higher income-to-needs ratios (M = 2.86 vs. 1.98, t = 3.61, p < .001), and reported slightly lower levels of depressive symptoms (M = 11.2 vs. 12.8, t = 2.12, p < .05) than those with missing data. They were also more likely to be living with a partner (87% vs. 75%, p < .001) and somewhat more likely to report that they planned to return to work at least part time during the study child's first year of life (62% vs. 51%, p < .05). Demographic data are summarized in Table 10.1.

Measures

Depression

Maternal reports of depressive symptoms were assessed at 1, 6, 15, 24, and 36 months with the Center for Epidemiological Studies–Depression (CES-D) scale (Radloff, 1977). Cronbach's alphas were high at each assessment (range = .88 to .91) and depression scores were moderately correlated over time (range = .41 to .58). In line with the work of Radloff and others (Myers & Weissman, 1980), a cutoff score of 16 or above was used to define poten-

TABLE 10.1. Sample Characteristics for Families Included in Depression Analyses

	n	%
Child ethnicity		
European American, non-Hispanic	950	78
African American, non-Hispanic	139	11
Hispanic	68	6
Other	58	5
Child sex		
Girls	592	49
Boys	623	51
Maternal education		
< 12 years	106	9
High school or GED	250	21
Some college	406	33
Bachelor's degree	268	22
Postgraduate	185	15
Husband/partner in the home	1,055	87
Child care plans at birth		
Full time	627	52
Part time	124	10
None	464	38

Note. n = 1,215. GED, General Equivalency Diploma.

tially serious depression. Only women with at least four out of five CES-D scores are included.

Demographics

Maternal education was operationalized as number of years in school at the time of recruitment. Family type was coded as two-parent versus other at the 1-month visit and was updated at each assessment. Family size was also updated at each assessment. An income-to-needs ratio was computed from maternal interview data collected at each home visit.

Social Support

Perceptions of the availability of social support were assessed at each home visit using the 11-item Relationships With Other People scale (Marshall & Barnett, 1993) in which the respondents rate their relationships over the past month. This scale has high internal consistency (alphas over .90 at each assessment) and moderate stability (range from $r = .52$ to $r = .63$).

Mother–Child Interaction

Mother–child interaction during play was observed at each assessment to obtain an age-appropriate but conceptually coherent index of maternal sensitivity and responsiveness, as well as child mood. At the 6- and 15-month home visits, mothers and infants were videotaped in 15-minute semistructured play interactions. At 24 and 36 months, mother–child interaction was observed in the laboratory.

The videotaped episodes of mother–child interaction from all 10 sites were sent to a central location for coding. Teams of six coders scored the videotapes at each age. All coders were blind to depression status and any other information about study families. At each age, 20% of the tapes, selected at random, were double-coded to obtain a measure of intercoder reliability. Reliability was monitored throughout the coding period and coders were unaware which of their tapes would be assigned to a second coder.

A composite free-play score of maternal sensitivity during play was created from observer ratings at each age. At 6, 15, and 24 months it reflected the sum of three 4-point ratings of sensitivity to nondistress, positive regard, and intrusiveness (reversed). At 36 months, three conceptually similar but more age-appropriate 7-point ratings made up the composite: supportive presence, respect for autonomy and hostility (reversed). At each age, the scales ranged from "not at all characteristic" to "highly characteristic" of the interaction. The 36-month ratings were recalibrated to 4-point scales to make them comparable to earlier ratings. Intraclass correlation (Winer,

1971) coefficients averaged across pairs of raters were .87 at 6 months, .83 at 15 months, .85 at 24 months, and .84 at 36 months. Cronbach's alphas were .75, .70, .79, and .78, respectively.

Child behavior was also rated from these videotapes of mother–child interaction. At 6, 15, and 24 months, child negative and positive mood were rated on 4-point scales ("not at all characteristic" to "highly characteristic"). At 36 months, child enthusiasm (which was conceptually related to positive mood) and child negativity were rated on 7-point scales. These 36-month scales were recalibrated to 4-point scales to make them comparable to the 6, 15, and 24 month ratings. Interrater reliability coefficients (intraclass correlations) ranged from .67 to .75 for positive mood and from .85 to .90 for negative mood.

CHILD OUTCOME MEASURES AT 36 MONTHS

Social–Emotional Outcomes

Maternal Reports of Behavior Problems and Social Competence

During the laboratory visit at 36 months, mothers completed two questionnaires describing their child's typical behavior at home. The 99-item Child Behavior Checklist–2/3 (CBCL; Achenbach, Edelbrock, & Howell, 1987) was used to assess problem behaviors.

Social competence and disruptive behavior were also assessed with the 30-item Adaptive Social Behavior Inventory (ASBI; Hogan, Scott, & Bauer, 1992). In this chapter, we combined the CBCL–2/3 scales and the ASBI Disrupt scale into one *behavior problem composite* and the ASBI express and comply scales into a *cooperative behavior composite* after conducting factor analyses (see NICHD Early Child Care Research Network, 1998a, for details). The score from each scale was standardized and summed to form the composites.

Observed Compliance

At the end of the free-play period, the assistant handed the mother containers for the toys and instructed her to have the child help to pick up the toys; no other directions were given to mother. (Details may be found in NICHD Early Child Care Research Network, 1998a.) Child and mother behaviors were videotaped for the next 5 minutes or until all toys had been placed in the containers. The child's behavior was rated on 5-point global scales developed for this study (1 = "not at all characteristic" to 5 = "very characteristic"). Compliance, assertive noncompliance (reversed), passive noncompliance (reversed), and dyadic cooperation made up the composite score *observed compliance* used in these analyses.

Cognitive and Language Functioning

Cognitive performance was assessed with the school readiness composite from the Bracken Scale of Basic Concepts (Bracken, 1984), administered during the 36-month home visit. The school readiness composite contains 51 items designed to measure five aspects of children's knowledge: color recognition, letter identification, number/counting skills, comparisons, and shape recognition. The standard score ($M = 10$, $SD = 3$) was used in the analyses.

Reynell Developmental Language Scale

Children's language competence was assessed with the Reynell Developmental Language Scale (Reynell, 1991), administered during the 36-month laboratory visit. The scale is composed of 67 items and yields two scores, verbal comprehension and expressive language. The correlation between expressive language and verbal comprehension was .76. Percentile scores were used in the analyses.

To ensure that data on both the Bracken and the Reynell were collected in a consistent and reliable manner across all 10 sites, examiners collected data only after they met prespecified criteria for administering the tests.

RESULTS

Definition of Depression

Women were placed in the "never depressed" group if they scored below 16 on the CES-D at every assessment ($n = 663$ or 54.5%). Women who scored 16 or above at least once but fewer than four times were considered "sometimes depressed" ($n = 460$ or 37.9%). Women with elevated CES-D scores on four or five assessments were considered "chronically depressed" ($n = 92$ or 7.6%). Paired comparisons indicated that each group differed from the other two ($p < .001$) at each assessment.

Depression Group Comparisons on Socioeconomic and Social Support Variables

Women in the three depression groups differed from one another in educational level, $F(2,1212) = 38.77$, $p < .001$ [never depressed ($M = 14.9$); sometimes depressed ($M = 13.9$); chronically depressed women ($M = 13.0$)]. A similar pattern was evident in the income-to-needs ratio, which changed little over the 36 months (M's averaged over the 1–36-month period = 4.0; 2.8; 1.9, $F(2,1210) = 41.09$, $p < .001$. The groups also differed with respect to the presence of a partner in the household at 1 month (never = 93%; sometimes

= 81%; chronic = 72%, $\chi^2(2)$ = 57.30, p < .001). These figures had changed only slightly by 36 months: 91%, 75%, and 67%. A linear relationship was found between depression group and plans to stay at home (never = 32%; sometimes = 44%; chronic = 52%, $\chi^2(2)$ = 19.88, p < .001). The three depression groups also differed in perceived social support, $F(1,4702)$ = 69.5, p < .001.

Overview of Analysis Strategy for Mother–Child Interaction

This set of analyses examined maternal and child behavior during the structured interaction at 6, 15, 24, and 36 months. A longitudinal Poisson regression analysis was conducted using the general estimating equations (GEE) approach (Liang & Zeger, 1986). Because of positive skewness in the data, the measures of maternal sensitivity and child positive and negative affect were subjected to log transformations.

The GEE analyses tested the extent to which the maternal and child variables from the mother–child interaction sessions over time varied as a function of maternal depression group and selected child and maternal characteristics. The group growth curve model included site as a fixed-effects control variable; child sex and birth order, maternal depression group, and maternal education as between-subjects fixed-effects predictors; and the presence of a partner in the household, maternal employment status (full time, part time, not working), income-to-needs ratio, and social support as time-varying fixed-effects predictors. The initial model included main effects for each of these seven predictors and interactions between maternal depression group and each other predictor. Nonsignificant interactions were omitted from the model iteratively to reduce the collinearity among the predictors. Interactions were included to test the moderating effects of socioeconomic risk factors and social support on the association between chronicity of depression symptoms and mother–child interaction.

Longitudinal Analyses of Mother–Child Interactions

Maternal Sensitivity

Mothers in the three depression groups showed different patterns of sensitivity in play with their children across the first 3 years, after adjusting for the other variables in the model. There were both significant differences among the three groups in terms of their overall level of sensitivity, $F(2,3439)$ = 12.12, p < .001, and patterns of change over time, $F(6,3439)$ = 2.42, p < .05. The group of women who were never in the clinical range on the CES-D tended to be more sensitive in interactions with their children than mothers in the other two groups. Women who showed chronically elevated CES-D scores demonstrated a different pattern of change over time than women in the other two groups; specifically, they showed more decline in sensitivity during the child's second year and some recovery at 3 years.

In addition, analyses indicated that income-to-needs moderated these associations, $F(2,3439) = 11.51$, $p < .001$. Pairwise comparisons indicate that income is more strongly related to sensitivity among the mothers reporting elevated symptoms of depression than among the mothers who never reported being depressed. Women who reported depressive symptoms and had low income-to-needs ratios were less sensitive than their more financially comfortable counterparts, and this was especially so for the women reporting chronic symptoms of depression.

Child Positive and Negative Mood

Children in the three maternal depression groups did not show different patterns of change over time in the amount of positive or negative mood displayed in structured interactions with their mothers. Neither the mean level averaged over time nor the patterns of those means over time were significantly different among the three groups, with demographic variables controlled. Income-to-needs, however, interacted with maternal depression group, $F(2,3439) = 3.60$, $p < .05$ in that child positive mood was more strongly related to income among children whose mothers reported being chronically depressed than among children in the other two groups. Table 10.2 presents means and standard deviations for mother–child interaction variables averaged across age.

TABLE 10.2. Means and Standard Deviations of Mother–Child Interaction and Child Outcomes by Maternal Depression Group

	Never		Sometimes		Chronic	
Variable	M	(SD)	M	(SD)	M	(SD)
Mother–child interaction						
Maternal sensitivity[a]	9.65	(1.08)	9.08	(1.30)	8.59	(1.30)
Child positive[a]	2.65	(.37)	2.62	(.37)	2.48	(.38)
Child negative[a]	1.40	(.40)	1.45	(.43)	1.53	(.48)
Child outcomes						
School readiness	9.51	(2.67)	8.55	(3.07)	7.95	(2.77)
Expressive language	98.61	(13.68)	95.79	(15.03)	89.68	(15.63)
Verbal comprehension	100.56	(14.83)	95.37	(16.49)	90.86	(15.42)
Compliance (observed)	0.06	(3.30)	−0.02	(3.23)	−0.03	(3.00)
Cooperation (reported)	0.37	(1.56)	−0.30	(1.74)	−1.19	(1.94)
Behavior problems (reported)	−1.09	(3.13)	0.93	(3.85)	3.24	(4.01)

Note. Means are unadjusted. School readiness refers to the school readiness composite from the Bracken Basic Concepts Scale; expressive language and verbal comprehension are subscales of the Reynell Developmental Language Scale.
[a]averaged across 6, 15, 24, and 36 months.

Child Outcomes at 36 Months

The final analyses examined the extent to which children in the three maternal depression groups differed on selected cognitive and social outcomes at 36 months. Analyses of covariance were conducted on each of the child outcomes. Table 10.2 presents descriptive statistics for child outcome measures as a function of maternal depression group.

In a first analysis, after controlling for site, child sex and birth order, and maternal educational level, children in the three maternal depression groups differed on five out of six child outcomes at 36 months: Bracken school readiness scores, $F(2, 1134) = 6.02$, $p < .01$; expressive language, $F(2, 1105) = 6.25$, $p < .01$; and verbal comprehension, $F(2, 1132) = 7.38$, $p < .001$; on the Reynell, and maternal reports of problem behavior, $F(2, 1150) = 64.63$, $p < .001$; and cooperation, $F(2, 1150) = 30.63$, $p < .001$. Groups did not differ on observed compliance in the laboratory. Pairwise comparisons were conducted and effect sizes ($d = [M_1 - M_2]/SD$) estimated as the difference between adjusted means divided by the estimated pooled standard deviation (root mean squared error) from that analysis.

These comparisons indicated that children of mothers who reported feeling depressed chronically or sometimes had significantly, albeit modestly, lower school readiness ($d = .25$ and $d = .21$, respectively) and verbal comprehension scores ($d = .35$ and $d = .20$, respectively) than did children whose mothers never reported feeling depressed. In addition, children whose mothers reported feeling chronically depressed had lower expressive language scores than did children whose mothers never ($d = .43$) or sometimes ($d = .33$) reported depressive symptoms. Maternal reports of problem behavior and cooperation differed among the three groups. Women who reported being chronically depressed rated their children as less cooperative ($d = .46$) and more problematic ($d = .62$) than women who reported depression some of the time who, in turn, rated their children as less cooperative ($d = .34$) and more problematic ($d = .52$) than did women who never reported feeling depressed. Compared with the women in the chronic group, the women in the never depressed group rated their children as displaying substantially more cooperative behaviors ($d = .81$) and fewer behavior problems ($d = 1.14$).

A second model added maternal sensitivity to test the hypothesis that maternal sensitivity mediated the observed depression group differences. Maternal sensitivity was a strong predictor of all six child outcomes at 36 months, over and above covariates and maternal depression symptoms (including observed compliance in the laboratory which had not varied with maternal depression group). Higher sensitivity was related to higher scores on measures of school readiness, $F(1,1133) = 71.27$, $p < 001$; expressive language, $F(1,1104) = 41.54$, $p < .001$; verbal comprehension, $F(1,1131) = 132.83$, $p < .001$; observed compliance in the laboratory, $F(1,1127) = 5.49$, $p < .01$; and to maternal reports of more cooperation, $F(1,1149) = 39.34$, $p <$

.001, and fewer behavior problems, $F(1,1149) = 4.65$, $p < .05$. Maternal sensitivity appears to mediate the effects of maternal depression group on school readiness, expressive language, and verbal comprehension. Once maternal sensitivity was added to the model, differences among the depression groups were no longer significant. The evidence for mediation was modest, however, accounting for less than 1% of the variance. The third model tested whether the magnitude of the association between maternal sensitivity and child outcomes varied by maternal depression group. Main effects for depression group paralleled the findings from Model 1 in regard to expressive language, and maternal reports of cooperation and behavior problems (see Table 10.2). In addition, maternal sensitivity interacted with maternal depression group in analyses of expressive language, $F(2,1102) = 4.18$, $p < .05$, and maternal reports of cooperative behavior, $F(2,1147) = 5.06$, $p < .01$. Maternal sensitivity was more strongly related to expressive language scores among children whose mothers reported feeling depressed some of the time than among children whose mothers never reported feeling depressed; maternal sensitivity was also more strongly related to ratings of compliance in both groups of depressed mothers. In general, when mothers were less sensitive and also reported feeling depressed their children had poorer expressive language and were rated as less cooperative.

DISCUSSION

We examined the impact of maternal reports of chronic depression and co-occurring risk factors on mother–child interaction and child functioning. Our data provide partial support for our explanatory model, highlighting associations between maternal depressive symptoms and other risk factors as well as differences in maternal sensitivity as a function of the chronicity of symptoms. We also found several associations between maternal reports of more chronic depressive symptoms and child outcomes, and consistent with the model, some of these were mediated by maternal sensitivity. Mothers who reported more symptoms of depression but who were still highly sensitive to their children buffered them from some of the potentially negative effects of depressive symptoms, whereas the combination of a mother who reported feeling depressed and who was also insensitive during play provided additional risk with respect to some cognitive and social outcomes.

Consistent with our model and with the results of prior studies of maternal depression (e.g., Campbell, Cohn, & Meyers, 1995; Teti, 2000), maternal sensitivity during play varied as a function of whether a woman reported elevated symptoms of depression consistently over the 36 months of the study, only some of the time, or never. In general, women who never reported feeling depressed were the most sensitive with their babies. Women who reported feeling chronically depressed were not only the least sensitive but also the only group to show a systematic decline in sensitivity between the 15-month and 24-month assessments, although their level of sensitivity increased again at 36 months.

The decline in sensitivity at 24 months among the chronically symptomatic mothers is of particular interest, not only because it demonstrates differences in both levels of sensitivity and patterns of sensitivity over time in the chronic group but because it may implicate developmental changes in children's behavior as contributing to these changes in maternal sensitivity. The 24-month visit is likely to coincide with marked developmental changes (from 15 months) in toddlers' mobility, verbal ability, and bids for autonomy, making even relatively undemanding play interactions more challenging for some mothers than they were at earlier ages when children were more compliant and less mobile, and at 36 months when autonomy bids may be less intense (Belsky, Woodworth, & Crnic, 1996; Crockenberg & Litman, 1990). It is well documented that child negativity peaks at about 24 months (Belsky et al., 1996; Kopp, 1989).

Family income acted as a moderator of the effects of depressive symptoms. Women with higher income-to-needs ratios who also reported chronic symptoms of depression were more sensitive at each assessment than were chronically symptomatic women with lower incomes, who tended to be the least sensitive. Conger, Conger, and Elder (1997) have reported that ongoing financial strains often lead to negative moods which, in turn, influence interactions in the family, including less skillful childrearing. McLoyd (1990) has also implicated financial need as one determinant of parental adjustment, with poor parental adjustment associated with less adept parenting. These data from studies primarily of school-age children and adolescents, appear to have applicability to infants and toddlers as well. Even though the women reporting chronic symptoms were the least sensitive, children's positive and negative mood during mother–child play did not vary systematically as a function of maternal reports of depression, once demographic covariates were controlled. Mirroring the interaction between financial resources and depression group for maternal sensitivity, however, children whose mothers reported more chronic depression and higher financial resources were more positive than were children of mothers with fewer financial resources who reported more chronic symptoms. In contrast to child mood in the mother–child interaction, the scores for child outcomes varied as a function of maternal depression group. In general, children whose mothers were never depressed did best on cognitive and linguistic measures and children whose mothers reported being depressed did more poorly. There also was a linear relation between maternal reports of cooperation and problem behavior and chronicity of self-reported depression.

Maternal sensitivity over the 6-to 36-month period was a particularly powerful predictor of children's development. As expected, maternal sensitivity accounted for some of the effects of depressive symptoms, in line with a mediational model. However, these effects were small, suggesting that feelings of depression and lack of sensitivity are both important in under-standing the results.

Children whose mothers reported being depressed some of the time performed better on a measure of expressive language when they had more sensitive mothers. Thus, for these children, maternal sensitivity appeared to compensate somewhat for maternal self-reported depression, possibly because more sensitive mothers talk more to their young children and encourage conversation. Similarly, more sensitive mothers in the two depression groups rated their children as showing more cooperation than did mothers who reported depression and were also less sensitive. Thus, maternal sensitivity in these women reporting elevated depressive symptoms appeared to reflect a positive mother–child relationship despite the presence of depressive symptoms, leading to more positive perceptions of child behavior and to better language development at 36 months.

11

—

The Interaction of Child Care and Family Risk in Relation to Child Development at 24 and 36 Months

NICHD Early Child Care Research Network

The role of extrafamilial contexts in compensating for, or contributing to, family risk in relation to child development has been of great interest for some time. Child care experiences have been examined in relation to both their potential benefits for children at high risk (Campbell & Ramey, 1994; Lazar, Darlington, Murray, Royce, & Snipper, 1982) and their possible harm for children who are either at low or high risk (Belsky, 1988, 1990b; Hojat, 1990; Leach, 1994; White, 1985). Available data provide evidence of the benefits of high-quality child care for children with risk factors (Burchinal, Campbell, Bryant, Wasik, & Ramey, 1997; Currie & Thomas, 1995; Peisner-Feinberg & Burchinal, 1997), while evidence also suggests that participation in child care can be detrimental for children without family or child risk (Greenstein, 1993), or that poor-quality child care might amplify other risks (Belsky, Woodworth, & Crnic, 1996; Burchinal, Peisner-Feinberg, Bryant, & Clifford, 2000; Howes, 1990; National Institute of Child Health and Human Development [NICHD] Early Child Care Research Network, 1996). However, these data are limited because of the absence of studies focusing on different types of risk in large and diverse samples.

We predicted that children from families at higher risk would have poorer developmental outcomes at 24 and 36 months of age than would children from families at lower risk. Further, we hypothesized that family

From *Applied Developmental Science*, 2002, Vol. 6, pp. 144–156. Copyright 2002 by Lawrence Erlbaum Associates. Reprinted by permission.

risk would interact with child care experiences to produce dual-risk, compensatory, and lost-resources effects. Specifically, (1) children with dual family and child care risks (i.e., low quality care or extensive hours in care) were expected to be especially vulnerable to poor developmental outcomes, (2) high-quality child care was expected to compensate for the effects of high family risk on children's development, and (3) low-quality child care and/or extensive hours in child care were expected to negatively affect the development of low-risk children.

METHOD

Participants

A detailed description of the participants can be found in Chapter 1. Of the original 1,364 participating children, 794 constituted the subsample for this study's analyses. Of these, 504 children were observed in nonmaternal care at both 24 and 36 months; 106 children were observed only at 24 months, and 184 children were observed only at 36 months. Children were included if they had been observed in nonmaternal care at either 24 or 36 months and had completed assessments of all the family risk factors and at least one 36-month outcome.

The reasons that children were not observed in nonmaternal care included caregiver refusal, child absence from child care, and recent changes in the child care setting (see NICHD Early Child Care Research Network, 1996).

Overview of Data Collection Procedure and Measures

Data for this report were collected from the time the child was 1 month of age through 36 months of age. When the child was 1 month old, basic demographic information on the child and family was gathered and mothers completed questionnaires during a home visit. Data on child care usage were collected through phone calls conducted every 3 months, and through face-to-face contacts with mothers at 6, 15, 24, and 36 months. Observations of nonmaternal child care and interviews with caregivers were conducted when children were 24 and 36 months of age. Data were gathered in the home on children's social–emotional and cognitive development, mother's psychological functioning, and mother–child interaction when children were 24 and 36 months of age.

Family Risk Variables

During the home interview, mothers reported on their own *ethnicity* (collected at 1 month), *education* (collected at 1 month) (reversed), and presence or absence of a *partner in the home* (collected at 24 and 36 months). Family income information was obtained during maternal interviews at 24 and 36 months. An *income-to-needs ratio* (reversed), an index of family economic resources, was computed at 24 and 36 months. It was calculated from U.S. Census Bureau tables as the ratio of family income to the appropriate poverty threshold for each household size and number of children under 18, with higher scores indicating greater financial resources in the household.

Maternal depressive symptoms were assessed at 24 and 36 months, using the Center for Epidemiological Studies–Depression (CES-D) scale (Radloff, 1977), a self-report measure designed to assess depressive symptomatology in the general population. Cronbach's alpha coefficients ranged from .88 to .91 in the present sample.

Social support (assessed at 24 and 36 months) (reversed) was measured using the 11-item Relationships with Other People questionnaire (Marshall & Barnett, 1991), in which the mother rated support over the past month. The measure was designed to assess the individual's general perception of the availability of social support. Cronbach's alphas indicated high internal consistency (over .90) at each time point.

Financial stress was measured at 24 and 36 months, using questions developed specifically for this study. This three-item self-report instrument assessed mothers' satisfaction with their financial situation, worry about financial matters, and predictability of income, using 5-point Likert scales. Internal consistency estimates ranged from alpha = .67 to .69 in the present study.

Marital quality (reversed) was assessed using the six-item Intimacy subscale of the Personal Assessment of Intimacy in Relationships (PAIR) inventory (Schaefer & Olson, 1981) which was completed during the 1- and 36-month home interviews with the mother. The subscale scores (based on an average of the six responses; Cronbach's alphas = .80 and .86 for 1 and 36 months, respectively) were standardized and reverse-coded such that higher scores indicated more risk.

Parenting stress was assessed with mothers at 24 and 36 months, using the 20-item Parenting Experiences Questionnaire (Marshall & Barnett, 1991). Internal consistency was high, with Cronbach's alpha = .79 for both 24 and 36 months.

Mother's personality aggregate (reversed), assessed at 6 months only, is a composite variable computed as the mean of three subscales taken from the Neuroticism Extraversion Openness (NEO) Personality Inventory (Costa & McRae, 1985): maternal neuroticism (reversed), maternal extraversion, and maternal agreeableness. The composite had moderate internal consistency (alpha = .63).

Child Care Variables

Amount of care was assessed as the average number of hours in nonmaternal care per week determined for the following age epochs: 4–6 months, 7–15 months, 16–24 months, 25–36 months. The latter two time points were utilized in the current analyses and are referred to as hours in care at 24 and 36 months.

Quality of care was assessed during two half-day visits to the child's primary nonmaternal care setting at 24 and 36 months. Only settings in which children spent 10 or more hours per week were observed. The quality-of-care measures used in the present analyses were obtained using the Observational Record of the Caregiving Environment (ORCE), a live observational instrument designed specifically for this study, to assess the caregiving received by the individual child (see Chapters 3 and 5). The composite variable for quality was generated at 24 months by computing the mean of five qualitative ratings (1 = not at all characteristic to 4 = highly characteristic) made at the end of each observation cycle: sensitivity/responsiveness to child's nondistress expressions; positive regard; stimulation of cognitive development; detachment (reversed); and flat affect (reversed) (see NICHD Early Child Care Research Network, 1996). At 36 months, two additional categories, fostering exploration and intrusiveness (reversed) were added to the composite. Note that this quality composite reflects an emphasis on child-centered, as opposed to adult-centered, care. Cronbach's alphas for the composite were .86 and .82 at 24 and 36 months, respectively. Inter observer reliability estimates (Pearson correlations) for the quality composite were .81, .80 (videotapes), and .89, .90 (live) at each age.

Child Outcomes

Behavior Problems

Both mother and caregiver reports of total child behavior problems (24 and 36 months) were taken from the Child Behavior Checklist–2/3 (CBCL; Achenbach, Edelbrock, & Howell, 1987). The total behavior problem scores from the 99-item CBCL–2/3 included externalizing (aggressive and destructive behavior), internalizing (social withdrawal and depression), sleep problems and somatic problems.

Prosocial Behavior

Both mother and caregiver reports of prosocial behavior (24 and 36 months) were calculated as the mean of the express and comply subscales of the Adaptive Social Behavior Inventory (ASBI; Hogan, Scott, & Bauer, 1992). In the current sample the 24/36-month coefficient alphas for these scales completed by mothers were .77/.76 for express, and .82/.82 for comply; and .82/.84 and .84/.87 for those completed by caregivers.

Reynell Developmental Language Scale

The Reynell Developmental Language Scale (RDLS; Reynell, 1991) was administered by an experimenter during the laboratory session at 36 months of age. The RDLS comprises two 67-item scales and yields two scores, verbal comprehension (receptive) and expressive language. The Verbal Comprehension scale was used, and the internal consistency was .93.

RESULTS

The analysis plan involved two steps. First, factor analyses of the risk variables were conducted. Second, analyses predicting child outcomes as a function of risk, child care, and interactions between risk and child care were conducted.

Factor Analyses

Principal component factor analyses with varimax rotation were performed to reduce the number of potential risk indicators for use in the substantive analyses and to identify empirically dimensions or types of risk. Risk variables at 24 and 36 months of age included income-to-needs ratio (reversed), maternal depressive symptoms, social support (reversed), financial stress, parenting stress, the maternal personality aggregate assessed at 6 months (reversed), marital quality (reversed), mother's education at 1 month (reversed), single-parent status, and maternal ethnicity (0 = European American, 1 = minority). The data for individuals with missing data (e.g., nonpartnered mothers who did not complete the measure of marital quality) could not be included in these factor analyses. When composites were computed based on these factor analyses, these individuals were included (see next paragraph).

The first of three factors, psychosocial risk, had high loadings for maternal depressive symptoms, lack of social support, parenting stress, the maternal personality aggregate, and low marital quality. The second factor, socioeconomic risk, had high loadings for income-to-needs (reversed), financial stress, and mother's education (reversed), with high scores indicating low income and low educational levels. The third factor had high loadings for single-parent status and minority status and was labeled sociocultural risk. At both time points, these three risk factors were moderately intercorrelated. The average intercorrelation between any two risk factors was .30, and the highest correlation was .37 (between psychosocial and socioeconomic risk at 24 months).

Factor-based risk scores were computed for all subjects based on these factor solutions. Using a loading of .40 as a cutoff for inclusion in the computation of scores, only one cross-loading was found. Financial stress loaded on psychosocial risk (.43) and socioeconomic risk (.51) in the 36-month solution. This variable was assigned to the socioeconomic risk composite, given its conceptual relation to other variables with high loadings on this factor. For individuals with missing data, such as nonpartnered mothers without a marital quality measure, the computation of psychosocial risk was based on an average of the other four risk variables in that composite.

Risk, Child Care, and Child Outcomes

Regression analyses examined the extent to which family risk and child care experiences were related to child outcomes at 24 and 36 months of age, and tested whether child care experiences moderated the relations between psychosocial risk and outcomes. The analysis models in these analyses included site, family risk, child care interactions, and interactions between family risk and child care experiences. The family risk block included the three factor scores labeled psychosocial risk, socioeconomic risk and socio-cultural risk. The child care block included the average hours of child care and the quality of care. Two blocks of interactions were included: child care hours × the three family risk variables and child care quality × the three family risk variables. Data collection site was included as a covariate. Effect sizes were computed when predictors were significantly related to outcomes.

Two types of analyses were conducted. A multiple regression analysis was used to examine predictors of receptive language that was assessed only at 36 months. The analysis model included site and blocks representing family risk, child care, and risk × child care. Repeated-measures mixed-model analyses were used to examine predictors of maternal and caregiver report of behavior problems and prosocial behaviors, collected at both 24 and 36 months. These analysis models added age and interactions between age and the other blocks of variables to the model listed above.

Effect sizes were computed based on Cohen's (1988) recommendations. Effect sizes were computed separately for the results from 24 and 36 months because there is not an overall R^2 in mixed-model analyses that includes more than one random variable.

Results from analysis of maternal report of behavior problems, shown in the first column of Table 11.1, indicate two blocks of variables adding significant increments of explained variance. The block of risk factors showed both a significant main effect ($F[3,481] = 44.16$, $p < .001$) and a significant interaction with time ($F[3,481] = 3.67$, $p < .01$). The Psychosocial Risk factor was the only risk factor significantly associated with maternal report of behavior problems. Overall, mothers who scored higher on the Psychosocial Risk factor (beta = 8.72, $p < .001$) tended to report more behavior problems when their children were both 24 and 36 months of age. Although a significant predictor at both ages, the magnitude of this association was even stronger when children were 36 months of age (beta = 9.88, $p < .001$) than at 24 months of age (beta = 7.56, $p < .001$). Thus there was a significant risk × age interaction. The associated effect size at 36 months, $f^2 = .19$, indicated a moderate association, but at 24 months, $f^2 = .05$ indicated a more modest association. The block of child care variables did not contribute significantly to this model as main effects or in interactions with age or risk factors.

The second column in Table 11.1 shows the results from the analysis of the caregiver's report of behavior problems. Two blocks of variables were significant: the block of family risk variables ($F[3, 376] = 5.60$, $p = .0009$),

TABLE 11.1. Results of Regression of 24- and 36-Month Outcomes on Risk and Child Care Predictors

	Behavior problems				Prosocial behavior					
	Mother-reported		Caregiver-reported		Mother-reported		Caregiver-reported		Language	
	β	SE	β	SE	β	SE	β	SE	β	SE
Risk	44.16***		5.60*		32.42***		2.97*		39.08***	
Psychosocial	8.72***	.87	2.00	1.24	−.11***	.01	−.02	.02	.35	.93
Socioeconomic	1.29	.86	2.82*	1.19	−0.02	.01	−.01	.02	−7.66***	.93
Sociocultural	.30	.87	.88	1.17	−0.01	.01	−.04*	.02	3.07**	.96
Child care	1.42		4.20*		2.34		13.83***		11.63***	
Quality	−.66	.40	−1.33*	.58	.01*	.01	.05***	.01	2.60***	.54
Hours	.10	.55	1.33	.82	−.02E-1	.01	.02	.01	−.02	.64
Risk × care quality	.88		1.20		3.71*		.29		.88	
Psysoc. × qual	.24	.59	.74	.87	.02	.01	.03E-1	.01	−.32	.80
Soceco. × qual.	−.87	.56	−1.47	.81	−.01	.01	−.01	.01	1.06	.71
Soccul. × qual.	.58	.60	.74	.84	.02*	.01	−.01	.01	.14	.77
Risk × care hours	1.21		.76		.14		.48		.38	
Psysoc. × hr.	−1.45	.88	1.40	1.36	.01	.01	−.01	.02	−.55	1.03
Soceco. × hr.	1.23	.85	−1.18	1.24	−.01	.01	−.01	.02	.88	1.03
Soccul. × hr.	.02	.75	1.06	1.09	.01E-1	.01	.01	.02	.25	.94
Age	−.38	.36	−.02	.66	.04***	.01	.03**	.01	—	
Risk × age	3.67*		1.54		1.12		2.24		—	
Psysoc. × age	1.16**	.43	−1.18	.72	−.01	.01	.03*	.01		
Soceco. × age	.14	.40	1.18	.67	−.00	.01	−.02	.01		
Soccul. × age	−.92*	.43	−.36	.70	−.01	.01	.01E-1	.01		
Child care × age	2.79		.66		1.97		.59		—	
Quality × age	.16	.32	−.45	.51	−.00	.01	−.01	.01		
Hours × age	.95*	.40	−.58	.71	−.01*	.01	.03E-1	.01		

Note. Values, in the first row of each block, are *F* statistics. All other table entries are parameter estimates with standard errors. Individual parameter estimates were interpreted only if the block test was significant.
* *p* < .05; ** *p* < .01; *** *p* < .001.

and the block of child care variables ($F[2, 376]$ = 4.20, *p* = .016). Caregiver report of more behavior problems was associated with higher socioeconomic risk (beta = 2.82, *p* = .018). This was a small association (f^2 = .01). In addition, caregivers reported fewer behavior problems when child care quality was higher (beta = 1.33, *p* = .022). The associated effect size, f^2 = .01, suggests a small association between child care quality and caregiver report of behavior problems.

Next, we analyzed the mother's report of prosocial behaviors. Prosocial behaviors were significantly related to the block of risk variables ($F[3, 482]$ = 32.42, *p* < .001) and the block of interactions between risk and child care quality (F[3, 482] = 3.71, p=.011). Psychosocial Risk was the only risk variable with a significant main effect, with an associated effect size of f^2 = .09. Mothers who reported more psychosocial risk described their children as displaying fewer prosocial behaviors. Though not showing a main effect, Sociocultural Risk also interacted with child care quality (f^2 = .008). Mother's prosocial behavior ratings were not related to Sociocultural Risk when child care quality was higher but were negatively related to Sociocultural Risk when quality was lower.

The caregivers' reports of prosocial behaviors showed a different pattern of associations with family risk and child care experiences (Table 11.1). The caregivers' reports of prosocial behaviors were significantly related to blocks of risk variables (F[3, 374] = 2.97, p = .032) and child care variables (F[2, 374] = 13.83, p < .001). Caregivers rated children as having fewer prosocial behaviors if their families had higher scores on the Sociocultural Risk variable (f^2 = .02). Children in higher-quality child care settings were rated as showing more prosocial behaviors than children in lower-quality child care settings (f^2 = .02). In addition, caregivers reported more prosocial behaviors at 36 months than at 24 months (a time main effect, beta = .77, p = .01).

The final analysis examined children's receptive language at 36 months, and results are shown in the fifth column in Table 11.1. Receptive language scores were related to both the family risk (F[3, 648] = 39.08, p < .001) and child care blocks (F [2, 648] = 11.63, p < .001). Higher language scores were predicted by lower socioeconomic risk (f^2 = .13), less sociocultural risk (f^2 = .02), and higher child care quality (f^2 = .05). The risk × child care interactions were not significant.

To determine the relative contributions of maternal ethnicity and partner status in the sociocultural risk composite, we conducted additional analyses. We replaced the risk composite variable in the longitudinal regression analyses with maternal ethnicity (1 = nonminority or 0 = minority) and partner status (1 = partnered or 0 = not partnered), and then examined the associated coefficients when the sociocultural risk factor was significant. When children with lower sociocultural risk were rated by caregivers as having significantly more prosocial behaviors, neither partner status (beta = .07, p = .097) nor mother's ethnicity (beta = .04, p = .26) were significantly related to caregiver report of prosocial behavior. The association between higher language scores and less sociocultural risk was more differential, with mother's ethnicity significantly related to language (beta = 7.96, p < .001), and partner status unrelated (beta = −.26, p = .89). Nonminority children scored higher on language measures than did minority children.

Next, we decomposed the one significant interaction involving sociocultural risk, the interaction between sociocultural risk and child care quality. The follow-up analyses showed that both the interaction of child care quality and ethnicity (beta = −.030, p = .08) and the interaction of child care quality and partner status (beta = −.030, p = .11) predicted mother's prosocial behavior ratings, but nonsignificantly.

DISCUSSION

Although interactions between child care and types of family risk were the primary and motivating focus of this inquiry, main effects of family risk and child care quality were the predominant findings. Family psychosocial risk was associated with more behavior problems and fewer prosocial behaviors as reported by mother. In contrast, 36-month vocabulary skills were predicted by both socioeconomic and sociocultural risks. This finding is consistent with previously reported NICHD study results (NICHD Early Child Care Research Network, 2000b) and with the research on the effects of socioeconomic resources (Lee & Burchinal, 1987; Sameroff, Seifer, Baldwin, & Baldwin, 1993) on children's intellectual development. The socioemotional results parallel the findings of Sameroff and Seifer (1983); they also support Amato and Ochiltree's (1986) contention that distinguishing types of risk may be important in examining environmental influences on children's outcomes. The examination of the relative contribution of ethnicity and partner status in predicting language showed that maternal ethnicity was more strongly associated with receptive language than partner status, such that higher language scores were associated with nonminority status.

Limited evidence was found to suggest child care experiences moderate the negative associations between family risk and child outcomes. Family risk interacted with child care quality in only one of the five analyses and did not interact with child care quantity in any of the analyses. One interaction of the dual-risk type was found. Specifically, sociocultural risk × child care quality predicted mother-reported prosocial behavior. This finding indicated that higher sociocultural risk was associated with less prosocial behavior when children were in low-quality, but not average or high-quality child care.

It was also expected that high-quality, stable child care would buffer some of the negative influences on outcomes typically found among children from high-risk environments. This study provided no evidence that high-quality care served such a compensatory function for children experiencing risk conditions. Similarly, none of our findings supported the suggestion that children from low-risk family environments might be susceptible to the adverse effects of extensive or low-quality child care. It should be noted that we tested the full, continuous interaction in the whole sample rather than between extreme groups.

Limitations of the current study's sample may have contributed to the lack of significant effects. By design, the selected sample excluded mothers who were at risk because of drug addiction, adolescent birth, and living in unsafe neighborhoods. Moreover, as mentioned previously, the study sample and the recruited sample differed in several significant ways (e.g., the study sample had higher education and income). These differences and the sampling plan probably contributed to an underrepresentation of families with many risk conditions and could have influenced our findings.

In addition, the lack of "lost resource" findings for children from low-risk family environments could be due, in part, to the fact that very few low-risk children were in low-quality child care settings. Similarly, the relatively small number of high-risk children in high-quality care could have contributed to the lack of significant compensatory effects of that care.

In addition to these sampling considerations, alternative interpretations of our findings need to be stated. The fact that mother-reported socioemotional outcomes were associated with mother-reported family psychosocial risk may have less to do with the child's behavior than with the mother's own psychological well-being and perceptions. This interpretation is strengthened by the fact that caregiver reported socioemotional outcomes were not related to family risk. Similarly, caregiver reports of child prosocial behavior were related to observed child care quality, but this relation could be due to a reporter bias—perhaps high-quality caregivers have more positive views toward the children in their care. It also could be that children behave differently in different settings, so mothers' reports more accurately portray children's behavior at home, and caregivers' reports reflect children's behavior in child care. The findings for verbal skills, however, are not subject to reporter bias and are not setting dependent and reiterate the conclusion of other reports that both family and child care environments contribute to the child's cognitive development.

IV

Child Care and Health

Among investigations in early childhood education that were published in the 1930s are several showing that rates of communicable illness in children attending nursery schools are lower than those in matched control cases. This evidence was used to argue that enrollment in group programs does not necessarily result in greater risk of illness for children than staying at home. But many of these nursery school programs had trained nurses on staff who could avert the spread of common communicable illness by examining the children at the beginning of each session and preventing contact with other children, when children became sick. In other instances, teachers received special training that enabled them to be effective screening agents, producing the same results.

The current world of child care ordinarily does not afford such intensive preventive health care as that found in laboratory nursery schools. Although health care criteria—in both provider training and everyday practice—are prominent in state and local child care licensing regulations, health care practice actually varies widely across various types of child care. The child care medical literature preceding the National Institute of Child Health and Human Development (NICHD) Study of Early Child Care includes numerous publications showing that children in child care experience more bouts of respiratory illness, otitis media, and diarrhea than do children reared exclusively at home. However, most of the earlier studies were cross-sectional, examined a single category of illness, focused on only one or two types of child care arrangements, and/or did not control for family or community factors known to be related to the illness. Neither did most of these studies address the relation between elevated rates of illness and children's cognitive, language, and social development (the exception were studies of otitis media and its relation to language development).

The NICHD Study of Early Child Care investigators sought to determine whether the findings in the medical literature would replicate in a large longitudinal study that permits controlling for family factors, that includes data about children in different types of child care arrangements, and that affords the possibility of studying the effects of illness on psychological functioning. In two published papers, both abridged for this section, the investigators show that contemporary rates of communicable diseases are greater among children enrolled in child care during the first 2 years of life than among those who are not, the difference lessening at 3 years but increasing again between 3 and 4½ years. The increase in rate of illness in the first 2 years of life bears little relation to other aspects of children's development except, perhaps, for a small increase in behavior problems. Children who were enrolled in child care with more than six other children experienced more bouts of upper respiratory tract illness between the ages of 3 and 4½. However, those who were enrolled in large-group care between 2 and 3 were somewhat *less* likely to become ill when attending child care after the age of 3 than those who were first enrolled in group care after that age, suggesting possible immunizing effects of early child care.

12

Child Care and
Common Communicable Illnesses

NICHD EARLY CHILD CARE RESEARCH NETWORK

Children who attend child care arrangements, especially those enrolled in child care centers, are exposed more often to common communicable illnesses (e.g., Louhiala, Jaakkola, Ruotsalainen, & Jaakkola, 1997; Paradise et al., 1997). The explanations most commonly offered for increased rates of illness among children in child care point to elevated levels of exposure to pathogens carried by other children in child care settings. The most vulnerable time for transmitted infections is immediately after entry into a new child care arrangement (Churchill & Pickering, 1997; Reves et al., 1993). Studies of upper and lower respiratory tract infections also point to increased exposure to other children (and the viruses they carry) as the primary risk factor for elevated rates of illness among children in child care settings (Anderson et al., 1988; Collier & Henderson, 1997; Ponka, Nurmi, Salminen, & Nykyri, 1991).

To our knowledge, there have been few prospective studies of communicable illness in children in relation to the many types of child care arrangements children now attend. Most studies have been cross-sectional, have examined only a single category of illness, have focused on only one or two types of child care arrangements, and have failed to control for other family and community factors known to be related to illness. A critical issue yet unresolved is whether the elevated rate of illness associated with child care is related to children's cognitive, language, and social development.

We reexamine associations between child care and common childhood infections, using data from approximately 1,200 children living in 10 different sites in the United States who are participating in the National Institute of Child Health and Human Development (NICHD) Study of Early Child Care (NICHD Early Child Care Research Network, 1997c). We investigate three key issues concerning the relationship between child care arrangements and three common childhood infections: enteric tract illness (GI), upper respiratory tract infection (URI), and ear infections or otitis media (OM). This study addresses (1) the pattern of these three common illnesses during the first 3 years of life for children in different types of nonmaternal care; (2) possible effects of child care experiences on the frequency of illnesses; and (3) the possible effect on later development in such areas as language, achievement, and social behavior. We hypothesize that rates of illness will be higher for children who have contact with large numbers of other children in child care. We also hypothesize that these increased rates of illness will not negatively affect other areas of children's development.

METHOD

Participants

For a detailed description of the sample participants, see Chapter 1.

Procedures

We obtained information from the mother about the parents, the child and child care arrangements using face-to-face interviews when the child was 1, 6, 15, 24, and 36 months of age and from telephone interviews done when the child was 3, 9, 12, 18, 21, 27, 30, and 33 months of age. All participating children were assessed at the study site in terms of their developmental outcomes at 15, 24, and 36 months of age.

Measures

Family Background and Child Characteristics

Four pieces of demographic information were used: mother's level of education, family size, presence of the father or another adult partner in the home, and family income (the income-to-needs ratio) (U.S. Department of Labor Women's Bureau, 1994). Child characteristics included ethnicity and sex. The Home Observation for Measurement of the Environment (HOME) Inventory was administered during a home visit when the child was 15 months of age (infant–toddler version); the early childhood version, at 36 months. HOME assesses the quantity and quality of stimulation and support available to the child in the home environment (Caldwell & Bradley, 1984).

Child Illness Histories

During the interviews held every 3 months, mothers were asked: "Since the last interview, has [child] had an ear infection? . . . a respiratory illness? . . . a gastrointestinal illness?"

Child Care Experiences

Child care information includes (1) type of care (center care, a child care home, care by a relative, or care in the child's own home by a nonrelative); (2) the total number of other children in all the child's nonmaternal care arrangements during a particular 3-month interval; (3) stability of care (the number of child care arrangements started during each 3-month interval); and (4) hours in care (how many hours the child spent on average each week in all forms of child care).

Child Developmental and Behavioral Outcomes

Children 3 years of age were assessed with the Bracken Basic Concept Scales (BBCS) and the Reynell Developmental Language Scales (RDLS). The BBCS (Bracken, 1984) is designed to assess a child's knowledge of basic concepts necessary for school readiness. The RDLS (Reynell, 1991) is composed of two 67-item scales: verbal comprehension and expressive language. When the children were 3 years of age, mothers completed the 99-item Child Behavior Checklist (CBCL; Achenbach, Edelbrock, & Howell, 1987). For the children in nonmaternal care, child care providers also completed the CBCL when the children were 3 years of age.

RESULTS

Statistical Analyses

To determine whether the prevalence of each illness varied throughout time and whether the illness varied as a function of background characteristics, family circumstances, and child care experiences, longitudinal logistic regression analyses were conducted using the generalized estimating equation approach (Liang & Zeger, 1986). To adjust for the dependency in the data caused by repeated measures, separate intercepts were estimated for each child. Time-invariant predictors (between-subject variables) included site, mother's education, ethnicity, and sex. Time-varying predictors included several measures of family, child, or child care experiences that were obtained at each of the 12 assessment points. These include child's age, child's age squared, type of interview (telephone or in-person), whether mother had a spouse or other adult partner present in the household, household size, average hours of all forms of child care during that 3-month assessment, whether the child changed child care arrangements during that period, whether the child attended a child care center during that period, whether the child attended a child care home during that period, whether the child was cared for by the father or grandparents or in the child's own home during that period, and the total number of children and adults summed across the various arrangements. The other two time-varying predictors were income (for children ages 1, 6, 15, 24, and 36 months) and HOME scores (children ages 15 and 36 months). Logistic regression models also included several interaction terms: age × each child care variable, and age × household size.

A multiple regression analysis was used to determine the relationship between child care experiences and rates of illness during the first 3 years of life and the child's developmental status at age 3 years. For each illness, a series of five regression analyses was run, one for each of the five 3-year child outcomes: Bracken school readiness, Reynell verbal comprehension, Reynell expressive language, CBCL externalizing problems, and CBCL internalizing problems. Each regression model included background, family, and child care factors as predictors. The time-invariant predictors included site, mother's education, ethnicity, and sex. The time-varying predictors were represented by the mean score for each family on each measure. Similarly, child care hours was represented as the average number of hours a child spent in all types of nonmaternal child care per week from birth through 3 years based on all 12 data collection points. There were three types of child care variables: (1) number of assessment periods the child was in center care; (2) number of periods the child was in a child care home; and (3) number of periods the child was cared for by relatives or at home by nonrelatives.

To determine whether a child's history of illness in child care affects the relation between experiences in care and developmental outcomes, we conducted a second series of regression analyses. Specifically, we added several statistical interaction terms involving the proportion of time a child had a particular illness and each child care experience factor.

Rates of Illness

Longitudinal logistic regression analyses indicated that the incidence of ear infections rises in the first year of life and peaks by age 1 year, then gradually declines during the next 2 years. Respiratory tract illness follows the same basic pattern, although the decline after age 1 year is much less pronounced. The rate of GI also rises in the first year of life, followed by a slow decline.

Child Care Experience and Illness History

Table 12.1 displays results from the longitudinal logistic regression analyses of each illness.

Hours per Week in Care

With two marginal exceptions, the number of hours per week children spent in child care had little to do with their likelihood of contracting a communicable illness. For OM, hours per week in care during the first year of life was related to the likelihood of acquiring the illness. For GI, hours per week during the third year of life increased the likelihood of contracting the illness.

Changes in Child Care Settings

Starting a new child care arrangement during an assessment period was associated with lower rates of OM and URI.

Number of Children in Child Care

The number of children present in nonmaternal child care arrangements was related to the frequency of URIs. The number of children was a significant predictor of both GIs and URIs. However, because the type of child care arrangement was controlled in the analysis, the findings may offer conservative estimates of the effect of number of children present in child care on the probability of acquiring an illness. Children in center care were exposed to an average of 10.3 other children at age 3 months, and 16.4 children at age 36 months. This contrasts with the average number of other children present in a child care home (2.3 children at age 3 months, and 3.8 children at age 36 months).

Type of Care

Compared with children in exclusive maternal care, those attending child care centers and family child care homes were more likely to acquire OM and URI. When examining rates of OM in these two settings, the effect of attending child care arrangements on rates of OM was much more pronounced during the child's first and second years of life than during the

**TABLE 12.1.   Results of Longitudinal Logistic Regression Analyses
for Otitis Media, Gastrointestinal Illness, and Respiratory Illness**

Model	Ear infections	Gastrointestinal illness	Upper respiratory tract illness
Child age	0.72 (0.65, 0.81)	1.16 (1.04, 1.30)	0.85 (0.76, 0.95)
Age squared[a]	0.64 (0.60, 0.68)	0.79 (0.75, 0.84)	0.80 (0.75, 0.84)
Background characteristics[b]			
Maternal education	0.98 (0.92, 1.05)	1.01 (0.95, 1.08)	1.01 (0.95, 1.07)
income-to-needs	1.07 (1.01, 1.13)	0.99 (0.92, 1.05)	0.99 (0.94, 1.05)
Father/partner present	0.85 (0.71, 1.01)	0.95 (0.80, 1.12)	0.98 (0.84, 1.14)
HOME inventory	1.06 (1.00, 1.13)	0.99 (0.94, 1.05)	1.03 (0.98, 1.08)
Household size			
12 mo	1.04 (0.98, 1.11)	0.94 (0.88, 1.00)	1.05 (0.99, 1.10)
24 mo	1.02 (0.96, 1.08)	0.98 (0.93, 1.04)	0.98 (0.93, 1.04)
36 mo	0.99 (0.90, 1.09)	1.03 (0.94, 1.13)	0.92 (0.85, 1.01)
Sex	1.15 (1.03, 1.29)	1.02 (0.92, 1.14)	1.02 (0.92, 1.12)
Ethnicity			
Hispanic vs. white	0.97 (0.76, 1.24)	0.94 (0.73, 1.21)	0.98 (0.78, 1.22)
Black vs. white	0.75 (0.60, 0.94)	0.62 (0.50, 0.77)	0.93 (0.77, 1.12)
Other vs. white	0.64 (0.48, 0.85)	0.71 (0.56, 0.91)	0.96 (0.76, 1.22)
Child care experiences			
Hours in child care			
12 mo	1.08 (1.01, 1.15)	1.04 (0.97, 1.11)	1.01 (0.95, 1.07)
24 mo	1.03 (0.97, 1.09)	0.96 (0.90, 1.01)	0.99 (0.94, 1.05)
36 mo	0.98 (0.88, 1.09)	0.88 (0.81, 0.97)	0.98 (0.90, 1.06)
Changes in child care	0.90 (0.82, 0.98)	0.98 (0.90, 1.07)	0.88 (0.81, 0.95)
Child care center			
12 mo	2.37 (1.81, 3.10)	1.15 (0.86, 1.53)	1.92 (1.44, 2.57)
24 mo	1.70 (1.37, 2.12)	1.04 (0.85, 1.27)	1.62 (1.31, 2.00)
36 mo	1.22 (0.86, 1.74)	0.95 (0.70, 1.29)	1.36 (0.99, 1.88)
Child care home			
12 mo	1.28 (1.09, 1.50)	1.05 (0.89, 1.25)	1.42 (1.20, 1.67)
24 mo	1.07 (0.93, 1.25)	1.05 (0.91, 1.21)	1.26 (1.09, 1.45)
36 mo	0.90 (0.70, 1.16)	1.05 (0.83, 1.31)	1.11 (0.89, 1.38)
Relative/in-home care			
12 mo	0.99 (0.88, 1.12)	0.94 (0.83, 1.07)	0.94 (0.83, 1.06)
24 mo	0.99 (0.88, 1.12)	1.06 (0.95, 1.19)	1.01 (0.91, 1.12)
36 mo	1.00 (0.82, 1.21)	1.20 (1.01, 1.43)	1.09 (0.93, 1.28)
Child care size			
12 mo	1.05 (0.95, 1.17)	1.09 (0.97, 1.22)	1.25 (1.09, 1.42)
24 mo	1.06 (0.98, 1.14)	1.10 (1.02, 1.18)	1.22 (1.12, 1.32)
36 mo	1.06 (0.95, 1.19)	1.11 (1.01, 1.21)	1.19 (1.06, 1.33)

Note. All values are represented as odds ratios (95% confidence limits). HOME indicates the total score from the Home Observation for Measurement of the Environment. Changes in child care indicates a new child care arrangement during a period (0 = no, 1 = yes). Relative/in-home care indicates care by a relative or by someone other than the child's parents in the child's home.
[a]Age squared is the quadratic term to examine curvilinear relationships.
[b]For ethnicity, White = 0; and Hispanic, African American, or other = 1; for sex, female = 0 and male = 1.

third year. Results showed higher rates of OM in center care during the first year of life followed by a gradual decline, so that by age 3 years, the rate among children in the four types of care were no longer different. The pattern for URI was similar, but the findings were not quite as strong. Results also showed that when children were being cared for by a relative, the risk of GI was lower in the first year of life but higher in the third year of life.

As Table 12.1 presents, we also computed the relative odds (odds of illness if the child was in particular type of care divided by the odds of illness if the child was not in that type of care) for the three illnesses at three ages: 12, 24, and 36 months. For OM, the odds ratio associated with center care at age 12 months was 2.37, but that declined to 1.22 by age 36 months (children in center care were more than twice as likely as home-reared children to contract an ear infection at age 1 year, but only 22% more likely by age 3 years). Likewise, for URI, the odds ratio associated with center care was 1.92 at 12 months, declining to 1.36 at 36 months. For GI, none of the odds ratios was greater than 1.20.

Illness and Child Developmental Outcomes

The final issue addressed by this study was whether the increased illness rate of children in child care settings is associated with poorer developmental and behavioral outcomes at age 36 months. Results from the 15 regression analyses run on the whole sample (three illness categories × five outcome variables) provide no evidence of an association between the frequency of acquiring a communicable illness and either language competence (not significant) or school readiness (not significant). By contrast, children who experienced higher rates of URI (beta = 2.64, SE = 0.81, p < .001) and GI (beta = 4.64, SE = 0.81. p < .001) were described by their mothers as having a modestly higher rate of internalizing problems. Similarly, children who experienced higher rates of OM (beta = 3.11, SE = 1.13, p < .006), URI (beta = 4.73, SE = 1.14, p < .001), and GI (beta = 6.04, SE = 1.15, p < .001) were reported by their mothers as developing slightly more externalizing problems. For children in child care, we reran the analyses using teacher reports of behavior problems. Results showed no relationship between children's rates of illness and teacher reports of behavior problems. The difference in results, depending on whether mothers or teachers reported on behavior problems, may reflect a common reporter bias on the part of mothers, as mothers were the only reporters on childhood illness.

There was little evidence that child care factors interact with illness histories to affect the course of a child's development. The only significant interaction involved mother-reported internalizing problems (hours in child care × the illness rate for URI); even this interaction was not significant when the child care provider's report of internalizing problems was analyzed.

DISCUSSION

Results of this longitudinal study confirm findings from cross-sectional studies with respect to the prevalence of ear infections, GI illnesses, and upper respiratory illnesses (Hoffman, Overpeck, & Hildesheim, 1996; National Center for Health Statistics, 1991). The likelihood of children acquiring common communicable illnesses during infancy is related to the type of child care they receive and to the number of other children in that care environment. This confirms findings from other studies of diarrheal illnesses (e.g., Churchill & Pickering, 1997) and OM (e.g., Collier & Henderson, 1997).

In contrast to reports stating that the likelihood of acquiring communicable illnesses increases with the amount of time spent in child care (Kotch & Bryant, 1990), we found little evidence that the number of hours of care per week resulted in increased illness rates for any of the three diseases examined. This finding, which contradicts results from some earlier studies, may have emerged because most of the children in this study spent more than 20 hours per week on average in nonmaternal care throughout the first 3 years of life. That is, most were in care for a sufficient amount of time to permit exposure to the other children in the setting.

Rates of infection for each illness studied rose during the first year of life, peaked in the second year, and then gradually declined. These data suggest that spending time in nonmaternal care may accelerate immunological responses to the pathogens that cause these illnesses. Although this study does not provide specific evidence of increased resistance to communicable illnesses by age 3 years because of early entry into child care, it may be that the children with more extensive early child care experience will show lower rates of communicable illnesses during kindergarten and first grade than children with no prior child care experience (Kramer, Wjst, & Wichman, 1999). Results clearly point to increased contagion as the primary reason for the frequency of each of the illnesses studied. Exposure to other children in nonmaternal child care arrangements increases the likelihood of contracting communicable illnesses, especially during infancy

When analyses were done within specific types of child care arrangements, the number of children present was significant only for URI and only for child care homes and care by relatives. This suggests that the pathogens connected to GI are so common and so virulent that exposure to even a very small number of other children is sufficient to increase the probability of contracting GI illnesses. The fact that the number of children present within each type of child care arrangement was not a factor associated with the rate of ear infections suggests that the number of children typically found in child care homes and relative care is too low to make a difference, and that the number of children typically found in child care centers is higher than the threshold (in effect, more in the range of 8–10 children). For children in child care, the number of children present in the child care arrangement seems to contribute less to the risk of GI infection with time. Although our results showed several small relationships between rates of illness and behavior problems, the absence of significant interaction effects between amount and type of child care and illness histories on child outcomes indicates that the effect of child care experience per se on infection is largely unrelated to children's behavior, to their language development, or to their school readiness. In effect, for children who attend child care there is little evidence that having a greater number of common communicable illnesses such as URI, GI, and OM during infancy significantly alters the normal progression of behavioral development.

Some caution should be exercised in applying the results from this study to children from high-risk families. The exclusion criteria used to select families for the study, coupled with slightly higher rates of participation among children from high socioeconomic backgrounds, limits the generalizability of the findings. Previous studies (Phillips, Voran, Kisker, Howes, & Whitebook, 1994) have shown that children from low socioeconomic status families are more likely to receive lower-quality child care and child care that is more sporadic, factors that may increase their risk of exposure to communicable illnesses.

13

Child Care and Common Communicable Illnesses in Children Ages 37–54 Months

NICHD Early Child Care Research Network

It is increasingly common for children older than 3 years to attend preschool programs, including children who have never been cared for outside the home as well as those who have been cared for only in informal, small-group settings (Shonkoff & Phillips, 2000). Relatively little is known about the illness histories of children who enter large-group care for the first time after age 3 years. Likewise, little is known about whether children who have had experience in large-group care prior to age 3 years may be at reduced risk for illness during the preschool years as a result of previous exposure to pathogens connected with respiratory tract and enteric illnesses (Ball, Holberg, Aldous, Martinez, & Wright, 2002).

Children who have never been in large-group care prior to age 3 years may be at increased risk of illness as they encounter elevated levels of exposure to pathogens carried by other children in child care settings (Churchill & Pickering, 1997). By comparison, children with previous experience in large-group care may have developed increased immunity to such pathogens, thus providing some resistance to exposure (Collier & Henderson, 1997). However, because there are so many serotypes of different viruses

From *Archives of Pediatrics and Adolescent Medicine*, 2003, Vol. 157, pp. 196–200. Copyright 2003 by the American Medical Association. Reprinted by permission. All rights reserved.

connected to the common cold, it is unclear whether exposure prior to age 3 years is sufficient to offset the level of exposure experienced by preschool children in large-group care. Findings from the few studies available are mixed, with some showing higher rates of illness among children newly entering care and some showing no difference (Ball et al., 2002; Nafstad, Hagen, Magnus, & Jaakkola, 1999).

In earlier reports (i.e., Chapter 12 of this volume), the National Institute of Child Health and Human Development (NICHD) Study of Early Child Care (NICHD Early Child Care Research Network, 2001a) suggested that children who entered child care during infancy had higher rates of gastrointestinal tract, upper respiratory tract, and ear infections during the first 3 years of life. In this chapter, we reexamine associations between attendance at child care and the same three common infections for children ages 37 to 54 months, a period when many children enter formal preschool programs but before nearly all go to kindergarten. Our data were obtained from approximately 1,100 children at 10 different data collection sites across the United States who were participating in the NICHD Study of Early Child Care.

We hypothesized, based on our previous study and results from other studies, that rates of respiratory tract, gastrointestinal tract, and ear infections would be higher for children who had contact with many other children in preschool or child care. This study extends the previous literature by examining these issues in a single prospective investigation involving a diverse sample of children from a variety of locations who were recruited at birth and who have experienced a full array of child care arrangements. The study also addresses the question whether children acquire some protection against infection as a result of prior experience in large-group care. Because the risk of infection appears to be a more direct function of the number of people to whom one is exposed rather than the type of care received, our study divides child care arrangements by size (> 6 vs. 6) rather than type (e.g., center care vs. child care homes) (Ball et al., 2002; Churchill & Pickering, 1997; Collier & Henderson, 1997; U.S. Department of Labor, Women's Bureau, 1994). Although any cutoff is arbitrary, the number 6 was selected for two reasons: (1) many states require that child care arrangements be licensed if more than 6 children are served in a setting, and (2) evidence shows that the risk of infections such as those examined does not rise steeply once the number of children in a setting exceeds six to eight (Collier & Henderson, 1997; NICHD Early Child Care Research network, 2001a; Paradise et al., 1997).

METHOD

Participants

A description of the study sample appears in Chapter 1 of this volume.

Procedure

We obtained information about parents and children using face-to-face interviews with the mother when the child was 1, 6, 15, 24, 37, and 54 months old and from telephone interviews done when the child was 3, 9, 12, 18, 21, 27, 30, 33, 42, 46, and 50 months old. We obtained information about the family context, changes in child care arrangements, the number of children in the child care arrangement, the amount of time the child spent in child care, and the child's health status and illnesses. The entire data collection protocol was reviewed by a steering committee supervised by the NICHD and was reviewed annually by the institutional review boards of the 10 participating institutions responsible for data collection.

Measures

Family Background and Child Characteristics

Four pieces of demographic information about families were used: mother's level of education, family size, presence of the father or another adult partner in the home, and family income (the income-to-needs ratio) (U.S. Department of Labor, Women's Bureau, 1994). Child characteristics included ethnicity and sex. Ethnicity was included as a factor in the statistical models to control for reporter bias. Previous studies, including the National Health and Nutrition Examination Survey II, have shown a tendency on the part of African American mothers to underreport common illnesses (Hoffman, Overpeck, & Hildesheim, 1996; NICHD Early Child Care Research Network, 2001a). The early childhood version of the Home Observation for Measurement of the Environment (HOME) Inventory (Caldwell & Bradley, 1984) was administered during home visits when the child was 6, 15, 37, and 54 months old. The HOME assesses the quantity and quality of stimulation and support available to the child in the home environment.

Child Illness Histories

During the face-to-face and telephone interviews, mothers were asked if the child had had at least one instance of an ear infection, respiratory tract illness, or gastrointestinal tract illness since the last interview.

Child Care Experiences

Child care information included total number of other children in all of the child's nonmaternal care arrangements during a particular data collection interval and hours in care (how many hours on average the child spent each week in all forms of child care).

RESULTS

Statistical Analyses

The focus of this study was on illnesses occurring between the ages of 37 and 54 months. To determine whether the prevalence of each illness varied across time and whether the illness varied as a function of background characteristics, family circumstances, and child care experiences, longitudinal logistic regression analyses were conducted using the generalized estimating equation approach (Liang & Zeger, 1986). Separate intercepts were estimated for each child. This approach adjusts for dependency in the data by using repeated measures. Time-invariant predictors (between-subject variables) included site, mother's level of education, ethnicity, sex, family income-to-needs ratio averaged from the 6- and 54-month assessments, total number of hours in child care from birth to 36 months, whether the child was in care with 6 or more other children (large-group care) during the first year of life (birth to age 12 months), whether the child was in large-group care during the second year of life (13–24 months), and whether the child was in large-group care during the third year of life (25–36 months). Site was used as a predictor to help control for heterogeneity in findings resulting from the use of 10 different locations for data collection. Time-varying predictors included several measures of family, child, or child care experiences that were obtained at each of the 4 assessment points (37–42 months, 43–46 months, 47–50 months, and 51–54 months). These included the child's age, child's age squared, presence of a spouse or other adult partner in the household, household size, average number of hours in all forms of child care during the target assessment interval, interaction between hours in care from birth to 36 months and hours in care during the target assessment period, and whether the child was in a child care arrangement with at least six other children during the target assessment period. Season (i.e., the proportion of months during an assessment interval that occurred during the winter flu season) was also used as a time-varying predictor. For the 37- to 42-month, 43- to 46-month, and 47- to 50-month assessment periods, the HOME measure was based on the mean HOME score from the 6-, 15-, and 37-month administrations of the HOME Inventory (first the scores were standardized, and then the mean was calculated). For the 51- to 54-month assessment period, the HOME measure was based on the mean HOME score from the 6-, 15-, 37-, and 54-month administrations of that instrument.

Table 13.1 indicates results from the longitudinal logistic regression analyses of each illness for the whole sample. It displays odds ratios with accompanying 95% confidence intervals for each aspect of child care experience examined, controlling for the family background and child characteristics described previously.

As expected, during the winter flu season, children were more likely to have each of the three illnesses examined (about 15% more likely to have

TABLE 13.1. Odds Ratios and 95% Confidence Intervals from Longitudinal Logistic Regression Analyses for Ear Infections, Gastrointestinal Tract Illness, and Respiratory Tract Illness

Model	Ear infections	Gastrointestinal tract illness	Upper respiratory tract illness
Child age	0.99 (0.97–1.01)	1.01 (0.99–1.03)	0.99 (0.98–1.01)
Age squared	1.00 (1.00–1.00)	1.02 (1.01–1.02)*	1.01 (1.00–1.01)
Background			
Maternal education level	0.99 (0.93–1.06)	0.98 (0.93–1.04)	1.03 (0.97–1.08)
Income-to-needs ratio	1.01 (0.96–1.07)	0.99 (0.95–1.03)	1.01 (0.97–1.05)
Father/partner	1.27 (0.86–1.88)	1.10 (0.81–1.51)	1.03 (0.77–1.42)
HOME inventory	1.00 (0.80–1.24)	1.13 (0.95–1.35)	1.14 (0.96–1.36)
Household size	0.99 (0.88–1.13)	1.04 (0.94–1.14)	0.96 (0.87–1.06)
Sex	0.98 (0.78–1.25)	1.02 (0.85–1.24)	0.97 (0.80–1.18)
Ethnicity			
Hispanic vs. European American	1.11 (0.64–1.94)	0.68 (0.41–1.11)	0.95 (0.61–1.49)
African American vs. European American	0.47 (0.29–0.78)*	0.48 (0.31–0.74)*	0.93 (0.65–1.32)
Other vs. European American	0.71 (0.40–1.28)	0.66 (0.40–1.09)	1.29 (0.76–2.19)
Season	1.28 (1.21–1.34)*	1.15 (1.09–1.20)*	1.33 (1.26–1.40)*
Child care experiences			
Hours in child care before age 3 yr	1.04 (0.90–1.21)	0.96 (0.85–1.10)	0.93 (0.81–1.05)
Hours in child care, current	0.98 (0.85–1.13)	0.97 (0.85–1.11)	1.08 (0.96–1.22)
Hours in child care before 3yr × hours in child care, current	1.10 (0.88–1.15)	0.99 (0.87–1.12)	0.90 (0.80–1.00)
≥6 other children in child care			
Year 1	0.87 (0.58–1.31)	1.10 (0.74–1.37)	0.81 (0.59–1.09)
Year 2	1.10 (0.70–1.47)	0.95 (0.71–1.28)	1.06 (0.80–1.42)
Year 3	0.88 (0.66–1.19)	0.76 (0.60–0.98)*	0.66 (0.52–0.83)*
≥6 other children in current child care	1.52 (1.20–1.92)*	1.40 (1.14–1.72)*	2.19 (1.80–2.69)*

Note. Data are presented as odds ratios (95% confidence intervals) for children ages 37–54 months. HOME, Home Observation for Measurement of the Environment.
*Statistically significant ($p < .05$).

gastrointestinal tract illness and 33% more likely to have an upper respiratory tract infection). Neither the number of hours spent in child care prior to age 3 years nor the number of hours per week children spent in child care from ages 37 to 54 months bore a relationship to the likelihood of contracting a communicable illness. The only two child-related conditions that mattered were whether the child was in a care arrangement with at least six other children during the assessment period (36–54 months) and whether the child was in large-group care (i.e., care with six or more other children) between ages 25 and 36 months. Children concurrently in large-group care were 2.2 times as likely to have an upper respiratory tract illness as children reared at home or in small-group care. Likewise, they were about 1.6 times as likely to have an ear infection and approximately 1.4 times as likely to have a gastrointestinal tract illness. Experience in large-group care during the first 2 years of life was not protective against contracting an illness during the period examined in this study (ages 37–54 months). However, children who were in large-group care in the third year of life had about a 34% decrease in the likelihood of contracting an upper respiratory tract illness between ages 37 and 54 months and a 24% decrease in the likelihood of contracting a gastrointestinal tract illness.

Finally, some research on the effects of child care has focused on the number of siblings rather than overall household size. Accordingly, we reran all analyses substituting number of siblings for household size. The results were essentially the same. That finding was not surprising in view of the $r = .88$ correlation between household size and number of siblings in this sample.

DISCUSSION

Findings from the NICHD Study of Early Child Care provide evidence that children's experience in nonmaternal care relates to common childhood infections during the first 3 years of life, especially if the child is enrolled in large-group care (NICHD Early Child Care Research Network, 2001a). Findings from this extension of the study showed two things. First, children who were in group care with 6 or more other children ages 24–36 months were less likely to contract a gastrointestinal tract or upper respiratory tract illness between the ages of 37 and 54 months compared with children who entered large-group care for the first time after age 3 years. On the other hand, experience in large-group care during the first 2 years of life had no effect on the likelihood of contracting communicable illnesses during that period. Thus, the findings are inconclusive regarding whether experience in child care during infancy confers only a short-term benefit or whether the results that emerged between ages 37 and 54 months represent the earliest stages of more long-term immunity. Findings from the Tucson Children's Respiratory Study showed that children who entered large-group care in infancy had more colds than home-reared children at age 3 years but had fewer colds than these children by age 6 years (Ball et al., 2002).

Second, children who were in large-group care between ages 37 and 54 months were generally at increased risk of upper respiratory tract illnesses, gastrointestinal tract illnesses, and ear infections (particularly upper respiratory tract illnesses) compared with children reared at home or those who participated in small-group nonparental care. On average, children in large-group care during the preschool years were about twice as likely to have a respiratory tract illness, approximately 1.5 times as likely to have a reported ear infection, and about 1.4 times as likely to have a gastrointestinal tract illness. In sum, our study partially confirms the findings reported by Hurwitz, Bunn, Pinsky, & Shonberger (1991) and partially contradicts those reported by Nafstad and colleagues (1999).

In contrast to reports that the likelihood of acquiring communicable illnesses increases with the amount of time spent in child care (Thacker, Addiss, Goodman, Holloway, & Spencer, 1992), we found little evidence that hours of care per week increased illness rates for any of the three diseases examined. This finding, which contradicts the results from some earlier studies, may have emerged because most of the children in our study spent more than 25 hours per week in nonmaternal care after age 3 years. In effect, most children were in care longer than the threshold amount of time needed to contract most communicable illnesses.

V

Child Care
and Mother–Child Relations

At the heart of the long-standing controversy over child care is the concern of scholars and parents that nonmaternal care may undermine the relationship between mothers and their young children, a relationship that is believed by many to be the cornerstone of healthy psychological development in childhood and adolescence. Although nonmaternal child care has been used to supplement maternal care throughout human history, in recent years, use of early child care has been largely the consequence of economic and demographic forces enabling women to work to support their families rather than the result of a need to enhance children's welfare.

Some experts in the area of early development now hold the view that mothers who separate themselves from their children for prolonged stretches of time do not achieve optimal relationships with their offspring. Mothers may not have sufficient opportunities to learn to detect and interpret the nonverbal cues that the young child uses with its caretakers and thus are not able to respond to their children in the most appropriate way. In these situations, babies are believed to experience either overstimulating or understimulating interactions with their mothers. They may find it hard to engage in interactions that are harmonious and that promote enjoyment of their interaction and exploration of their physical surroundings. Other experts fear that mothers who do not provide a continuous maternal presence deprive their babies of the opportunity to grow to trust the availability and sensitivity of their mothers. These babies would be less likely to be securely attached to their mothers, a condition that would interfere with their socioemotional and cognitive development. Still other experts argue that daily exposure to multiple caretakers diffuses the infant's expectations and communications with adults, thereby interfering with effective social development. Nevertheless, a sizable body of expert opinion continues to support the broad use of nonmaternal care owing to the belief that negative

191

effects on mother–child relationships do not outweigh the benefits that maternal employment provides to families and to children. Specifically, in addition to the increase of material resources that maternal employment brings to the family and to the children in it, maternal time with children is not diminished as much as one would think. Mothers give up on their personal time and spend time with their children when they are not working. Moreover, fathers are more involved with childrearing when mothers are employed.

In this section, we examine the links between characteristics of child care (e.g., child care quality, quantity, and type) and social relations between children and their mothers. Mother–child relations were observed during episodes designed to assess the child's attachment to the mother and also during interactions in which mother and child had a variety of toys available.

The findings presented in Chapter 14 reveal that child care quality, quantity, age of entry, stability, and type of care do not predict attachment security or avoidance at 15 months of age when examined as main effects. These results show, however, that when maternal sensitivity was low, these variables did, indeed, predict attachment security: Infants are less likely to be securely attached when low maternal sensitivity/responsiveness is combined with poor-quality child care, more than minimal amounts of child care, or more than one care arrangement. When children were 36 months old, a similar pattern occurred. When maternal sensitivity was low, more hours of child care per week was associated with increased risk of insecure–ambivalent attachment. As at 15 months, the quantity, quality, or type of care by themselves did not predict the security of attachment when the children were 36 months of age.

When children spent more hours in child care their mothers were less sensitive and the children were less engaged with their mothers during videotaped play recorded over the first 3 years of life (see Chapter 17). Higher child care quality, however, was linked to greater maternal sensitivity. Follow-up analyses of the links between early child care and both maternal sensitivity and child engagement when the children were 3, 4½, and in first grade provide a somewhat more complex picture (see Chapter 18). For all children, however, the negative associations between hours spent in child care and maternal sensitivity diminished over time.

Finally, after researchers statistically controlled for mothers' childrearing beliefs, they found that mothers who engaged in more "partnership behaviors" with their child care providers were more supportive and sensitive with their children (Chapter 16).

Taken together, the findings show that extensive child care is associated with lower levels of maternal sensitivity. The link between child care and mother–child relations is not the same for all children, however, and its net effect (after controlling for other predictors) is smaller than that of family predictors.

14

The Effects of Infant Child Care on Infant–Mother Attachment Security

NICHD Early Child Care Research Network

The prospect that routine nonmaternal care in the first year of life might have an adverse effect on the security of the infant's attachment to mother has been a subject of much discussion and debate (Belsky & Steinberg, 1978; Fox & Fein, 1990; Karen, 1994; Rutter, 1981). Evidence linking institutional rearing in the early years of life with affective and cognitive deficits led to early concerns that the experience of maternal deprivation posed hazards for the emotional well-being of young children (Bowlby, 1973). Later, these same concerns were voiced about day care. Indeed, Barglow, Vaughn, & Molitor (1987) interpreted findings linking child care with elevated rates of insecure attachment, especially insecure–avoidant relationships, as evidence that babies experience daily separations as maternal rejection. Others drew attention to the possibility that nonmaternal care might affect proximal processes of mother–infant interaction and thus interfere with the infant–mother attachment relationship (Jaeger & Weinraub, 1990; Owen & Cox, 1988). Time away from baby, Brazelton (1985) argued, might undermine a mother's ability to respond sensitively to the child, which would itself reduce the probability that a secure relationship would develop, and Sroufe (1988) suggested that daily separations might both cause the infant to lose confidence in the availability and responsiveness of the parent and reduce the opportunities for "ongoing tuning of the emerging infant-caregiver interactive system" (p. 286).

From *Child Development*, 1997, Vol. 68, pp. 860–879. Reprinted with permission of the Society for Research in Child Development.

Irrespective of the mechanisms responsible, it is noteworthy that several multistudy analyses have documented statistically significant associations between routine nonmaternal care in the first year and elevated rates of insecure attachment as measured in the Ainsworth & Wittig (1969) Strange Situation (Belsky & Rovine, 1988; Clarke-Stewart, 1989; Lamb & Sternberg, 1990). Examining child care in context is important because even these multistudy analyses documenting elevated rates of insecurity among groups of infants with early and extensive child care experience do not suggest that insecurity in inevitable. It is also important to assess the validity of the Strange Situation classifications in the case of children experiencing routine child care because Clarke-Stewart (1989) has highlighted the possibility that the apparent elevated rates of insecurity might be a result of the fact that children who have experienced the multiple separations associated with child care are not especially stressed by the Strange Situation and thus this procedure may not be a valid measure of attachment for these children.

The aims of this investigation were fourfold: (1) to determine if attachment classifications made on the basis of Strange Situation behavior were equally valid for infants with and without extensive child care experience in the first year of life; (2) to identify differences in the probability of attachment security in infants with varying child care experience (in terms of quality, amount, age of entry, stability, and type of care); (3) to identify the combination of factors (mother/child and child care) under which child care experience was associated with increased or decreased rates of attachment security; and (4) to determine whether early child care experience was associated specifically with insecure–avoidant attachment.

METHOD

Participants

Chapter 1 describes recruitment of participants and the sociodemographic characteristics of the sample. Strange Situation data for 1,153 infants (84.5% of the 1,364 recruited) are included in the major analyses in this report. (The Strange Situation was administered to 1,201 dyads; 6 were uncodable due to technical errors; 42 cases were eventually excluded because they received an Unclassifiable "U" code.) Table 14.1 presents characteristics of these families. The 211 mother–infant dyads who did not contribute Strange Situation data were compared with the rest of the sample on seven variables measured when the infants were 1 month old. There were no differences between the two groups on income-to-needs ratio, maternal depression, and mother's or child's race (European American vs. non-European American). However, those who did not contribute Strange Situation data, compared with those who did, were more likely to have boys (61.7% vs. 50.6%, likelihood chi-square ratio = 5.74, $p < .02$), to be single

**TABLE 14.1. Sample Characteristics of
Participants Included in Attachment Analyses**

Characteristics	%
Child ethnicity	
European American, non-Hispanic	81.5
African American, non-Hispanic	11.9
Hispanic	5.7
Other	0.9
Child sex	
Girls	49.4
Boys	50.6
Maternal education	
< 12 years	8.4
High school or GED	20.2
Some college	34.2
BA	21.9
Postgraduate	15.3
Husband partner in the home	86.9
Child care plans at birth	
Full time	53
Part time	23
None	24

mothers (22.9% vs. 12.9%, likelihood chi square = 14.45, $p < .001$), and to have more positive attitudes about the benefits of maternal employment for children (20.0% vs. 19.1%, $F(1, 1279) = 10.19$, $p < .002$).

Overview of Data Collection

Visits to the families occurred when the infants were 1, 6, and 15 months old. Observations in child care arrangements were conducted when the infants were 6 and 15 months old. The Strange Situation assessment of infant attachment security (Ainsworth, Blehar, Waters, & Wall, 1978) was conducted in a laboratory playroom visit when the infants were 15 months old (± 1 month). Telephone interviews to update maternal employment and child care information were conducted when the infants were 3, 9, and 12 months old, and phone calls to update information on child care and to schedule the 6- and 15-month observations occurred when the infants were 5 and 14 months old.

At all home visits, mothers reported on a variety of factors, including household composition and family income. In addition, at the 1-month visit, mothers completed a modified Attitude toward Maternal Employment Questionnaire (Greenberger, Goldberg, Crawford, & Granger, 1988). At 6 months, they completed a modified Infant Temperament Questionnaire (ITQ; Carey & McDevitt, 1978), and selected scales of the Neuroticism Extraversion Openness (NEO) Personality Inventory (Costa & McCrae, 1985), and at 1, 6, and 15 months, the Center for Epidemiologic Studies–Depression (CES-D) scale (Radloff, 1977). At the 6- and 15-month home visits, mothers and infants were videotaped in a 15-minute semistructured play interaction adapted from a procedure used by Vandell (1979), and the home visitor completed the Infant/Toddler Home Observation for Measurement of the Environment (HOME) Inventory (HOME; Caldwell & Bradley, 1984).

Infants in child care at 6 and 15 months were observed for 2 half days in the child care arrangement in which they spent the most time, using the Observational Record of the Caregiving Environment (ORCE) developed for this project (see Chapters 3, 5, and 6).

Overview of Measures

Control Variables

Control variables included an income-to-needs ratio and a measure of the mother's beliefs about the benefits of maternal employment. The income-to-needs ratio is an index of family economic resources, with higher scores indicating greater financial resources per person in the household (see Chapter 7). This variable was averaged across the three assessments at 1, 6, and 15 months to create an overall average income-to-needs ratio. The beliefs about benefits of maternal employment measure was created by summing five 6-point items from the Attitude toward Maternal Employment Questionnaire administered at the 1-month visit (Greenberger et al., 1988). Cronbach's alpha was .80. Higher scores reflected the belief that maternal employment was beneficial for children.

Child and Family Measures

Composite variables were created from the mother and child measures.

A composite measure of the mother's psychological adjustment was created by summing the average of the three CES-D scores (reverse-scored) from the three ages plus scores on three scales of the NEO Personality Inventory: neuroticism (reverse-scored), extraversion, and agreeableness. Cronbach's alpha was .80.

Two composite measures of maternal sensitivity were included. The first was constructed on the basis of ratings of videotaped episodes of mother–child play at 6 and 15 months. A composite variable was created by summing the individual scales for sensitivity to nondistress, positive regard, and intrusiveness (reverse-scored). Cronbach's alphas were .75 and .70 for the 6- and 15-month composites, respectively. These two scores were averaged to create the overall sensitivity in play composite used in these analyses.

The second composite measure was constructed on the basis of data obtained from the Infant/Toddler HOME (Caldwell & Bradley, 1984). A composite score was computed by summing the positive involvement factor score (Cronbach's alphas = .52 at 6 months and .56 at 15 months) and the lack of negativity factor score (Cronbach's alphas = .50 at 6 months and .54 at 15 months). The 6- and 15-month scores were averaged to create the sensitivity in the HOME score used in these analyses (Cronbach's alphas = .60 and .64).

A measure of infant temperament based on 55 6-point items from the ITQ was administered at 6 months. The composite measure, difficult temperament, was created by calculating the mean of the nonmissing items, with appropriate reflection of items, so that numerically large scores consistently reflected a more "difficult" temperament. Cronbach's alpha was .81.

Child Care Variables

At 5 and 14 months, information about the child care setting was obtained. This information was used to classify the type of care of the arrangement observed at 6 and 15 months: mother (i.e., those children not in any regular child care), father, other relative, in-home nonrelative, child care home, and child care center. A composite measure of amount of care was created by computing the mean hours per week from the monthly care average from 4 through 15 months. Children who received no regular nonmaternal care through 15 months received scores of "0." On the basis of maternal reports, two additional measures were generated. One was age of entry into routine child care (1 = entered care at 0–3 months, 2 = entered care at 4–6 months, 3 = entered care at 7–15 months, 4 = children who had not entered care by 15 months when the Strange Situation procedure was conducted). The second was frequency of care starts, a measure of stability of care, which reflected the number of different arrangements the child experienced through 15 months.

Observations of the child care settings were conducted on 2 half days that were scheduled within a 2-week interval. During these sessions, observers scored child care quality using the ORCE (see Chapters 3, 5, and 6). ORCE observers recorded the occurrence of specific behaviors directed by the caregiver. These behaviors focused on positive caregiving and included the following: positive affect, positive physical contact, response to distress, response to vocalization, positive talk, asking questions, other talk, stimulation of cognitive or social development, facilitation of the infant's behavior. At each age a composite variable was created by summing standardized scores for these behavior scales.

ORCE observers also made qualitative ratings of the observed caregiving. A second composite was thus based on 4-point qualitative ratings of the same dimensions of caregiving behavior that were rated for the mothers in the structured play task with their infants. This composite also had good internal consistency (alphas of .89 at 6 months and .88 at 15 months).

Both positive frequency scores and qualitative ratings had adequate interobserver reliability with "gold standard" videotapes and with live reliability partners at 6 and 15 months (.86 to .98).

Attachment Security

The Strange Situation is a 25-minute procedure containing brief episodes of increasing stress for the infant, including two mother–infant separations and reunions. It is designed to elicit and measure infants' attachment behavior. Attachment behaviors may be categorized as secure (B) or insecure (A, C, D, or U; Main & Solomon, 1990). When stressed, secure (B) infants seek comfort from their mothers, which is effective and permits the infant to return to play. Avoidant (A) infants tend to show little overt distress and turn away from or ignore the mother on reunion. Resistant (C) infants are distressed and angry, but ambivalent about contact, which does not effectively comfort and allow the children to return to play. Examples of disorganized/disoriented (D) behaviors are prolonged stilling, rapid vacillation between approach and avoidance, sudden unexplained changes in affect, severe distress followed by avoidance, and expressions of fear or disorientation at the entrance of the mother. A case that cannot be assigned an A, B, C, or D classification is given the unclassifiable (U) code. The U classifications (3.5% of the sample) have been eliminated from the major analyses in this report.

The Strange Situation was administered according to standard procedures (Ainsworth et al., 1978) by research assistants who had been trained and certified according to a priori criteria to ensure that the assessments were of very high quality. These research assistants were trained so that the child's child care status was not discussed during the Strange Situation (so as not to bias coders). Videotapes of the Strange Situation episodes from all sites were shipped to a central location (different from the one responsible for coding mother–child interaction) and rated by a team of three coders who were blind to child care status. The three workers, all with a minimum of 4 years' previous experience coding Strange Situations from a variety of low- and high-risk samples, received additional training using master-coded tapes (including tapes coded by Mary Main), and intensive supervision continued during formal scoring to maintain expertise. Before beginning formal scoring, coders also passed the University of Minnesota Attachment Test Tapes for ABC classifications.

Distress during the three mother-absent episodes was rated with a 5-point scale for each episode. A rating of 1 reflected no overt distress and no attenuation of the child's exploration. A rating of 5 reflected immediate, high distress resulting in termination of the separation. These ratings were summed across episodes to create a total distress score, which could range from 3 to 15. Cronbach's alpha was .84.

The three coders double-coded 1,201 Strange Situation assessments. Disagreements were viewed by the group and discussed until a code was assigned by consensus. Across all coder pairs, before conferencing, agreement for the five-category classification system (ABCDU) was 83% (kappa = .69) and agreement for the two-category classification system (secure/insecure) was 86% (kappa = .70). Distress was coded by a single worker based on the written notes by all coders. A second worker coded 47 cases from the notes for reliability. Pearson correlations between the two ratings ranged from .93 for Episode 6 to .96 for Episode 7.

RESULTS

Assessing the Validity of the Strange Situation

The issue of the internal validity of the Strange Situation was addressed for children with routine separation experience by investigating two extreme groups of children: those with less than 10 hours of child care per week every month from 0 to 15 months ($n = 251$) and those with 30 or more hours per week in every month from 3 to 15 months ($n = 263$). One theoretical challenge to the validity of the Strange Situation for children with extensive child care would be if it were found that children with extensive child care showed less distress in the mother absent episodes of the Strange Situation than did the children with no child care.

Results of a 2 (high/low child care intensity) × 5 (attachment classification) analysis of variance (ANOVA) for the distress rating provided no support for the hypothesis that the Strange Situation was a less valid measure of attachment for children with extensive child care experience. The mean distress level of children in high-intensity child care was 6.5, and in low-intensity child care was 6.0. (For cell means, see NICHD Early Child Care Research Network, 1997b.)

Effects of Child Care on Attachment Security

Analysis Plan

Two parameterizations of attachment categories were selected: secure (B) versus insecure (A, C, and D), and secure (B) versus insecure–avoidant (A). The secure–insecure dependent variable afforded the testing of child care effects at the most global level of adaptive versus maladaptive child outcomes. The secure–avoidant dependent variable provided a means for testing the proposition that infant child care experiences were specifically related to the incidence of insecure–avoidant attachment.

Due to the categorical, binary nature of the dependent variables, logistic regression analyses were employed (with secure = 1 and insecure = 0, or avoidant = 0). In a series of analyses, the dependent variable (secure–insecure or secure–avoidant) was predicted from (1) one of five characteristics of the mother (psychological adjustment, sensitivity in play, sensitivity in the HOME) or the child (difficult temperament, sex), (2) one of five characteristics of child care (positive caregiving frequency, positive caregiving rat-ings, amount of care, age of entry, and frequency of care starts), and (3) the interaction between the two selected (mother/child and child care) vari-ables. Alpha was set at .05 for all analyses, rather than adjusting alpha for the number of analyses, because of a concern regarding Type II errors.

The order of entry of predictor variables was guided by our theoretical rationale and our major hypotheses. In each analysis, control variables reflective of selection effects (income-to-needs ratio, beliefs about the bene-fits of maternal employment) were entered into the regression equation first, and then the main effect of a mother or child characteristic was tested. The main effect of a child care variable was tested next, and then the inter-action between (i.e., the product of) the mother/child variable and the child care variable. When these two-way interactions proved significant, subse-quent analyses were undertaken to determine whether they could be clari-fied by considering selected additional child care predictors within the con-text of the two-way interaction.

After analyses of continuous child care variables were completed, atten-tion was turned to the categorical variable of type of child care. Chi-square analyses were performed to determine whether attachment security was related to type of care at 5 and at 14 months, and additional logistic regres-sion analyses were used to evaluate the effects of child care variables on attachment outcomes within types of care. Table 14.2 presents unadjusted descriptive statistics for predictor variables by attachment classification (ABCD).

Secure–Insecure Analyses

Tables 14.3 and 14.4 present results of the secure–insecure analyses. These tables show the association of attachment security with each mother and child predictor (top panel of Table 14.3), each child care predictor (bottom panel of Table 14.3), and each interaction term (Table 14.4). The Wald chi square for each variable indicates the effect of adding that variable follow-ing entry of prior variables; the odds ratio is the ratio of the probability that an event will occur to the probability that it will not (i.e., the closer to 1.00, the smaller the effect).

Among the five mother/child variables, two were significant predictors of attachment security: psychological adjustment and sensitivity in the HOME. As expected, mothers who exhibited greater sensitivity and respon-siveness toward their infants and mothers who had better psychological adjustment were more likely to have securely attached infants.

None of the five child care variables, entered after the mother/child variables, significantly predicted attachment security.

Of the 25 interaction terms included in the logistic regression analyses (Table 14.4), six were significant predictors of attachment security: (1) maternal sensitivity in play × positive caregiving ratings, (2) maternal sensi-

TABLE 14.2. Descriptive Statistics for Mother, Child, and Child Care Variables, by ABCD Classification

			Classification									
	A			B			C			D		
Predictor	n	M or %	(SD)	n	M or %	(SD)	n	M or %	(SD)	n	M or %	(SD)
Mother variables												
Psychological adjustment	156	-.44	(3.05)	700	.14	(2.76)	101	-.10	(3.05)	174	-.28	(2.86)
Sensitivity–play	161	-.25	(.56)	711	.06	(.79)	102	.21	(.78)	177	-.08	(.88)
Sensitivity–HOME	161	-.22	(.87)	710	.05	(.58)	102	.03	(.56)	177	-.02	(.58)
Child variables												
Temperament	157	3.16	(.44)	705	3.18	(.40)	101	3.16	(.38)	175	3.19	(.37)
Sex (%)												
Boys	94	16.12		352	60.38		58	9.95		79	13.55	
Girls	68	11.93		360	63.16		44	7.72		98	17.19	
Child care variables												
Positive caregiving frequency	111	-.20	(2.70)	422	-.01	(2.58)	53	.78	(2.43)	107	.30	(2.52)
Positive caregiving ratings	111	14.36	(2.84)	420	14.74	(2.59)	53	15.66	(2.70)	107	14.79	(2.67)
Amount of care (hr/week)	162	25.42	(18.06)	712	22.97	(18.33)	102	19.42	(17.27)	177	23.80	(18.02)
Age of entry[a]	162	1.84	(1.11)	712	1.85	(1.14)	102	1.80	(1.13)	177	1.83	(1.12)
Frequency of care starts	162	2.37	(1.91)	712	2.56	(2.01)	102	2.25	(1.82)	177	2.76	(2.13)
Type of care–5 months (%)												
Mother	47	11.24		259	61.96		40	9.57		72	17.22	
Father	20	15.04		79	59.40		17	12.78		17	12.78	
Other relative	38	21.23		106	59.22		11	6.15		24	13.41	
In-home nonrelative	9	10.00		56	62.22		8	8.89		17	18.89	
Child care home	31	14.69		137	64.93		15	7.11		28	13.27	
Child care center	11	10.78		67	65.69		9	8.82		15	14.71	
Type of care–14 months (%)												
Mother	44	13.10		204	60.71		36	10.71		52	15.48	
Father	27	16.17		103	61.68		10	5.99		27	16.17	
Other relative	28	17.61		89	55.97		14	8.81		28	17.61	
In-home nonrelative	14	13.86		60	59.41		12	11.88		15	14.85	
Child care home	34	14.47		147	62.55		18	7.66		36	15.32	
Child care center	11	7.97		97	70.29		11	7.97		19	13.77	

[a] 1 = 0–3 months, 2 = 4–6 months, 3 = 7–15 months, 4 = not entered in care by 15 months.

TABLE 14.3. Mother/Child and Child Care Predictors (Main Effects) of Secure (B) versus Insecure (A, C, D) Attachment

Predictor	n	Wald χ^2	Odds ratio
Mother/child variables			
Psychological adjustment	1,129	3.90[*]	1.05
Sensitivity–Play	1,149	2.82	1.14
Sensitivity–HOME	1,148	7.25[**]	1.32
Temperament	1,136	.26	1.08
Sex	1,151	.77	1.11
Child care variables			
Positive caregiving frequency	692	2.24	.96
Positive caregiving ratings	690	.64	.98
Amount of care	1,151	.06	1.00
Age of entry	1,151	.01	.99
Frequency of care starts	1,151	.82	1.03

Note. In all analyses, income-to-needs ratio and work beliefs were entered first as control variables. For ease of presentation, reported Wald chi-square values for child care predictors reflect the main effect of each variable on attachment security, following entry of control variables. In fact, child care variables were entered following control variables and mother/child variables, yielding nonsignificant results similar to those reported above.
[*]$p < .05$; [**]$p < .01$.

tivity in the HOME × positive caregiving ratings, (3) maternal sensitivity in play × positive caregiving frequency, (4) maternal sensitivity in the HOME × amount of care, (5) maternal sensitivity in play × care starts, and (6) child sex × amount of care. Although significant (see Wald chi squares), these interaction effects were relatively small (see odds ratios).

To explore the nature of the significant interactions in as simple a way as possible, categorical groupings were formed from the variables involved. For maternal sensitivity and quality-of-care variables, the continuous variables were transformed into categories reflecting low, moderate, and high sensitivity or quality. Participants who were in the highest quartile on any variable were in the "high" group, and participants in the lowest quartile were in the "low" group. The "moderate" group comprised participants in the middle 50% of the distribution. For amount of care, three categories were formed: full-time care (> 30 hours/week), part-time care (10–30 hours/week), and minimal or no care (10 hours/week). For care starts, the categories were 0, 1, and more than 1 start.

The significant maternal sensitivity × child care quality interactions indicate a consistent pattern related to low maternal sensitivity and low-quality child care. The lowest proportion of secure attachment was obtained when both maternal sensitivity and child care quality were low. For these three interactions, the proportions of secure children among those receiving low scores on both maternal sensitivity and positive caregiving were .44, .45, and .51; the mean proportion of secure attachment for the rest of the

TABLE 14.4. Child Care × Mother/Child Interactions Predicting Secure (B) versus Insecure (A, C, D) Attachment

Predictor	n	Wald χ^2	Odds ratio
Psychological adjustment × . . .			
Positive caregiving frequency	683	1.10	1.01
Positive caregiving ratings	681	.05	1.00
Amount of care	1,129	.14	1.00
Age of entry	1,129	2.67	1.03
Frequency of care starts	1,129	.06	1.00
Sensitivity–play × . . .			
Positive caregiving frequency	629	4.28*	.93
Positive caregiving ratings	690	3.92*	.93
Amount of care	1,149	.00	1.00
Age of entry	1,149	.05	.98
Frequency of care starts	1,149	3.88*	1.08
Sensitivity–HOME × . . .			
Positive caregiving frequency	692	.84	.95
Positive caregiving ratings	690	4.09*	.89
Amount of care	1,148	4.52*	1.01
Age of entry	1,148	1.34	.91
Frequency of care starts	1,148	1.97	1.07
Temperament × . . .			
Positive caregiving frequency	689	.12	1.03
Positive caregiving ratings	687	2.49	1.14
Amount of care	1,136	.36	1.00
Age of entry	1,136	.28	1.07
Frequency of care starts	1,136	.17	.97
Sex × . . .			
Positive caregiving frequency	692	.20	1.03
Positive caregiving ratings	690	.01	1.00
Amount of care	1,151	4.19*	1.01
Age of entry	1,151	.07	.97
Frequency of care starts	1,151	.71	1.05

Note. In all analyses, income-to-needs ratio and benefits of work were entered first as control variables, followed by the mother/child variable, then the child care variable, and then the interaction term. The main effects of the mother/child variables when all terms were included in the model were as follows: sensitivity–play, positive caregiving frequency analysis: Wald $\chi^2 = 2.97$, $p = .08$, odds ratio = 1.20; sensitivity–play, positive caregiving ratings analysis: Wald $\chi^2 = 5.12$, $p > .05$, odds ratio = 3.42; sensitivity–play, frequency of care starts analysis: Wald $\chi^2 = .24$, $p > .10$, odds ratio = .94; sensitivity–HOME, positive caregiving ratings analysis: Wald $\chi^2 = 6.25$, $p = .01$, odds ratio = 7.67; Sensitivity HOME, amount of care analysis: Wald $\chi^2 = .04$, $p > .10$, odds ratio = 1.03; sex, amount of care analysis: Wald $\chi^2 = 1.16$, $p > .10$, odds ratio = .81.
*$p < .05$.

children, collapsed across all the other cells, was .62. For purposes of this article, this and similar patterns will be referred to as "dual-risk" effects.

The dual-risk pattern was evident but less pronounced for the interactions between the mother's sensitivity in the HOME and the amount of care, and for the mother's sensitivity in play and the number of care starts.

A different pattern was evident for the sex × amount of care interaction. The proportion of security was lowest among boys in more than 30 hours of care per week and girls in less than 10 hours of care per week.

Some evidence was also found for a compensatory interaction pattern in relation to high-quality child care. The proportions of secure attachment for children with less sensitive and responsive mothers were higher if the children were in high-quality child care (.53, .63, .58) than if they were in low-quality child care (.44, .45, and .51), and a linear increase in security as child care quality increased was observed in two of the three analyses. However, a compensatory effect was not found for amount of child care. The less time children of less sensitive and responsive mothers spent in child care, the more likely they were to be securely attached.

A final pattern, one that was unanticipated, is that the proportions of secure attachment show that, for children in low-quality child care, security proportions were higher if the mother was highly sensitive (.73, .72, .69) than if she was insensitive (.44, .45, .51), whereas for children in high-quality child care, maternal sensitivity did not appear to be related to attachment security (proportions ranged from .53 to .63 regardless of maternal sensitivity).

Secure–Insecure Follow-Up Analyses

For the secure–insecure analyses yielding significant two-way interactions, we sought to determine whether consideration of additional child care conditions would further illuminate the dual-risk pattern of results. Although significant two-way interactions were obtained, we did not find evidence that these interactions were moderated by additional features of child care.

Secure–Avoidant Analyses

The set of logistic regression analyses used to predict secure–insecure attachment was repeated for secure–avoidant attachment. Two of the five mother/child predictors were significant: sensitivity in play, Wald $\chi^2(1, n = 871) = 7.16$, $p < .01$, odds ratio = 1.36, and sensitivity in the HOME, Wald $\chi^2(1, n = 870) = 10.54$, $p < .01$, odds ratio = 1.51. Infants whose mothers were more sensitive and responsive toward them were more likely to be securely attached than insecure–avoidant. Paralleling the results of the secure–insecure analyses, none of the five child care variables was significant as a main-effect predictor of secure–avoidant attachment. Only one of the 25 interaction terms was significant—sensitivity in play × care starts, Wald $\chi^2(1, n = 871) = 6.24$, $p < .05$, odds ratio =1.17.

Type-of-Care Analyses

Chi-square analyses were performed on attachment security × type of care at 5 months and at 14 months of age. The results indicated that type of care was not significantly related to secure–insecure or secure–avoidant attachment at either age.

Additional analyses were performed to determine whether various aspects of child care quality, amount, age of entry, and care starts were related to attachment security within types of care. None of these yielded significant results.

DISCUSSION

Validity of the Strange Situation

The first purpose of the present study was to evaluate the internal validity of the Strange Situation assessment procedure. This was necessary because concerns have been raised about the appropriateness of using the separation-based Strange Situation to assess the attachment of infants in child care, who presumably have had more experience with absences from their mothers. No significant differences in ratings of infants' distress during mothers' absence in the Strange Situation were observed between children with less than 10 hours of care per week vs. children with more than 30 hours of care over the first year of life. Thus, there was no evidence of differential validity for the Strange Situation as a function of child care experience.

Main Effects of Mother and Child Characteristics

Children's attachment security was related to the mother's sensitivity and responsiveness, especially observed in the natural setting of the home, and to her overall positive psychological adjustment. These findings are consistent with a substantial theoretical and empirical literature linking infants' attachment security to their mothers' psychological adjustment (e.g., Spieker & Booth, 1988; for a review, see Belsky, Rosenberger, & Crnic, 1995) and sensitive and responsive caregiving (e.g., Ainsworth et al., 1978; for reviews, see Belsky & Cassidy, 1994; Clarke-Stewart, 1988).

Main Effects of Infant Child Care

After selection effects were taken into account, along with child effects (i.e., temperament, and sex) and mother effects (i.e., psychological adjustment, and sensitivity), results pertaining to main effects of child care were clear and consistent: There were no significant differences in attachment security related to child care participation. Even in extensive, early, unstable, or poor-quality care, the likelihood of infants' insecure attachment to mother did not increase, nor did stable or high-quality care increase the likelihood of developing a secure attachment to mother.

It is unclear why the results of this inquiry are different from those of past studies. Comparison of our results with those of earlier studies must give substantial weight to the present findings because of the advantages of this study—its methodological strengths, its control for family selection effects, its recency, and its "quality control" (in which, for example, Strange Situation coders were highly trained, reliable, and blind to the child's care arrangement). Nevertheless, it should be noted that the present study shares a limitation with previous studies, namely, that it was not possible to conduct observations in all eligible child care arrangements. Approximately 16% of the care providers contacted at 6 and 15 months were unwilling, unable, or unavailable to be observed.

Interaction Effects with Child and Mother Characteristics

Although analyses revealed no significant main effects of child care, it was not the case that child care was totally unrelated to attachment security. A consistent pattern observed across five of the six significant interactions supported the proposition that children's attachment is affected by a combination of maternal and child care factors. Children with the highest rates of insecurity with their mothers experienced conditions that could be considered to constitute a dual risk. This was most clearly demonstrated by children whose mothers and caregivers were least sensitive and responsive to their needs and behavior. Children who received less sensitive and responsive caregiving in child care as well as less sensitive and responsive care from mothers had the highest rates of insecurity. Parallel but less pronounced effects were observed for children who experienced the dual risks of less sensitive and responsive mothering combined with more time spent in child care or more care arrangements over time. These results support a dual-risk model of development (see Belsky & Rovine, 1988; Werner & Smith, 1992).

Beyond the dual-risk effects, other significant interactions were observed. For children in low-quality child care, the probability of a secure attachment was low if the mother was less sensitive and responsive and high if she was highly sensitive and responsive. For children in high-quality care, the security proportions were moderate regardless of the mothers' behavior.

A second pattern pertains to the interaction between maternal sensitivity and amount of child care. Children whose mothers exhibited less sensitive and responsive behavior toward them in the HOME observation and interview were more likely to be securely attached if they spent more time with mother (and less time in child care). Our tentative explanation is that there may be a "dosage effect" for maternal sensitivity and involvement:

Children with less involved mothers may need more time with them in order to develop the internalized sense that the mother is responsive and available, whereas children with more sensitive and responsive mothers may require less time to develop confidence in the mother's availability.

A third interaction pattern suggested different developmental processes for boys and girls. Whereas more time in child care was associated with a somewhat higher rate of insecurity for boys, less time in care was associated with a somewhat higher rate of insecurity for girls.

The interaction analyses provided evidence that high-quality child care served a compensatory function for children whose maternal care was lacking: The proportion of attachment security among children with the least sensitive and responsive mothers was higher in high-quality child care than in low-quality care. However, there was no evidence that amount of time in child care compensated for the mother's lack of sensitivity and involvement, because the proportion of secure attachment among the children with the least sensitive and responsive mothers was higher in minimal hours of child care than in many hours of care.

Effect of Child Care on Avoidance

Previous studies (compiled by Belsky & Rovine, 1988; Clarke-Stewart, 1989) suggested that effects of child care were most likely to increase the rate of one particular form of insecurity—insecure avoidance. In contrast to the results of earlier research, there was no evidence that child care experience is associated with avoidance per se.

CONCLUSION

The results of this study indicate that child care by itself constitutes neither a risk nor a benefit for the development of the infant–mother attachment relationship as measured in the Strange Situation. However, poor-quality, unstable, or more than minimal amounts of child care apparently added to the risks already inherent in poor mothering, so that the combined effects were worse than those of low maternal sensitivity and responsiveness alone. Such results suggest that the effects of child care on attachment, as well as the nature of the attachment relationship itself, depend primarily on the nature of ongoing interactions between mother and child (Ainsworth, 1973; Sroufe, 1988).

15

—

Child Care and Family Predictors of Preschool Attachment and Stability from Infancy

NICHD Early Child Care Research Network

This chapter addresses two concerns regarding the relations between child care experience and child–mother attachment at 36 months as assessed by the MacArthur coding system (Cassidy, Marvin, & MacArthur Attachment Working Group. 1992). First, in a large, normative sample of children, this study uses a comprehensive set of maternal, family, child, and child care factors to predict attachment quality in preschool, with a particular focus on the extent to which features of child care predict attachment classification after maternal, family, and child factors are controlled. Second, acknowledging differential measurement of child–mother attachment in infancy and preschool, the study analyzes associations of child care predictors with patterns of stability and instability in attachment security from 15 to 36 months while controlling for mother, family, and child factors.

It has been argued that hours away from the mother during the first year of life may adversely affect the proximal processes of mother–child interaction and ultimately the attachment relationship (Belsky, 1999; Jaeger & Weinraub, 1990; Owen & Cox, 1988), and this argument can also be used to hypothesize that more time in child care will be associated with insecurity after infancy. On the other hand, time away from the mother per se may not

From *Developmental Psychology*, Vol. 37, 847–862. Copyright 2001 by the American Psychological Association. Reprinted by permission.

be associated with attachment insecurity in the preschool years: Rather, the quality of that experience away from the mother may be the feature of child care associated with security. Children in high-quality care could learn communication skills that could be used in shared plans with the mother, an essential component of secure interaction (goal-corrected partnership) in the preschool years (Marvin, 1977).

Given the longitudinal nature of the National Institute of Child Health and Human Development (NICHD) Study of Early Child Care and the repeated assessment of attachment at 15 and 36 months, the present study presents an opportunity to examine not only the prediction of attachment at 36 months but also the extent and correlates of stability in attachment classification at 15 and 36 months. Meta-analytic studies of attachment across time support the notion of continuity from infancy through adolescence (Fraley, 1999; van IJzendoorn, Schuengel, & Bakermans-Kranenburg, 1999). Whether stability in attachment from infancy to the preschool period will be observed is still open to question. Crittenden (2000) suggested that some instability during this period is normative. In addition to the increase in experience in nonfamilial contexts and new threats to safety to which the preschooler is exposed, Crittenden proposed that developmental maturation itself may be a cause of instability during this period. She argued that increasing cognitive and linguistic competence makes possible the expression of new, more complex attachment organizations in the preschool period. On the basis of her dynamic–maturational model of attachment, Crittenden specifically predicted an increase in the use of coercive (Type C) attachment patterns. In this pattern, aspects of the resistant behavior are organized into a strategy that compels the attachment figure to comply with the child's needs (Teti & Gelfand, 1997). Indeed, there is some empirical support for this hypothesis (Bohlin & Hagekull, 2000; Fagot & Pears, 1996; Teti, Gelfand, Messinger, & Isabella, 1995).

Instead of asking simply about the extent of attachment stability, we examined family, maternal, and child factors associated with continuity and discontinuity. From infancy to the preschool period in particular, such factors are likely to be related to changes in the quality of the parent–child relationship (Sroufe, Carlson, Levy, & Egeland, 1999). It is also important to examine the direction of change for unstable dyads, especially for studies of the effects of child care, in which child care is hypothesized to have either positive or negative effects. For instance, Egeland & Hiester (1995) suggested, "It may well be that many of the children in day-care who were classified as securely attached at 12 months of age will be insecurely attached by preschool age because of the inconsistency in care resulting from repeated separations" (p. 482). They also hypothesized, however, that for initially insecure pairs, early child care may support a shift toward security: "[E]arly day-care may provide some mothers, particularly those who are single heads of household, with the relief they need to cope better and provide better care" (p. 482). Thus, Egeland & Hiester articulated hypotheses that related amount and stability of child care in infancy to (1) a shift from security in infancy to insecurity in the preschool years and (2) a shift from insecurity in infancy to security in the preschool years for children being raised in single-parent, low-income families.

METHOD

Participants

A description of the participants in the NICHD Study of Early Child Care is provided in Chapter 1.

Table 15.1 presents characteristics of the families included in the analyses examining child attachment outcomes at 36 months.

Child attachment security data at 15 and 36 months were available for 1,153 and 1,150 children, respectively, and 1,060 children provided attach-

TABLE 15.1. Sample Characteristics of Participants Included in Multinomial Logistic Regression Analyses of 36-Month Attachment Security

Characteristic	Whole sample (1,140 families)		Observed sample (869 families)	
	n	%	n	%
Child gender				
Female	558	48.9	428	49.3
Male	582	51.1	441	50.7
Child ethnicity				
White	851	74.6	636	73.2
Black	157	13.8	119	13.7
Hispanic	74	6.5	65	7.5
Other	58	5.1	49	5.6
Maternal education				
Less than high school diploma	101	8.9	60	6.9
High school graduate	233	20.4	178	20.5
Some college	378	33.2	293	33.7
College graduate	252	22.1	192	22.1
Postgraduate work	176	15.4	146	16.8
Income-to-needs ratio				
0–1 (poverty)	172	15.1	102	11.8
> 1–1.8 (near poverty)	152	11.7	114	13.1
> 1.8 (nonpoor)	814	71.5	651	75.1
Average no. of hours per week in care	22.83	(16.02)	27.67	(14.04)

Note. Numbers in parentheses in last row are standard deviations.

ment data at both time points. Compared with families that remained in the study through 36 months, families that did not contribute attachment data at 36 months were more likely to have mothers who were nonwhite or Hispanic (31.9% vs. 18.8%); mothers with less education (13.4 years vs. 14.3 years), more depressive symptoms (13.0 vs. 11.2), and more separation anxiety (72.8 vs. 70.0); and households with fewer two-parent families (73.1% vs. 86.4%) and lower income-to-needs ratios (2.1 vs. 2.8). All comparisons noted were significant at $p < .05$.

Overview of Data Collection

Information about the timing, location and other aspects of data collection conducted during the children's first 3 years of life can be found in Chapter 1.

Measures

This presentation of measures is organized to reflect the way in which variables functioned in the analyses. We first present measures used as dependent variables in the substantive analyses of the effects of child care. Next we describe covariates in the analyses of child care effects, and then we describe child care measures. Composites were used to reduce both the number of variables and the complexity of the analyses being performed as well as to increase measurement reliability.

Attachment Measures

This report includes measures of child attachment security at 15 and 36 months. The Strange Situation (Ainsworth, Blehar, Waters, & Wall, 1978) was conducted during the 15-month laboratory visit (see Chapter 14 for a description of the procedures at 15 months). At 36 months, a modified Strange Situation (Cassidy et al., 1992) was conducted during a laboratory visit.

36 Months

A modified Strange Situation procedure based on recommendations by Cassidy and colleagues (1992) was used to assess attachment security at 36 months. In this procedure, designed to be moderately stressful for the child, the mother and child were invited to make themselves comfortable in a room containing a basket of toys, a beanbag chair, a chair for the mother, and a schoolhouse with small plastic figures. After 3 minutes, the mother was signaled to leave. The first separation lasted 3 minutes unless the child was distressed. After a 3-minute reunion, the mother left again, and the second separation lasted for 5 minutes unless the child was distressed, in which case the mother returned to the room early. The assessment was terminated after 3 minutes of the second reunion. Research assistants at the 10 sites were trained and certified to conduct this modified Strange Situation according to standard procedures.

The child's behavior during the assessment was classified according to the system developed by the MacArthur Working Group on Attachment (the MacArthur system; Cassidy et al., 1992). Videotapes were shipped to a central location and rated by a team of three coders who were blind to child care status, maternal sensitivity ratings, and previous attachment classification. The three coders were trained and certified by Jude Cassidy to code using the MacArthur system. All coders had passed the minimum 75% agreement at the level of ABCD classifications with Jude Cassidy on a set of 21 test tapes.

The MacArthur coding system classifies preschoolers as secure (B) or insecure (A, C, and D). Secure (B) children are able to resolve the stress of the separation and resume calm, comfortable interaction with the parent. Insecure–avoidant (A) children maintain extreme neutrality toward the parent and even after reunion rarely express either positive or negative emotion toward the parent. Insecure–ambivalent (C) children show fussy, helpless, whiny, and/or resistant behavior toward the parent. They may seek contact but find it unsatisfactory. Insecure–controlling/insecure–other (D) children either are controlling or show combinations of strategies, such as avoidance and ambivalence or avoidance and controlling behavior, during the reunions. Controlling children take charge of the reunion, usually in either a caregiving (role reversal) or punitive manner. A child showing more than one type of controlling behavior is classified as controlling–general. Coders also make a global 9-point security rating. A team of three coders conducted the coding. Reliability was calculated based on 867 randomly paired cases. Disagreements were discussed, and a consensus code was assigned. Intercoder agreement (before conferencing) on the four-category ABCD classifications was 75.7% (kappa = .58). The average correlation between paired coders on the 9-point security rating was .73. An examination of the 4×4 reliability contingency table revealed that coders were less likely to confuse B with A, B with C, B with D, and A with C (p's < .002) and more likely to confuse A with D ($p < .06$) and C with D ($p < .15$). Thus, distinguishing among the insecure groups (A, C, and D) in these analyses was supported.

Mother/Family/Child Measures

Demographic Variables

The income-to-needs ratio (details about the formula is given in Chapter 14) was averaged across 0–36 months to create an average income-to-needs ratio. Higher income-to-needs ratios were associated with greater security at 36 months, more cumulative child care hours, and greater child care quality. Maternal education was represented by five levels determined when the child was 1 month old (for details, see Chapter 7). More education was associated with higher security scores, more child care hours, and greater child care quality at 36 months. Two-parent status (either married or partnered) was determined from interviews at 1, 3, 6, 15, 24, and 36 months. The cumulative variables used in the analyses had three levels: 0 = never lived in a two-parent household, 1 = sometimes lived in a two-parent household, and 2 = always lived in a two-parent household. Seventy percent of the children consistently lived in a two-parent household through 36 months.

Maternal Well-Being

Maternal psychological functioning was a composite formed by averaging the standardized scores of depressive symptoms (reverse scored) at 1, 6, 15, 24, and 36 months on the Center for Epidemiologic Studies–Depression (CES-D) scale (Radloff, 1977) and at 6 months on three scales of the Neuroticism Extraversion Openness (NEO) Personality Inventory (Costa & McCrae, 1985): Neuroticism (reverse scored), Extraversion, and Agreeableness. Cronbach's alpha was .80. (More details about this measure can be found in Chapter 14.)

Parenting Behavior

Four observational measures of parenting included the ratings from both concurrent (36 months) and 6–36-month averages of *maternal sensitivity* (described below) and *responsiveness in the home* as measured by the Infant/Toddler Home Observation for Measurement of the Environment (HOME) Inventory (Caldwell & Bradley, 1984) at 6 and 15 months and the Preschool HOME at 36 months. The Positive Involvement factor score and the Lack of Negativity factor score were summed and then standardized and averaged across age.

Mother–child interaction was videotaped in semistructured 15-minute observations at each age. The observation task at 6 months had two components. In the first 7 minutes, mothers were asked to play using any toy or object available in the home or none at all; for the remaining 8 minutes, mothers were given a standard set of toys they could use in play with their infants. At 15, 24, and 36 months, the observation procedures followed a "three boxes" procedure in which mothers were asked to show their children age-appropriate toys in three containers in a set order (see Vandell, 1979). The mother was instructed to have her child play with the toys in each of the three containers and to do so in the order specified.

At each age, a *maternal sensitivity* composite based on three of the ratings was constructed. At 6, 15, and 24 months, it comprised the sum of three 4-point ratings, sensitivity to nondistress, positive regard, and intrusiveness (reverse-scored). At 36 months, three 7-point ratings formed the composite: supportive presence, respect for autonomy, and hostility (reverse scored). Intercoder reliability on the composite was .87 at 6 months, .83 at 15 months, .85 at 24 months, and .84 at 36 months. Internal consistencies were .75, .70, .79, and .78, respectively. The composite scores were moderately stable across time (r's ranged from .39 to .48). Composites across age periods (from 6 to 36 months and from 24 to 36 months) were computed by standardizing the scores at each age and averaging them across time.

Parenting Attitudes

Mothers reported about their *authoritarian beliefs* about childrearing at 1 month on the Modernity Scale (Schaefer & Edgerton, 1985). Higher scores indicated more traditional beliefs. Cronbach's alpha was .90. *Maternal attitudes toward separation* were also measured at 1 month using the 21 items from subscale I, Maternal Separation Anxiety, of the Separation Anxiety Scale (Hock, Gnezda, & McBride, 1983). A high score on this scale indicates that a mother experiences worry, sadness, and guilt when separated from her child. It also reflects adherence to beliefs about the value of exclusive maternal care. Internal consistency exceeded .90.

Child Measures

Child positive engagement of mother was the average of composites of child behavior from the 15-, 24-, and 36-month mother–child interaction observations. At 15 and 24 months, positive engagement was the sum of 4-point ratings of child engagement of mother and positive mood; at 36 months, positive engagement was formed from the sum of 7-point ratings of child affection toward mother and negativity (reverse-scored). Cronbach's alphas for the positive engagement composites were .58, .74, and .78. Intercoder reliabilities of the composite ratings computed according to Winer (1971) were .74, .70, and .77 at 15, 24, and 36 months, respectively. The scores at each age were standardized and averaged across time.

Child compliance, reflecting compliance and cooperation with the mother and the absence of assertive and passive noncompliance, was rated at 36 months from videotaped observations in the laboratory of the child's response to the mother's request to have her child pick up toys following a 15-minute toy-play period. Five-point ratings of compliance, assertive noncompliance, passive noncompliance, and dyadic cooperation were completed by centralized coders who were unaware of other information on the children. Reliabilities of the ratings according to Winer's (1971) procedure ranged from .79 to .93 (see NICHD Early Child Care Research Network, 1998a). These ratings were standardized and combined to create the final composite.

Mother-reported behavior problems were measured with the 99-item Child Behavior Checklist—2/3 (Achenbach, 1992). Mothers rated how characteristic each behavior was of the child over the last 2 months (0 = *not true*, 1 = *sometimes true*, 2 = *very true*). The two broadband factors, Externalizing (aggressive and destructive behavior problems) and Internalizing (social withdrawal and depression), were standardized and summed (see NICHD Early Child Care Research Network, 1998a).

Child social competence at 36 months was assessed with the Adaptive Social Behavior Inventory (Hogan, Scott, & Bauer, 1992). Mothers respond to the scale's 30 items in terms of frequency of occurrence (1 = *rare*, 2 = *sometimes*, 3 = *almost always*). The Express scale (13 items) taps sociability and empathy; the Comply scale (10 items) measures prosocial engagement and cooperation. Coefficient alphas for the Express and Comply scales were .76 and .82. These two subscales were standardized and summed (see NICHD Early Child Care Research Network, 1998a).

Child Care Variables

At 3-month intervals, starting when the infants were 3 months old, mothers were telephoned and asked about their current child care arrangements, from which information was obtained about amount of care, number of arrangements, type of care, and age at entry. Amount of care was the average of the weekly hours in care from 0 to 36 months. Number of arrangements, a measure of stability of care, was a count of the number of times the mother reported that the child started a new child care arrangement, cumulated from 0 to 36 months. Mothers' telephone reports were also used to create three classifications for type of care at 36 months: mother care, relative care, and all others (center care and child care home).

Analysis of covariance was conducted to determine if concurrent type of care at age of outcome was associated with attachment security. There were no differences in security ratings across any of the three categorizations for type of care and no further type-of-care analyses were conducted.

Age at entry into child care was trichotomized. The age at which the child began averaging at least 10 hours/week of child care was categorized into one of three categories: before 15 months, between 16 and 35 months, and never.

A measure of child care quality was obtained from observations of the child care settings at 6, 15, 24, and 36 months for children spending at least 10 hours/week in a regular nonmaternal care arrangement. Observations of the sensitivity, involvement, and stimulation provided by caregivers in the child care arrangement were conducted on 2 half days during a 2-week interval. The Observational Record of the Caregiving Environment (ORCE; see Chapter 6) was used during these visits.

RESULTS

Preliminary Analyses

We sought to determine whether the classifications of 36 months attachment in this sample, in which the majority of the children had child care experience and thus were routinely separated from their mothers, had construct validity. Validation involved determining that child attachment classification was associated with non–child care measures in a manner consistent with past work in attachment research and attachment theory.

We expected secure children (coded as B) to have mothers with greater psychological adjustment, greater sensitivity in play and home observations, and fewer authoritarian childrearing attitudes. We expected secure children to be more positive in interactions with their mothers, to be more compliant during the laboratory toy cleanup, and to have fewer mother-reported behavior problems and more mother-reported social competence. We expected children coded as D to have the most problematic scores on these measures. To test these propositions, we computed one-way analyses of variance (ANOVAs). All the tests of association were significant, although the indices of association were modest. All *post hoc* significant differences were found for secure versus various insecure groups (two for B vs. A, six for B vs. C, and nine for B vs. D). None of the comparisons between the insecure groups reached significance. Thus, for secure versus insecure, at least, attachment classifications from the MacArthur coding scheme for preschool Strange Situation assessments are related to maternal and family antecedents and concurrent child outcomes in a manner consistent with previous research and attachment theory. In support of the hypothesis that the D group would be the most extreme, the greatest number of differences was found between the B and D groups. (A table is available upon request.)

Relations of Family and Child Covariates with Attachment

Selection (Control) Variables

A set of covariates referred to as selection variables was first identified in order to control for bias in child care usage. Unless these selection variables were controlled, effects could be attributed to child care variables that were really associated with factors that affected both child care usage and child attachment outcomes. The selection variables were income-to-needs ratio, maternal education, and maternal attitudes toward separation. Families with more maternal education and higher income-to-needs ratios had children who began child care at younger ages and for more hours. They chose higher-quality care. More of their children were securely attached, compared with children from families with lower maternal education and lower income-to-needs ratios. Families with mothers who reported more separation anxiety had children who started child care at older ages and for fewer hours. They chose lower-quality care. More of the children of mothers with higher separation anxiety scores were insecurely attached.

Mother/Family/Child Covariates

In addition to controlling for selection effects, we controlled for other maternal and child factors that have been shown to be associated with child attachment security. The mother and family variables included maternal depressive symptoms, maternal sensitivity, and two-parent status. Mothers who reported more depressive symptoms had more children who were insecurely attached, compared with mothers who reported fewer depressive symptoms. More children of sensitive mothers were securely attached, compared with children of less sensitive mothers. Finally, more children of two-parent families were securely attached, compared with children of single-parent families. We also included child gender as a covariate because it was a moderator of child care effects on attachment at 15 months (Chapter 14). Although it showed no relations with the dichotomous secure–insecure variable at 36 months, it was associated with the four-way ABCD variable.

Relations between Child Care and Attachment Classification at 36 Months

Multinomial logistic regression (Hosmer & Lemeshow, 1989) was used to examine the associations between child care and the preschool Strange Situation attachment classification. The categorical dependent variable (A, B, C, or D) was predicted from control variables reflective of selection effects (income-to-needs ratio, maternal education, and maternal attitudes toward separation), mother/family/child characteristics (maternal sensitivity, maternal depressive symptoms, family status, child gender), and four child care variables (hours per week, number of arrangements, age at entry, and quality). All predictors were entered into the analyses at the same time. Table 15.2 presents unadjusted descriptive statistics for predictor variables by attachment classification (A, B, C, or D) at 36 months.

It was impossible to include all participants in a single analysis because some of the child care variables (hours per week, number of arrangements, and age at entry) involved the total sample, whereas child care quality was available only for those children observed in child care. Thus, the multinomial logistic regressions were conducted twice, once for the total sample and once for the sample observed in care.

The overall multinomial logistic regression model for the full sample was significant, $\chi^2(36, n = 854) = 75.1$, $p < .001$, and likelihood ratio tests on individual variables revealed that one selection and two mother/family/child variables were significant predictors of attachment classification: income, maternal sensitivity, and child gender. None of the three child care

TABLE 15.2. Descriptive Statistics for Selection, Mother/Family/Child, and Child Care Variables by ABCD Classification at 36 Months

	Attachment classification											
	A			B			C			D		
Predictor	n	M or %	SD	n	M or %	SD	n	M or %	SD	n	M or %	SD
Selection variables												
Income-to-needs ratio	55	2.87	2.70	701	3.55	2.72	196	3.18	2.34	186	3.21	3.13
Maternal education (years)	55	13.71	2.39	701	14.62	2.41	197	14.03	2.50	187	13.96	2.65
Maternal separation anxiety	55	69.05	13.51	693	68.90	13.14	196	71.24	13.16	185	71.81	13.49
Mother/family/child variables												
Maternal depression	55	-0.12	0.71	701	-0.08	0.72	197	-0.01	0.73	187	0.18	0.88
Maternal sensitivity	55	-0.08	0.78	701	0.11	0.67	197	-0.09	0.77	187	-0.29	0.92
Always two parents (%)	55	65.45		701	74.47		197	67.51		187	58.82	
Child gender (% girls)	55	33.18		701	46.79		197	50.25		187	58.82	
Child care variables												
Hours per week	55	20.35	15.69	701	23.32	16.19	197	22.09	16.32	187	22.52	15.14
No. of arrangements	55	5.51	3.41	701	5.04	3.50	197	4.99	3.52	187	4.99	3.25
Entry into 10 hours/week by 36 months (%)	52	90.38		658	91.34		184	87.50		174	93.68	
Quality	40	0.20	0.76	540	0.05	0.81	148	-0.09	0.80	141	-0.04	0.83

Note. A, insecure–avoidant; B, secure; C, insecure–ambivalent; D, insecure–controlling/insecure–other.

predictors available for the whole sample significantly predicted any attachment classification. That is, variations in the amount of care, the frequency of care arrangements, or the age of entry did not increase or decrease a child's chances of being in a particular attachment classification after we controlled for all selection and mother/family/child variables.

When the analysis was performed on the sample of children observed in child care, the results were essentially the same, $\chi^2(39, n = 643) = 70.1, p < .01$. Boys experiencing many hours of care (30+ hours/week) and girls experiencing minimal amounts of care (<10 hours/week) were somewhat less likely to be securely attached. Therefore, instead of testing all possible mother/family/child by child care interactions, in the present study these four interactions (maternal sensitivity × quality; maternal sensitivity × hours per week; maternal sensitivity × number of arrangements; and hours per week × child gender) were tested, one at a time, in the multinomial logistic regression models.

Only one interaction, maternal sensitivity × hours per week, added significantly to the models, $\chi^2(3, n = 854) = 8.3, p < .05$. As hours in care increased, children with more sensitive parents were more likely to be classified as B, and children with less sensitive parents were more likely to be classified as C.

Relations between Child Care and Stability of 15-Month Attachment Classification

We examined prediction from, and the stability of, Strange Situation ABCD classifications at 15 months in several ways. First, using a binomial test, we determined whether the proportions of children in the A, B, C, and D categories differed significantly between 15 and 36 months. There were no differences in the proportions of B ($p > .45$) and D ($p > .15$) classifications at the two ages. However, at 36 months there were significantly fewer A classifications ($p < .001$) and significantly more C classifications ($p < .001$) than there were at 15 months.

Second, the categorical ABCD variable at 15 months (ABCD15) was included in a multinomial logistic regression model. ABCD15 accounted for significant variance, $\chi^2(9, n = 650) = 21.2, p < .05$, when mother/family/child factors measured between the two assessments were controlled. The individual parameter estimates (Table 15.3) indicated that attachment classification at 15 months accounted for variance in four of the six attachment category contrasts at 36 months when all other predictors were controlled. Children in the B or C categories at 15 months were more likely to be in the B category at 36 months than the A category, and children in the C category at 15 months were less likely to be classified as D at 36 months than to be classified as B. Children classified as C at 15 months were more likely to remain classified as C at 36 months than to be classified as D or A. The same effect of ABCD15 was found when child care quality was included in the model with ABCD15, $\chi^2(9, n = 515) = 21.1, p < .05$.

TABLE 15.3. Parameter Estimates for Multinomial Logistic Regression Model Relating Child Care to ABCD Attachment at 36 Months (ABCD36), with ABCD Attachment at 15 Months (ABCD15) Included, Full Sample Only

Significant contrast	Wald χ^2	β	SE	Odds ratio	Confidence intervals
ABCD36: A vs. B					
Maternal sensitivity	NS				
Child gender = boy	NS				
ABCD15 = B	4.10*	−0.88	0.43	0.42	0.18–0.97
ABCD15 = C	3.99*	−2.70	1.40	0.01	0.00–0.95
ABCD36: C vs. B					
Maternal sensitivity	6.75**	−0.39	0.15	0.68	0.51–0.91
Child gender = boy	6.30*	−0.55	0.22	0.58	0.38–0.89
ABCD15	NS				
ABCD36: D vs. B					
Maternal sensitivity	17.62***	−0.65	0.15	0.53	0.39–0.71
Child gender = boy	5.17*	−0.53	0.23	0.59	0.37–0.93
ABCD15 = C	4.55*	−1.17	0.55	0.31	0.11–0.91
ABCD36: A vs. D					
Maternal sensitivity	NS				
Child gender = boy	3.53†	0.74	0.40	2.10	0.97–4.55
ABCD15	NS				
ABCD36: C vs. D					
Maternal sensitivity	NS				
Child gender = boy	NS				
ABCD15 = C	8.15**	1.75	0.61	5.74	1.73–19.04
ABCD36: A vs. C					
Maternal sensitivity	NS				
Child gender = boy	3.83*	0.76	0.39	2.14	1.00–4.58
ABCD15 = B	3.78†	−0.98	0.50	0.38	0.14–1.01
ABCD15 = C	5.62*	−3.28	1.38	0.00	0.00–0.57

Note. A, insecure–avoidant; B, secure; C, insecure–ambivalent; D, insecure–controlling/insecure–other.
†$p < .10$; *$p < .05$; **$p < .01$; ***$p < .001$.

Third, to clarify these stability findings, we analyzed the contingency table of the ABCD classifications at the two ages. Overall stability between 15 and 36 months was significant but modest. There was significant stability in the A and C categories from 15 to 36 months and it was significantly unlikely that a child classified in the C category at 15 months would be classified in the A category at 36 months.

Finally, to examine whether child care variables were related to the attachment instability for the secure–insecure dichotomies observed at 15 and 36 months, we used logistic regression to predict security or insecurity at 36 months within both the initially secure and initially insecure groups. By proceeding in this manner we were in a position to determine, on the one hand, why some children who were initially secure remained that way over time whereas others did not, and, on the other hand, why some children who were initially insecure remained that way whereas others did not. The predictor variables in these logistic regression analyses were the same selection, mother/family/child, and child care variables used in the first analyses except that they were averaged over the interval of interest, from 16 to 36 months, rather than over the lifetime of the child. The age-at-entry variable was dichotomized to reflect those who entered an average of 10 hours/week of child care between 16 and 35 months and those who did not (either because they entered care earlier or not at all). Thus, we were capturing change in status with this variable. In these analyses, as before, all mother/family/child variables and child care variables were included in the analyses, which were conducted on both the total sample and the observed-in-care sample, with the four interaction terms entered one at a time.

Initially Secure

The results, for the whole sample, for the children who were classified as secure at 15 months ($n = 480$) show that 65% were classified as secure at 36 months. Children who changed from a secure classification at 15 months to an insecure classification at 36 months had families with higher income-to-needs ratios and mothers with less education and lower sensitivity at 24–36 months (whole sample only). Girls were more likely than boys to change from secure to insecure from 15 to 36 months (40% vs. 31% for girls and boys, respectively; whole sample). Starting at least 10 hours/week of care between 16 and 36 months was associated with changing from secure to insecure, a finding that was significant for the observed-in-care sample (p .05). Of the 38 secure children who were observed in care at 36 months and who had begun care sometime between 15 and 35 months, 50% became insecure, compared with 34% of secure children who had entered care before 15 months or not at all. Using the effect size formula recommended by Rosnow and Rosenthal (1988), we computed the effect size, r_p, to be .09. None of the interactions involving child care variables was significant.

Initially Insecure

The results, for the whole sample, for the children who were classified as insecure at 15 months ($n = 307$) show that 41% were classified as insecure at 36 months. The shift to security was associated with greater maternal sensitivity in both the whole and observed-in-care samples. Child care factors did not account for change from insecure to secure attachment. None of the interaction terms was significant.

DISCUSSION

This study addressed two research questions. The first was the extent to which cumulative child care experience was related to preschool attachment classification when selection and mother/family/child factors were statistically controlled. The second question focused on whether maternal, family, child, and child care factors related to stability of attachment security from 15 to 36 months.

Relations between Child Care and Attachment Classification at 36 Months

Features of child care were not associated with attachment classification at 36 months as main effects. As at 15 months, the amount of, type of, number of arrangements for, age at entry into, and quality of child care experienced by children in this sample were not associated with attachment classification at 36 months. These results are consistent with more recent work on child care and infant and toddler attachment (e.g., Roggman, Langlois, Hubbs-Tait, & Rieser-Danner, 1994; Symons, 1998) and with an older body of research on preschool-age children (Moskowitz, Schwarz, & Corsini, 1977; Portnoy & Simmons, 1978; Roopnarine & Lamb, 1978). However, across the two reports on child care and attachment produced by the NICHD Study of Early Child Care, associations between child care and attachment did occur under conditions of insensitive mothering. In the present report, the association is specifically for the group with Type C attachment, children who have ambivalent relationships with their parent.

Relations between Child Care and Stability of 15-Month Attachment Classification

We found modest stability for ABCD attachment classification from 15 to 36 months, in contrast to the overall stabilities reported in Fraley's (1999) and van IJzendoorn and colleagues' (1999) recent meta-analyses. In our study, the four-category ABCD classification revealed a bit of lawful association between the two time points (kappa = .057). This lawfulness appeared to be due to a higher number of cases than expected in the A to A and C to C cells and fewer cases than expected in the C to A and C to D cells, associations that would be obscured if the analysis included only the secure-insecure dichotomy. Although the most "stable" group was secure infants who remained secure (64%), in fact this proportion was about what would be expected by chance, because rates of security at both ages were about 62%. Overall, at 36 months the likelihood of being classified a C increased and the likelihood of being classified an A decreased, although the overall likelihood of being secure remained constant. This move to C was predicted by Crittenden (2000), although for a different preschool coding system. Our findings are consistent with her speculation that preschoolers will tend to use the more coercive strategies that are available to them.

The associations of attachment classification with maternal sensitivity were, in general, as predicted, with low or decreased sensitivity from 24 to 36 months predicting the change from security to insecurity, and higher sensitivity from 24 to 36 months predicting the change from insecurity to security. These results are compatible with the interpretation that a decline in maternal sensitivity in the third year of life, or the lack of appropriate maternal adjustment to the changing demands of parenting a preschooler, could contribute to a shift from security to insecurity between 15 and 36 months. Frodi, Grolnick, and Bridges (1985) reported a similar finding in their study on stability of attachment within infancy. So there is evidence in this and other studies that aspects of the caregiving environment may be associated with a failure to find the expected stability in attachment security. In our study, in accordance with the predictions articulated in Egeland and Hiester's (1995) report, children who moved from security to insecurity were more likely to have entered into at least 10 hours per week of child care during the interval between 15 and 35 months than were children who remained secure. The effect was not strong, but it did suggest that some children respond to entry into nonmaternal care in the toddler and pre-school years with behaviors indicative of insecurity.

16

Caregiver–Mother Partnership Behavior and the Quality of Caregiver–Child and Mother–Child Interactions

MARGARET TRESCH OWEN
ANNE M. WARE
BILL BARFOOT

Despite theoretical support and professional and popular acceptance of the importance of communication between parents and child care providers, there has been little empirical study of assumptions and practices regarding cooperative relations between this aspect of parent–caregiver partnerships and benefits for children. The research has focused more on general attitudes of parents toward their child care providers and the general attitudes of providers toward parents (Galinsky, 1988; Kontos & Dunn, 1989; Kontos & Wells, 1986) but has rarely addressed the relationship between parent–caregiver dyads as "partners" in the child's care. An exception in this regard is the work of Elicker in the specification and measurement of various characteristics of the parent–caregiver relationship (Elicker, Noppe, Noppe, & Fortner-Wood, 1997).

In this chapter, we examine the association between mother–caregiver communication, particularly concerning the behavior and experiences of the child, and the child's experience of growth-promoting interactions with

From *Early Childhood Research Quarterly*, 2000, Vol. 15, pp. 413–428. Copyright 2000 by Elsevier. Reprinted by permission.

caregivers in child care settings and with mother. We focus particularly on caregiver–parent partnership behavior involving sharing and seeking of information about the child as an index of collaborative problem solving or a "caregiving partnership" between caregiver and parent.

Parent–caregiver communication about the child is a means of linking the home and child care contexts of the child's experience. Seeking and sharing information about the child's experiences and behavior should contribute to greater knowledge and perceptiveness about the child and thereby influence sensitive caretaking of the child. If parents share their unique knowledge about their children and their children's family experiences with child care providers, and providers inform parents about the child's behavior and achievements while under their care, child care providers and parents should each be better equipped to provide supportive and sensitive care of the child (Elicker & Fortner-Wood, 1995; Powell, 1978). In addition, such information can be important in formulating plans for the child that build on experiences in both the home and child care settings and thereby provide positive linkages between the two.

The following questions were examined in an investigation of how positive linkages between child care and home settings may be associated with children's experience of positive interactions with their mothers and caregivers: (1) Is communication between the mother and her child care provider, particularly pertaining to the seeking and sharing of information about the child's behavior and experience, related to more positive caregiver–child interaction in the child care setting and more positive mother–child interaction? (2) Does communication about the child by both the mother and the caregiver add to the predictions of positive caregiver–child and mother–child interaction? (3) Does mother–provider partnership behavior contribute uniquely to positive interactions after controlling for potential confounds of mother and provider childrearing beliefs?

METHOD

Participants

Participants in the study were 53 mothers and their children's 53 primary child care providers when the children were three years old. The families were participants in the Wisconsin site of the National Institute of Child Health and Human Development (NICHD) Study of Early Child Care because the measure of parent–caregiver partnership behavior was administered only to participants at this site. Families in the present study were restricted to those who used regular nonmaternal child care at 36 months and had data collected in the child care setting and with the mother in the lab visit.

At recruitment, when the children were born, the mean age of the mother was 28.8 years (range = 19–46 years) and their mean family income was \$33,000 (range = \$2,500–\$122,500; *SD* = \$25,000). Most of the mothers were white (96.2%), were married (83.0%), and had at least some college education. Among the child care providers, 20 were from child care centers and 33 were nonrelative family day home or in-home child care providers. Their mean age was 31.7 years (range = 19–63 years). Most caregivers were white (93.8%) and had some college education. Years of caregiving experience ranged from less than 1 year to 25 years.

Procedures

All measures in the present study were collected within 2 months of the child's third birthday through interviews, questionnaires, and live and video-taped observations conducted in home, lab, and child care visits. Although observational and questionnaire data were collected from multiple caregivers when the child was in center-based care, the data from only a single caregiver per child was examined in the present study. Caregiver data were included only if the caregiver was designated as "primary" and she had completed the partnership questionnaire.

Measures

Partnership Behavior of Caregiver and Mother

Partnership behavior was measured with parallel forms of the Caregiver–Parent Partnership Scale (Ware, Barfoot, Rusher, & Owen, 1995) administered to the parents and child care providers. The partnership scale was based on descriptions of mother–caregiver interaction (Kontos, 1987; Powell, 1989) and measures various self-reported interactions between parents and their child care providers. The 16 items of the scale are rated on 5-point Likert scales, with higher scores indicating more frequent partnership-relevant behavior. Most items could be grouped into one of three categories: (1) communications that shared information about the child ("discuss what makes child angry, happy, or sad"), (2) communications that sought information about the child or the child's experiences ("ask about feelings shown by child during the day/at home"), and (3) behavior relevant to adult support ("share your talents or skills at day care"). Three-factor solutions from principal components factor analyses with varimax rotations of the parent and of the child care provider responses confirmed the *a priori* grouping of items for parents and for caregivers. Three composites of the questionnaire items were formed for the parents' and the providers' responses; analogous parent and caregiver items were averaged in forming the composites: sharing information (five items, alphas = 0.88 and 0.86 for caregivers and mothers, respectively); seeking information (three items, alphas = 0.73 and 0.84 for caregivers and mothers); and adult relations (six items, alphas = 0.80 and 0.81 for caregivers and mothers). Adult relations was not included in the analyses because of our focus on the exchange of child-related information between parent and caregiver.

The correlation between caregiver seeking and sharing was moderately strong ($r = 0.56$) as was the correlation between mother seeking and sharing ($r = 0.63$). Thus, mothers' seeking and sharing scores and caregivers' seeking and sharing scores were each summed for composite ratings of communication with each other about the child. The resulting composite variables, mother partnership behavior and caregiver partnership behavior, were not significantly correlated ($r = 0.06$).

Quality of Caregiver–Child Interaction in Child Care

Observations of the child care arrangements were made on two half-day visits using the Observational Record of the Caregiving Environment (ORCE; see Chapters 2 and 5 for details). In the present study quality of caregiver–child interaction was indexed by a composite based on the sum of seven of the 4-point qualitative ratings of the child's primary caregiver: sensitivity to nondistress signals, stimulation of cognitive development, positive regard expressed to the child, detachment (reverse scored), fostering exploration, intrusiveness (reverse scored), and flatness of affect (reverse scored).

Quality of Mother–Child Interaction

The quality of mother–child interaction was measured from videotaped 15-minute observations conducted in a lab visit when the child was 36 months. (For details of the procedure, see Chapter 17.) Mother–child interaction was rated with 7-point global rating scales. An *a priori* composite of the individual scales was formed from the sum of supportive presence, respect for autonomy, and stimulation of cognitive development. Cronbach's alpha indicated high internal consistency of the composite scores (0.80) in the present sample. Intercoder reliability of the maternal positive caregiving composite was 0.83 as calculated by the intraclass correlation (Winer, 1971).

Nonauthoritarian Childrearing Beliefs

Measures of maternal and caregiver childrearing beliefs were included as covariates in analyses of the relation between mother–caregiver partnership behavior and the quality of mother–child and caregiver–child interaction. Childrearing beliefs were measured with the Modernity Scale (Schaefer & Edgerton, 1985; see Chapter 15) administered to the mothers when their child was 1 month and administered to the child care providers when the child was 36 months.

RESULTS

On average, most mothers and caregivers reported frequent seeking and sharing of information about the child and the child's experiences with each other. To examine differences in maternal and caregiver Partnership Behavior and the relation of partnership behavior to type of child care (center-based vs. less formal care), a 2×2 repeated-measure multivariate analysis of variance (ANOVA) was run with partnership behavior as a within-subjects measure (caregiver partnership behavior and maternal partnership behavior) and type of care as a between subjects measure. Mothers reported significantly more partnership behavior (seeking and sharing of information) than caregivers reported ($F [1, 51] = 12.43$, p .001), but there was no significant effect of type of care or interaction between respondent (mother/caregiver) and type of care.

Bivariate relations between the predictors (partnership behavior and childrearing beliefs) and between the predictors and the quality of caregiver–child and mother–child interaction were examined in correlational analyses. Table 16.1 shows correlations between the measures. As expected, caregiver nonauthoritarian childrearing beliefs were positively correlated with more caregiver partnership behavior and with positive caregiver–child interaction. Similarly, mothers with more nonauthoritarian childrearing beliefs reported more partnership behavior and were rated more positively in mother–child interaction. Mothers' and caregivers' reported partnership behaviors were each significantly correlated with caregiver–child interaction quality, so that more partnership behavior of both mother and caregiver was associated with more positive caregiver–child interaction. Mothers' partnership behavior was also significantly related to more positive mother–child interaction, but caregivers' reported partnership behavior was unrelated to mother–child interaction.

TABLE 16.1. Correlations between Partnership Behavior, Positive Interactions with Child, and Childrearing Beliefs for Mothers and Caregivers

	M partner	Cg beliefs	M beliefs	Cg–child interaction	M–child interaction
Cg partnership behavior	.06	.48***	.20	.38**	.11
M partnership behavior		.12	.32*	.51***	.41**
Cg childrearing beliefs			.19	.35**	.09
M childrearing beliefs				.24	.41**
Cg–child positive interactions					.44**

Notes. Cg, caregiver; M, mother.
*p < .05; **p < .01; ***p < .001.

Predictions of positive caregiver–child interaction and of positive mother–child interaction from partnership behavior of mother and caregiver were examined in multiple regression models, controlling for maternal and caregiver nonauthoritarian childrearing beliefs. The regression model was significant in the prediction of positive caregiver–child interaction from partnership behavior, controlling for caregiver and maternal beliefs, explaining 40% of the variance in caregiver–child interaction ($F[4, 52] = 8.09$, $p < .001$). Both caregiver and mother partnership behavior were significant predictors of positive caregiver–child interaction. The regression model predicting mother–child interaction from partnership behavior was also significant, explaining 25% of the variance ($F[4, 52] = 4.06$, $p < .05$). In this model, mother partnership behavior was a significant predictor of positive mother–child interaction.

DISCUSSION

The hypothesized relation between partnership behavior of mothers and their child care providers and more positive caregiver–child interaction was supported in the present study. When mother and caregiver reported more frequent communication with each other about the child and the child's experiences, by seeking and sharing information about the child, the caregiver's interactions with the child were observed to be more sensitive, supportive, and stimulating, indicative of higher-quality caregiving. The mother's seeking and sharing of information about the child and her caregiver's seeking and sharing of information each significantly added to the prediction of more positive caregiver–child interaction. Partnership behaviors of both mother and caregiver with each other were associated with positive caregiver–child interactions even when controlling for mothers' and caregivers' childrearing beliefs. In addition, higher-quality mother–child interaction was observed when mother reported more partnership behavior with the caregiver.

The findings are consistent with the view that adults are better equipped to foster children's new exploration and enhance the appropriateness and meaningfulness of children's experiences when they have knowledge of the child's behavior and experiences in other settings. A fundamental basis for the emphasis on a partnership relationship between child care provider and parent is the potential for discontinuity in young children's experiences that can stem from a lack of connection between the settings (Powell, 1989). These findings advance understanding of how parent–caregiver communication is related to the developmental potential of the child's environmental settings in several ways. First, the few previously existing empirical studies of relations between parent–caregiver partnership behavior and caregiving quality in child care have linked caregiver partnership behavior and child care quality at a general classroom level, not at the level of individual children's experiences. The present findings provide evidence connecting communications of caregiver–parent dyads, as partners in the child's care, and the quality of care the child experienced with the caregiver. Second, to our knowledge, the relation between caregiver and parent partnership behavior and the interactions of the mother with her child has not previously been examined, nor has evidence for a positive link been reported. Third, the prediction of positive mother–child and caregiver–child interactions from communications between caregiver and mother about the child was examined while controlling for the potentially confounding relations of caregiver and parent nonauthoritarian childrearing beliefs, offering some control for potential confounds of individual characteristics of mother and caregivers that could explain such a link.

In summary, the importance of supportive linkages between children's home and child care experiences was demonstrated in finding positive associations with the quality of interactions with the child in child care and in the home. The present study adds support to the current professional emphasis on communication between parent and caregiver as a feature of high-quality child care programs.

17

Child Care
and Mother–Child Interaction
in the First 3 Years of Life

NICHD EARLY CHILD CARE RESEARCH NETWORK

A focus on the associations of child care with mother–child interaction is important for two reasons. First, it addresses child care effects on both the child's and the mother's side of the relationship. Second, because mother–child interaction is an important predictor of a range of developmental outcomes (e.g., Bornstein & Tamis-LeMonda, 1989; Pianta & Egeland, 1994; Rogoff, Mistry, Goncu, & Mosier, 1993), examining the associations between child care and mother–child interaction may illuminate linkages between child care and development.

Hypothesized effects of early child care on the quality of mother–child interaction have focused primarily on how the amount of child care experience and the associated separation relate to the mother–child relationship. It has been suggested that nonmaternal child care, particularly when initiated early in infancy, can be negatively associated with the quality of mother–child interaction because the amount of child care correspondingly reduces the amount of time mother and child spend together. A sufficient amount of time is considered necessary in the early months for the mother

From *Developmental Psychology*, 1999, Vol. 35, pp. 1399–1413. Copyright 1999 by the American Psychological Association. Reprinted by permission.

to learn her infant's signaling patterns and rhythms (e.g., Brazelton, 1986; Sroufe, 1988; Vaughn, Gove, & Egeland, 1980) and to respond with sensitivity to the infant's needs (Lamb & Easterbrooks, 1981). Nonmaternal care may be more strongly associated with poorer-quality mother–child interaction when it occurs early rather than later in the preschool years, because infancy may be a time when dyadic affective attunement is more difficult to achieve because of the limited ability of the infant to communicate. Similar arguments, however, also support hypothesized negative effects of the amount of child care on the quality of mother–child interaction past infancy. Greater amounts of nonmaternal care could be associated with poorer communication between mother and preschooler, because the mother–child relationship requires an increasingly sophisticated signaling system in the preschool years that may be hindered when time together is reduced due to child care.

The National Institute of Child Health and Human Development (NICHD) Study of Early Child Care provided an opportunity to examine relations between early child care and mother–child interactions in a longitudinal study encompassing a large, diverse sample of families. Approximately 1,300 families from 10 sites across the United States were followed from the children's birth through first grade in order to address the nature and effects of early child care on young children and their families. Features of child care use were tracked every 3 months, and observations of the quality of child care experiences were made at four major data collection ages in the first 3 years of life. Demographic and attitudinal characteristics of the families were measured repeatedly, beginning when the infants were 1 month of age. This procedure allowed for the control of features of the family related both to child care use and to the outcomes in question.

Measurement of mother–child interaction was conducted at four ages across the first 3 years of life. The semistructured observations of mother–child interaction involved similar constructs at each age, but procedures were modified to allow age-appropriate observations of the mother's supportiveness of her child's play and exploration and the child's engagement with the mother during these interactions.

To examine the relation between rearing conditions of young children and the mother–child relationship, we used data from the NICHD Study of Early Child Care to address three related questions: (1) Does the amount of child care and the instability of child care negatively predict—and the quality of child care positively predict—qualities of mother–child interaction over the first 3 years of life? (2) Are associations between child care and mother–child interaction similar across the first 3 years of life or do they change over time? (3) Do relations between child care and mother–child interaction differ for families who vary by income or by mothers' symptoms of depression?

METHOD

Participants

A description of the participants is available in Chapter 1. Mother–child interaction data collected when the children were 6, 15, 24, and 36 months old were available for 1,272, 1,240, 1,150, and 1,139 families, respectively. Compared with families with at least one observation of mother–child interaction, those who dropped out following the 1-month recruitment visit had lower maternal education and higher maternal separation anxiety; they were also more likely to be without partners and African American. Compared with families who completed all four observations ($n = 989$), those who were missing one to three observations ($n = 242$) had less income and maternal education, had more maternal symptoms of depression and separation anxiety, perceived their infants to be more difficult, were less likely to be married or living with a domestic partner, and were more likely to be an ethnic minority (African American or Hispanic). All comparisons noted were significant at $p < .01$.

Children who spent 10 or more hours per week in nonmaternal care were eligible to be observed in child care. Of those eligible, 78.6% were observed at 6 months, 77.4% at 15 months, 85.8% at 24 months, and 90.3% at 36 months. Compared with those who were eligible but not observed in child care (all differences were significant at $p < .01$), families in the observed sample had higher incomes, the mothers had higher education, and the children experienced more hours of care and were more likely to be in less formal child care.

Overview of Data Collection

An overview of data collection is available in Chapter 1.

Dependent Measures

Mother–Child Interaction

Mother–child interaction was videotaped in semistructured 15-minute observations at each age. The observation task at the 6-month visit had two components. In the first 7 minutes, mothers were asked to play with their infants and were told that they could use any toy or object available in the home or none at all; for the remaining 8 minutes, mothers were given a standard set of toys they could use in play. At 15, 24, and 36 months, the observation procedures followed a three-boxes procedure in which mothers were asked to show their children age-appropriate toys in three containers in a set order (see Vandell, 1979).

Data were collected across the 10 sites by research assistants who attended a common training meeting prior to the visits at 6, 15, 24, and 36 months. Each data collector passed certification procedures based on a common certifier's review of videotapes of the data collector administering the procedures. The videotapes of mother–child interaction were shipped to a central, non–data collection location for coding. Coders were blind as to other information about the families.

Mother–child interaction at 6, 15, and 24 months was rated on 4-point global rating scales developed for this study; 7-point rating scales were used at 36 months. To reduce the number of variables analyzed and to characterize mother–child interaction parsimoniously, we formed *a priori* composites of maternal care and child engagement of mother from the individual ratings.

The maternal sensitivity composite was formed at 6, 15, and 24 months from the sum of sensitivity to nondistress, intrusiveness (reverse-scored), and positive regard. The maternal sensitivity composite at 36 months was formed from the sum of supportive presence, hostility (reverse-scored), and respect for autonomy. Composite scores ranged from 3 to 12 at 6, 15, and 24 months and from 4 to 21 at 36 months. Cronbach's alphas for the maternal sensitivity composites were .75, .70, .74, and .78 at 6, 15, 24, and 36 months, respectively.

The child positive engagement composite at 15 and 24 months was the sum of child engagement and positive mood. At 36 months the child positive engagement composite was the sum of child affection to mother and negativity (reverse-scored). Cronbach's alphas for the child engagement composites at 15, 24, and 36 months were .58, .74, and .78, respectively.

Intercoder reliability was determined by assigning two coders to 19–20 % of the tapes randomly drawn at each assessment period. Coders were unaware of which tapes among their assignments were assigned to second coders, and reliability assessments were made throughout the period of coding. Intercoder reliability was calculated as the intraclass correlation (Winer, 1971). Correlations for the maternal sensitivity composites were .87, .83, .84, and .84 at 6, 15, 24, and 36 months, respectively. Correlations for the child composites were .74, .70, and .77 at 15, 24, and 36 months.

Stability of Dependent Variables over Time

Correlations between maternal sensitivity composites at different ages were moderately strong and ranged from .39 (from 6 months to 15 months) to .48 (from 24 months to 36 months). The correlation between maternal sensitivity composites at 6 and 36 months was .42; the correlation between 15 and 36 months was .41. All correlations were highly significant (p's < .0001). The correlation between child engagement composites at 15 and 36 months was .15; at 15 and 24 months, .25; and at 24 and 36 months, .27. These correlations were also all highly significant (p's < .0001) but indicated only modest relations over time.

Correlations between maternal sensitivity and child engagement were moderately strong at each age (correlations ranged from .43 at 15 months to .60 at 36 months). Despite the strength of these relations between maternal and child behavior, we examined maternal and child behavior in separate analyses of the effects of child care to determine whether associations between child care and mother–child interaction may derive from effects on the child's or mother's behavior.

Child Care Predictors

At 3-month intervals, starting when the infants were 3 months old, mothers were telephoned and asked about their current child care arrangement; information from this call was gathered about the amount and stability of care. For amount of care, averages for weekly hours of care were determined for the following age epochs: 0–6 months, 7–15 months, 16–24 months, and 25–36 months. Children who received no child care during an epoch received scores of zero. The variable of interest was labeled "hours." Stability of nonmaternal care arrangements was indexed by mothers' reports of arrangements that were started across the epochs of interest. The variable of interest was labeled "starts."

Quality of child care was assessed at 6, 15, 24, and 36 months for children spending at least 10 hours per week in a regular, nonmaternal care arrangement. Observations of the sensitivity, involvement, and stimulation provided by caregivers in nonmaternal care settings were conducted on 2 half days that were scheduled within a 2-week interval. During these sessions, observers used the Observational Record of the Caregiving Environment (ORCE; see NICHD Early Child Care Research Network, 1996). Chapter 3 describes data collection using the ORCE. Quality of care was indexed by a composite denoting positive caregiving on the basis of the sum of five of the 4-point qualitative ratings: sensitivity to nondistress signals, stimulation of cognitive development, positive regard expressed to the child, detachment (reverse-scored), and flatness of affect (reverse-scored), with fostering exploration and intrusiveness (reverse-scored) added to the 36-month composite. The quality-of-care index was formed from this composite and was averaged over the four cycles of observation at each age. Cronbach's alphas for the quality composites were .89, .88, .86, and .82 at 6, 15, 24, and 36 months, respectively. The quality composites had very good interobserver reliability with "gold standard" videotapes (.94, .86, .81, and .80) and with other observers in the field at all ages (.90, .89, .89, and .90).

Covariates

Covariation between child care parameters and outcomes could be an artifact of the association between family selection factors and both child care and outcome variables. In the present analyses, we used covariates to minimize this confound. We examined three forms of covariates: selection, child, and family variables.

Selection (Control) Variables

These variables had to meet two criteria: (1) significant correlations with at least two of the three child care dimensions (hours, quality, starts) and one of the two dependent measures at 6, 15, 24, and 36 months and (2) conceptual distinctness. Two out of eight candidate variables met our criteria for selection variables: income-to-needs ratio and maternal education (measurement of these constructs is described in Chapter 7).

Family and Child Covariates

We also controlled for child and family factors that have been demonstrated to be associated with mother–child interaction. Our interest was in estimating the increment of variance in mother–child interaction associated with child care features over and above variance attributable to these predictors. Child variables included the mother's report of difficult child temperament at 6 months and child gender. Family variables included marital/partnered status, maternal depressive symptoms, and maternal separation anxiety. Chapter 7 contains information concerning these measures. Table 17.1 presents means and standard deviations for all measures included in the analyses.

RESULTS

Data Analysis

Controlling for selection, child, and family variables, we analyzed the relations between features of child care and mother–child interaction at 6, 15, 24, and 36 months by means of a repeated-measures general linear mixed-model analysis (Jenrich & Schluchter, 1986; Laird & Ware, 1982). We tested the extent to which mother and child interaction qualities varied as a function of selected demographic, child, family, and child care factors and whether those patterns of association changed over time. The repeated-measures analyses fit a separate regression model to the outcome variable at each age under the assumption that there was a common covariance structure over time. For example, the first regression model analyzing maternal sensitivity described the relations between the predictors and maternal sensitivity as measured in the first 6 months, the second model described the relations between the predictors and maternal sensitivity as measured between 6 and 15 months, and so on. We tested whether parameter estimates for each predictor varied significantly over time and, if they did not, computed the main-effect parameter estimates for each predictor as the

TABLE 17.1. Means of Variables in Longitudinal Regression Analysis: Whole Sample and Sample Observed in Child Care

| | \multicolumn{8}{c}{Child age (in months)} | | | | | | | |
| | 6 | | 15 | | 24 | | 36 | |
Measure	M	SD	M	SD	M	SD	M	SD
\multicolumn{9}{c}{Whole sample}								
Dependent variables								
Maternal sensitivity	9.21	1.78	9.41	1.64	9.44	1.73	17.32	2.72
Child engagement	—		5.01	1.11	5.61	1.22	11.18	1.99
Selection variables								
income-to-needs ratio	3.67	3.11	3.71	3.20	3.81	3.07	3.71	3.10
Maternal education	14.31	2.50	14.36	2.48	14.50	2.43	14.53	2.44
Child variables								
Child gender	0.52	0.50	0.51	0.50	0.51	0.50	0.51	0.50
Temperament	3.18	0.40	3.18	0.40	3.16	0.40	3.16	0.40
Family variables								
Marital/partnered status	0.86	0.35	0.86	0.35	0.87	0.34	0.85	0.35
Maternal depression	8.98	8.31	9.02	8.14	9.33	8.62	8.88	8.06
Separation anxiety	66.40	13.82	64.94	13.51	63.15	13.66	63.28	13.67
Child care								
Hours[a]	15.19	14.10	24.02	18.81	25.11	18.59	25.48	18.64
\multicolumn{9}{c}{Sample observed in child care}								
Dependent variables								
Maternal sensitivity	9.29	1.83	9.53	1.56	9.59	1.67	17.42	2.55
Child engagement	—		5.07	1.11	5.64	1.18	11.20	1.96
Selection variables								
Income-to-needs ratio	4.39	3.30	4.28	3.40	4.38	3.29	4.17	3.45
Maternal education	14.82	2.46	14.74	2.45	14.89	2.35	14.77	2.48
Child variables								
Child gender	0.52	0.50	0.52	0.50	0.50	0.50	0.50	0.50
Temperament	3.14	0.37	3.15	0.38	3.13	0.38	3.12	0.37
Family variables								
Marital/partnered status	0.88	0.32	0.87	0.34	0.88	0.33	0.84	0.36
Maternal depression	8.35	7.52	8.19	7.18	8.97	8.24	8.71	8.09
Separation anxiety	62.99	13.05	62.49	12.91	60.61	12.54	61.47	12.78
Child care								
Hours[a]	23.80	11.22	34.03	14.79	33.52	15.21	33.21	15.39
Quality	14.92	2.82	14.67	2.85	14.12	2.80	19.66	3.27
Starts[b]	1.80	1.02	1.37	1.37	1.15	1.22	1.56	1.53

Note. Dashes indicate that child engagement was not rated at 6 months.
[a]Mean hours of care across epochs: 0–6 months, 7–15 months, 16–24 months, 25–36 months.
[b]Number of child care arrangements started across epochs: 0–6 months, 7–15 months, 16–24 months, 25–36 months.

average of the age-specific parameters for that predictor. This main-effect parameter for each predictor reflects the across-time association between that variable (e.g., child care hours) and the mother–child interaction variable (e.g., maternal sensitivity) when all other predictors are at their mean values.

Results are presented separately for the whole sample (Table 17.2) and for the sample observed in care (Table 17.3). For the whole sample (including children with less than 10 hours per week of child care) and for the sample observed in care, both maternal sensitivity (at 6, 15, 24, and 36 months) and child positive engagement (at 15, 24, and 36 months) were predicted with the models described previously. In Tables 17.2 and 17.3, the statistical tests and estimates of effects are organized by blocks pertaining to the selection, child, family, and child care variables. The test at the block level tested the joint contribution of all the variables in that block in this simultaneous regression. The individual parameter estimates were interpreted only if the overall block test was significant. Results at the block level (F and p values) appear in bold typeface. At the level of individual parameters, coefficients for a given variable were averaged across age and are presented in Tables 17.2 and 17.3. The F and p values are also reported for the terms representing the interactions of the predictors with time (e.g., time × income-to-needs) that reflect whether the relation of that parameter and the dependent measure differed across the time points at which assessments were made. In the case of a significant interaction involving time, the parameter estimates at each time period are reported in the text, and the results of pairwise contrasts between parameters are described. In follow-up analyses, we determined that there were no significant interactions of child care variables with maternal depressive symptoms or income-to-needs; these are not discussed further.

Tables 17.2 and 17.3 also report the coefficients when all variables in the analyses were standardized to have a mean of 0 and a standard deviation of 1 across time. Thus, coefficients can be interpreted in terms of the relative magnitude they reflect in predicting the mother–child interaction dependent measures in the presence of the other predictors in the model.

Child Care and Mother–Child Interaction in the Whole Sample

Table 17.2 reports results involving analyses of the whole sample; results are shown for maternal sensitivity and for child positive engagement. Final model coefficients are reported for models including the selection, child, family, and child care variables. Data collection site and time (i.e., age of assessment) were also included in all models as covariates.

For maternal sensitivity, there were significant effects, at the block level, for the selection, child, family, and child care blocks. There was a sig-

TABLE 17.2. Results of the Repeated-Measures Regression Model for the Whole Sample

Variable	Maternal sensitivity			Child positive engagement		
	F	β	*SE*	*F*	β	*SE*
Site	4.33***			0.84		
Time	0.63			0.26		
Selection	**31.93***			**7.73***		
Income-to-needs ratio		.082***	.020		.066***	.023
Maternal education		.250**	.020		.102***	.024
Time × income	.014			2.57		
Time × education	1.29			0.56		
Child	**3.00**			**4.47***		
Gender (male)		−.063***	.017		−.082***	.019
Temperament		.051**	.018		−.032	.020
Time × gender	1.22			1.85		
Time × temperament	0.25			2.50		
Family	**7.84***			**5.59***		
Maternal depression		−.048**	.015		−.062**	.019
Marital/partnered status		.088***	.017		.043***	.021
Separation anxiety		−.088***	.018		−.081***	.021
Time × depression	1.76			1.89		
Time marital/partnered status	2.63*			4.95*		
Time × separation anxiety	2.06			0.33		
Child care	**3.45***			**3.35***		
Hours		−.048**	.017		−.062**	.020
Time × hours	2.17			0.30		

Note. Results at the block level appear in **boldface**.
* $p < .05$; ** $p < .01$; *** $p < .001$.

nificant main effect for hours of care. Controlling for site, time, selection, child, and family predictors, we found that mothers were more sensitive when their children were in fewer hours of child care. The child care hours × time interaction was not significant.

Significant effects within the selection, child, and family blocks of variables indicated that mothers were more sensitive when families had greater income-to-needs ratios, mothers were more educated, children were female and were described as having easier temperaments, mothers were less depressed and had less separation anxiety, and mothers had a spouse or a domestic partner. There was a significant interaction between time and marital/partnered status in predicting maternal sensitivity such that there was a significant relation between having a spouse or domestic partner and higher sensitivity at 15, 24, and 36 months (betas = .093, .093, and .134, respectively), whereas the relation between marital/partnered status and sensitivity at 6 months (beta = .030, NS) was significantly less than that at 36 months. Results for child positive engagement were very similar (see Table 17.2).

Child Care and Mother–Child Interaction in the Sample Observed in Child Care

The next set of analyses involved the subsample of children with more than 10 hours per week (on average) of nonmaternal care who were observed in their child care arrangements. These analyses differed from those just reported in that child care features included hours, quality, and number of arrangements, as well as interactions between child care hours and quality. Table 17.3 reports results involving analyses of the observed-in-care sample.

For maternal sensitivity, there were significant effects, at the block level, for the selection, family, and child care blocks but not for the child variables. For the prediction of maternal sensitivity from the features of

TABLE 17.3. Results of the Repeated-Measures Regression Model for the Observed-in-Care Sample

Variable	Maternal sensitivity			Child positive engagement		
	F	β	SE	F	β	SE
Site	3.39***			0.90		
Time	1.14			1.06		
Selection	**17.71***			**4.37***		
Income-to-needs ratio		.077**	.024		.073*	.028
Maternal education		.237***	.026		.084**	.031
Time × income	0.28			1.13		
Time × education	1.58			1.07		
Child	**0.89**			**1.73**		
Gender (male)		−.040	.022		−.046	.025
Temperament		−.031	.024		−.014	.027
Time × gender	0.37			1.13		
Time × temperament	0.42			2.42		
Family	**4.53***			**2.31***		
Maternal depression		−.049*	.021		−.065*	.027
Marital/partnered status		.080***	.021		.019	.027
Separation anxiety		−.076**	.024		−.065*	.029
Time × depression	3.35*			0.51		
Time × marital/partnered status	0.25			1.01		
Time × separation anxiety	0.80			1.23		
Child care	**1.73***			**1.95***		
Hours		−.050	.027		−.080*	.031
Starts		−.035	.019		−.040	.025
Quality		.050*	.023		.038	.028
Quality × hours	2.64			0.08		
Time × hours	0.83			1.23		
Time × number	0.24			2.00		
Time × quality	1.44			0.70		
Time × hours × quality	0.56			0.11		

Note. Results at the block level appear in **boldface**.
* $p < .05$; ** $p < .01$; *** $p < .001$.

child care, higher observed quality of child care was related to more maternal sensitivity. Child care hours and starts were not significant; however, it should be noted that the coefficient estimate for hours of care, though not significant in this subsample (beta = –.050), $t(1458) = 1.89$, $p = .059$, was nearly identical to the coefficient estimate for hours of care predicting maternal sensitivity in the whole sample (beta = –.048), $t(3260) = 3.61$, $p = .005$. Interactions of child care features with time of measurement were not significant, nor was the interaction between child care hours and child care quality.

The significant selection and family predictors of maternal sensitivity indicated that mothers were more sensitive when the family income-to-needs ratio was greater, maternal education was higher, maternal depressive symptoms and separation anxiety were lower, and mothers were married or living with a domestic partner. There was a significant interaction between time and maternal depressive symptoms in predicting maternal sensitivity such that there was a significant negative relation between maternal depressive symptoms and sensitivity at 36 months only (beta = –.106, $p < .05$), and the relation between maternal depressive symptoms and sensitivity at 6 months (beta = .054, NS) was significantly less than at 36 months.

For child positive engagement (see Table 17.3), the selection, family, and child care blocks added significant increments in explained variance, as they did for maternal sensitivity. In the significant prediction from child care variables, children were more positively engaged with their mothers when they attended child care for fewer hours. Child care quality and number of arrangements were not significant predictors of child positive engagement, nor were any of the interaction terms involving time and the child care variables.

According to the significant selection and family variables, children were more positively engaged with their mothers when the family income-to-needs ratio and maternal education were higher and maternal depressive symptoms and separation anxiety were lower. The mother's status as married or living with a domestic partner was not related to child engagement in the subsample observed in care. There were no significant interactions involving time with any of the selection, child, or family variables, nor were there any significant interactions between child care variables and maternal depressive symptoms or income-to-needs.

Type of Care

The aforementioned analyses of the subsample observed in care were rerun with type of care as a covariate in order to examine the extent to which the setting in which the child received nonmaternal care qualified the findings reported above. Type of care (child care home, center, and relative in home) was dummy-coded and entered in the model with the remaining variables. In no case did the presence of type of care change the findings reported earlier.

Ethnicity

The primary longitudinal analyses described above for the relations between features of child care and mother–child interaction were also rerun to examine whether the model results were different for white, non-Hispanic families and nonwhite, non-Hispanic families. The results reported earlier for the relations between child care and mother–child interaction are consistent across white, non-Hispanic and nonwhite, non-Hispanic families.

Relative Magnitude of Effects

To aid in interpreting the regression results, we computed predicted values for maternal sensitivity and child engagement in their original metrics from contrasting levels of child care hours and quality to illustrate differences in the mother–child interaction measures at similar levels of quality and hours. Predicted values for maternal sensitivity and child engagement were computed from child care hours and quality when they were significant in the regression models, adjusting in each case for all other variables in the models. For the whole sample, values for maternal sensitivity and child engagement were computed in terms of z-score units comparable to 0 and 40 hours of child care. For the observed-in-care sample, values were computed in z-score units comparable to 20 and 40 hours of child care (the child care sample all had more than 10 hours per week in child care); levels of quality were computed at –1 and +1 (standardized). We chose +1 and –1 standard deviations because there was no *a priori* level established for good- or poor-quality child care. The levels chosen for hours of care represented no care, part-time care, and full-time care.

We also computed predicted values of sensitivity and child engagement at comparable levels of maternal education, depressive symptoms, and child difficult temperament to allow comparisons of child care with predicted differences associated with each of these predictors. For example, we computed predicted means at the levels of maternal education of 11.2 and 16.9 years because these values had z scores in the sample distribution that were comparable to the z scores for child care hours of 0 and 40.

Table 17.4 shows the predicted adjusted means in the original metric for the sensitivity and child engagement measures from each predictor. The predicted values are presented for the 6-month and 36-month maternal sensitivity measures and for the 36-month child engagement measure (there was no 6-month engagement measure); recall that the significant child care predictors in the earlier regression analyses did not differ significantly by age.

TABLE 17.4. Predicted Adjusted Means of Mother–Child Interaction Associated with Selected Differences in Levels of Child Care Hours and Quality and Comparable Differences in Other Maternal and Child Predictors

Variable	Child care	Maternal		Child difficult temperament
		Education	Depression	
		Whole sample		
Sensitivity	Hours			
6 months				
0 hr	9.34	9.76	9.34	9.35
40 hr	9.10	8.52	9.10	9.09
36 months				
0 hr	17.52	18.17	17.52	17.53
40 hr	17.15	16.27	17.15	17.14
Child engagement	Hours			
36 months				
0 hr	11.34	11.38	11.26	11.28
40 hr	11.04	10.88	11.04	11.10
		Observed sample		
Sensitivity	Quality			
6 months				
– 1 quality	9.05	8.63	9.05	9.09
+ 1 quality	9.28	9.70	9.27	9.23
36 months				
– 1 quality	17.05	16.41	17.06	17.12
+ 1 quality	17.40	18.04	17.40	17.33
Child engagement	Hours			
36 months				
20 hr	11.23	11.37	11.22	11.20
40 hr	11.04	11.16	11.07	11.17

Note. Estimates were made for child care features that were significant in the repeated measures regressions. Estimated values were in the original scoring of the mother–child interaction variables (e.g., translated back to the maternal sensitivity scale at 6 months and the sensitivity and child engagement scales at 36 months).

DISCUSSION

In analyses controlling for family and child factors related both to the selection of child care and to qualities of mother–child interaction, child care features (hours and quality) were significant predictors in the present sample of mother–child interaction during the children's first 3 years of life. Before discussing and interpreting these findings, we note that the size of the sample provides considerable power for the detection of fairly small effects. Our analyses describing predicted values for mother–child interaction at varying levels of child care hours or quality attest to the small magnitude of the significant effects reported, particularly relative to mothers' education. The meaningfulness of these effects rests on the extent to which such small degrees of difference in maternal sensitivity or the child's engagement with the mother relate to meaningful differences in children's developmental outcomes at these and later ages. They may not. Nonetheless, when selection, child, and parental factors are taken into account, the findings indicate nonchance associations between child care hours and quality and aspects of mother–child interaction through the first 3 years of life.

Small, nonchance associations indicating that more hours in child care were related to less positive aspects of mother–child interaction are consistent with our hypotheses and with findings from some less well-controlled studies and studies with smaller samples that focused on the first year of life (e.g., Campbell, Cohn, & Meyers, 1995; Clark, Hyde, Essex, & Klein, 1997; Owen & Cox, 1988). The present study expands this pattern of results through 3 years of age. It is important to note that these associations did not differ significantly across ages of assessment.

Additional features of child care—specifically, the observed quality and stability of the care—could be examined for the children who were in child care more than 10 hours per week and observed in those arrangements. In this subsample, with the addition of these features of child care to the tested models, the effects of hours of care were examined with effects of quality and stability of care held constant. For children in regular child care, their interaction with their mothers was again somewhat less positive when they spent more hours in nonmaternal care. Maternal sensitivity was not significantly associated with child care hours in this subsample as it was in the whole sample. Thus, for children in more than 10 hours of care per week, variation in the amount of care related to the quality of mother–child interactions primarily as a function of the child's engagement with the mother and not of the mother's behavior toward the child.

That high-quality child care was associated with a small degree of increased maternal sensitivity but not with more positive child engagement suggests that the use of higher-quality child care may provide the mother with positive role models for involved caregiving (e.g., Cotterell, 1986; Edwards, Logue, Loehr, & Roth, 1986) or emotional support (Barnett, Marshall, & Singer, 1992) that in turn allow her to be more emotionally sensitive to her child. These findings confirmed our expectations of a positive association between child care quality and quality of mother–child interaction.

Stability of care has rarely been studied in relation to mother–child interaction, and in this study it was not related to maternal sensitivity or to child engagement. It should be noted, however, that the stability of child care can be measured in many ways. We focused on the number of child care arrangements the child experienced over time. This measure was not sensitive to changes in caregivers within arrangements. These small but significant associations obtained between child care quantity and quality and aspects of mother–child interaction apply to economically advantaged and disadvantaged families and to those in which mothers are more and less depressed.

Finally, to contextualize the relative importance of child care hours and quality, we compared these predictors with other well-known predictors of mother–child interaction. Maternal education was clearly a much stronger predictor of maternal sensitivity than either child care hours or child care quality. The estimated differences obtained in maternal sensitivity from high and low levels of maternal education comparable to 0 and 40 hours of care represented an approximate 12% relative change in maternal sensitivity, compared with an approximate 2% relative difference attributable to 40 hours of child care. It should be noted that the child care effects on mother–child interaction (for the behavior of mothers and children alike) were on the same order of magnitude as other child and maternal factors (child difficult temperament and maternal depressive symptoms) known to be reliable associates of mother–child interaction processes.

Implications of these findings should also be considered in light of other reports from the NICHD Study of Early Child Care pertaining to the mother–infant relationship (NICHD Early Child Care Research Network, 1997b). Child care, in and of itself, neither adversely affected nor promoted infants' attachment security with their mothers at 15 months of age. Thus, the negative relation between the amount of child care and maternal sensitivity and child engagement with mother reported here is apparently not of a sufficient magnitude to disrupt the formation of a secure infant attachment.

The small differences in mother–child interaction related to child care, although in keeping with theoretical predictions regarding the importance of time together and the value of higher-quality child care for the mother–child relationship, reflect relatively small variations in mother–child interaction. The ultimate long-term impact of such modest effects on children's functioning remains to be determined as these children are followed through their school years.

18

Early Child Care
and Mother–Child Interaction
from 36 Months through First Grade

NICHD EARLY CHILD CARE RESEARCH NETWORK

It is not surprising, in view of the importance attributed to mother's care in cultural ideals and scientific theories (McCartney & Phillips, 1988), that high rates of nonmaternal care usage—beginning in infancy and continuing throughout the preschool years—have fostered disagreement about how such early experience may affect the developing mother–child relationship (e.g., Belsky, 1986, 2001; Clarke-Stewart, 1988). Two bodies of research have emerged addressing this issue, one focused on the security of infant–mother attachment and the other on patterns of mother–child interaction. This chapter focuses on patterns of mother–child interaction, not just because it addresses both the child's and mother's side of the relationship but because mother–child interaction patterns prove to be significant predictors of a variety of developmental outcomes (e.g., Bornstein & Tamis-LeMonda, 1989; Pianta & Egeland, 1994; Rogoff, Mistry, Goncu, & Mosier, 1993). Most research on child care and mother–child interaction has focused on the amount of nonmaternal care that children experience. This is because several developmentalists have theorized that time away from the child may undermine the mother's capacity to get to know her child well and thus provide sensitive, responsive, and growth-facilitating care (Brazelton, 1986; Sroufe, 1988; Vaughn, Gove, & Egeland, 1980). The most comprehensive investigation of this issue to date was carried out as part of the National Institute of Child Health and Human Development (NICHD) Study of Early Child Care (Chapter 17). The primary purpose of this chapter is to extend this research and ask whether the effects of early child care on mother–child interaction discerned through age 3 are maintained, amplified, or attenuated as children experience the transition to school.

Despite widespread appreciation of the importance of high-quality child care for promoting child well-being, the relation between this dimension of child care experience and mother–child interaction has rarely been a focus of inquiry. Nevertheless, prevailing views regarding the consequences of higher- and lower-quality child care on both children and parents lead to the expectation that more sensitive, supportive mothering and more positive child responsiveness should be associated with higher-quality of child care experience. Specifically, especially as children develop and become increasingly active contributors to the mother–child dyad, better-quality early child care experience could enhance patterns of mother–child interaction via its effect on children's developing competencies (NICHD Early Child Care Research Network, 1999a, 2002a) and perhaps via contributions to children's expectations of responsive care from adults. Benefits of higher-quality child care for mother–child interaction may also ensue when caregivers offer particularly good models of sensitive and supportive nurturance of the children in their care. We found support for the hypothesis that quality of child care matters for mother–child interaction in our earlier examination of mother–child interaction across the child's first 3 years (Chapter 17). Although we did not find instability of child care to be related to mother–child interactions in children's first 3 years in our earlier report, longer-term benefits or risks of child care experiences may relate to the stability of the early child care arrangements.

Early child care could have positive effects on family processes in some families and negative effects in others (e.g., Bronfenbrenner & Crouter, 1982; Desai, Chase-Lansdale, & Michael, 1989; Hoffman, 1989). Although there was no clear evidence in our earlier report through age 3 for differential effects of child care by maternal depression, low income, or child ethnicity, this chapter examines whether these indicators of family risk moderate the longitudinal effects of early child care experiences in the first 3 years on mother–child interaction across the transition to school.

In summary, to examine the relation between early child care experiences of young children and the mother–child relationship, data from the NICHD Study of Early Child Care were used to address three related questions: (1) Do children's child care histories with respect to amount, quality, and stability of child care in the first 3 years predict qualities of mother–child interaction from age 3 through first grade? (2) Are associations between cumulative early child care experience ages 0–3 and mother–child interaction through first grade similar across this period that crosses the transition to school, or do they change over time? (3) Are associations between early child care and mother–child interaction across the transition to school moderated by maternal depressive symptoms, low family income, and child ethnicity?

METHOD

Participants

A detailed description of the participants is provided in Chapter 1. For families included in the present analyses, mean years of mothers' education was 14.43 years (SD = 2.46). Average income-to-needs ratio was 3.47 (SD = 2.47) when the child was 3 years old and 3.72 (SD = 2.50) when the child was in first grade. The vast majority of families had a male partner living in the home (84% when the child was 3 and 81% when the child was in first grade); at first grade, 78% of the children were white, non-Hispanic and 22% were nonwhite (11% African American, 6% Hispanic, and 5% other). Number of hours per week in child care across the child's first 3 years ranged from 0 to more than 50. Among families whose child was in child care for at least 10 hours per week (74% of the study participants in the infant's first year), amount of child care averaged 24 hours per week from 0 to 6 months, 34 hours from 7 to 15 months, 34 hours from 16 to 24 months, and 33 hours from 25 to 36 months.

Mother–child interaction data at 36 months, 54 months, and in first grade were available for 1,148, 1,027, and 992 families, respectively. Compared with families with at least one observation of mother–child interaction at these ages, those not observed had lower maternal education, income, and higher maternal separation anxiety and depressive symptoms; they were also more likely to be without partners (26% vs. 12%) and nonwhite (35% vs. 22%). The families that were not included in the present study analyses did not differ from those included in terms of maternal sensitivity at 6 months, child temperament at 6 months, or child gender.

Children who spent 10 or more hours per week in nonmaternal care at major data collection periods were observed in child care at those ages to assess child care quality. Of those eligible to be observed, 78.6% were observed at 6 months, 77.4% at 15 months, 85.8% at 24 months, and 90.3% at 36 months. Compared with those who were eligible but not observed in child care, families in the observed sample had higher incomes, the mothers had higher education, and the children experienced more hours of care and were more likely to be in less formal child care.

Mother–Child Interaction Measures

Mother–child interaction was videotaped in semistructured 15-minute observations at each age. In the observation task at 36 months mothers were asked to show their children age-appropriate toys in three containers in a set order. The mother was instructed to have her child play with the toys in each of the three containers. At 54 months and in first grade, interaction activities included two tasks that were too difficult for the child to carry out independently and required the parent's instruction and assistance. In addition, a third activity was included that encouraged play between mother and child. The videotapes of mother–child interaction were shipped to a central, non-data collection location for coding. Coders were blind to other information about the families. Mother–child interaction was rated using 7-point global rating scales. The maternal rating scales included mothers' supportive presence, respect for the child's autonomy, stimulation of cognitive development, quality of assistance, and hostility. Child behavior rating scales included enthusiasm/agency in the tasks, negativity (expressed toward the mother), persistence (orientation to the tasks in the session), affection for mother (at 36 months and first grade; positive orientation to mother and sharing of positive affect), positive experience of the session (at 54 months; child's positive feelings of doing well and having a good relationship with parent), and affective mutuality (reciprocated, shared feelings support mutuality in the dyad). Coders rated both maternal and child behavior from a single viewing.

A *priori* composites of maternal sensitivity and child engagement of mother were formed from the individual ratings. The maternal sensitivity composite represented affectively positive, nonintrusive, respectful, responsive and supportive maternal care. It was formed at each age from the sum of the ratings for supportive presence, hostility (reverse-scored), and respect for autonomy. Cronbach's alphas for the maternal sensitivity composites were 0.78 at 36 months, 0.84 at 54 months, and 0.82 at first grade.

The child positive engagement composite at 36 months was the sum of child affection to mother and negativity (reverse-scored). At 54 months it was the sum of experience of the session, felt security, and negativity (reverse-scored). The child positive engagement composite from first-grade ratings was the sum of affection to mother, felt security, and negativity (reverse-scored). Cronbach's alphas for the engagement composites at 36 months, 54 months, and first grade were 0.78, 0.82, and 0.80, respectively. Intercoder reliability for the maternal sensitivity composites (intraclass correlations) was 0.84, 0.88, and 0.91 at 36 months, 54 months, and first grade, respectively. Reliability for the child composites were 0.77, 0.82, and 0.80.

Stability of Dependent Variables over Time

Correlations between maternal sensitivity composites at different ages were moderately strong and ranged from .49 to .52, which were somewhat higher correlations than found among sensitivity ratings across the child's first 3 years (Chapter 17). The correlations over time for the child positive engagement composites ranged from .22 (between 36 months and first grade) to .32 (between 54 months and first grade). Correlations of child engagement composites over time in the first 3 years ranged from .15 to .27. All reported stability correlations are highly significant ($p < .001$). Correlations between maternal sensitivity and child engagement were moderately strong at each age (r's ranged from .60 at 36 months to .62 in first grade).

Child Care Variables

Although the substantive findings in this chapter pertain to the study of early nonmaternal care experiences, which include father care among the types of child care, results of follow-up analyses excluding father care from the measures of child care are also provided. The *amount* of child care across the child's first 3 years was the mean hours of nonmaternal child care per week during each month from 0 to 36 months gathered from maternal report. *Instability* of child care in the first 3 years was indexed by the mother's report of the number of nonmaternal care arrangements that were started from 0 to 36 months. *Quality* of child care experienced over the child's first 3 years was assessed from observations of nonmaternal child care at 6, 15, 24, and 36 months for children spending at least 10 hours per week in a regular nonmaternal care arrangement using the Observational Record of the Caregiving Environment (ORCE; see Chapters 3 and 6 for a detailed description). Quality of care was indexed by a composite denoting positive caregiving based on the sum of five of the 4-point qualitative ratings: sensitivity to nondistress signals, stimulation of cognitive development, positive regard expressed to the child, detachment (reverse-scored), and flatness of affect (reverse-scored), with fostering exploration and intrusiveness (reverse-scored) added to the 36-month composite. In analyses for this chapter, quality of child care was the mean quality of child care from 6 to 36 months from these ORCE quality composite ratings.

Covariates

Covariates included were the same set used in the earlier report of relations between child care experience and mother–child interaction (see Chapter 17). Covariates included were site of data collection, family income, maternal education, marital/partnered status of the mother, maternal depressive symptoms, maternal separation anxiety, child gender, difficult temperament, and ethnicity.

RESULTS

Data Analysis Plan

Relations between features of child care in the first 3 years and mother–child interaction at 36 and 54 months and in first grade, controlling for child and family variables, were analyzed using a repeated-measures general linear mixed-model analysis (Jenrich & Schluchter, 1986; Laird & Ware,

1982). We tested the extent to which mother and child interaction qualities varied as a function of selected demographic, child, family, and early child care factors and whether those patterns of association changed over time (36 months, 54 months, and first grade). Separate intercepts were estimated for each individual, with the assumption that across-time assessments are correlated. Separate variances and correlations for each repeated assessment were estimated. The model included both time-varying predictors (income, depressive symptoms, marital/partner presence in household) and between-subject predictors (site, maternal education, child gender, child temperament, child ethnicity, maternal separation anxiety, early child care hours, early child care quality, and early child care instability). Covariates in the model are similar to those tested in the earlier report of mother–child interaction in the first 3 years with the exception of the addition of child ethnicity.

Interactions among certain variables were tested by adding them simultaneously to the model: quality × hours of child care, maternal depressive symptoms × each child care variable, income × each child care variable, and child ethnicity × each child care variable.

Results are presented for maternal sensitivity (Table 18.1) and for child positive engagement of mother (Table 18.3) separately. Two samples were tested, the whole sample ($n = 1,180$), which includes children with no early child care experience, and the subsample (895 of 1,180) of children who were observed in child care in their first 3 years. Results are reported in detail only from the analyses of the subsample observed in early child care. Findings with respect to associations with amount of care in the whole sample analyses (the only child care parameter examined in the whole sample analyses) are described to provide comparison and elaboration to findings with respect to the amount of early child care reported from the child care sample analyses. Associations between mother–child interaction and the family and child covariates were very similar across the sets of analyses and thus are reported only for the child care sample analyses.

In the tables presenting these results, the statistical tests and estimates of effects are organized by blocks pertaining to the demographic, child, and family covariates and the child care variables. The child care block is presented at the top of the tables. Tests at the block level tested the joint contribution of all the variables in that block with all other variables in the model controlled in this simultaneous regression. At the level of individual parameters, coefficients for a given variable are presented over time and for each age predicted. F and p values are reported for tests of main effects of each predictor and of interactions of the predictors with time (e.g., time × maternal depression). In the case of a significant interaction with time, the results of pairwise contrasts between parameters at the different ages are indicated in the table and described below. When interactions with time were not significant, tests of significance for the parameter at each age are not indicated. For interactions between hours and quality of care, and between depression and child care, income and child care, and child ethnicity and child care variables, only significant interactions are shown in the tables.

Tables report the coefficients when all variables in the analyses are standardized to have mean = 0 and standard deviation = 1 across time. Thus, coefficients can be interpreted in terms of the relative magnitude they reflect in predicting the mother–child interaction dependent measures in the presence of the other predictors in the model.

Child Care and Maternal Sensitivity

Amount of Early Child Care

Although hours of early child care in the first 3 years, as a main effect, did not predict maternal sensitivity (after controlling for other predictors) in the sample observed in child care, a significant interaction between hours and ethnicity was found in the prediction of maternal sensitivity (which was not further qualified by time). Regression coefficients indicated a significantly positive effect of hours of care on maternal sensitivity through first grade for nonwhite children, but no significant association of sensitivity with hours for the white sample. Thus, for the non-white sample, more time in child care in the first 3 years significantly predicted greater maternal sensitivity through first grade.

In the analysis of the whole sample, a significant main effect of hours of early child care was found ($F[1, 1, 163] = 3.91$, $p < .05$) as well as an interaction between hours of care and child ethnicity ($F[1, 1, 163] = 6.71$, $p < .01$), though inspection of regression coefficients revealed a somewhat contrasting pattern of results relative to the sample observed in child care. In the case of the whole sample, more time in nonmaternal care predicted less maternal sensitivity for the whole sample (beta = –0.04, $SE = 0.02$, $p < .05$), but more hours in early child care was related to less maternal sensitivity only for white children (beta = –0.07, $SE = 0.02$, $p < .01$) and not for nonwhite children (beta = 0.05, $SE = 0.04$, Ns).

To follow up the significant interactions between hours of care and child ethnicity and to examine patterns of associations between hours of early child care and sensitivity for African American and Hispanic children, the two largest nonwhite groups in the sample, we reran the models classifying child ethnicity as white, African American, Hispanic, and other. The interaction between child ethnicity and hours of child care was again significant in the analyses of the sample observed in early child care ($F[1, 871] = 2.92$, $p < .05$) but nonsignificant in the whole sample.

To further illustrate these predictions of maternal sensitivity from hours of care by child ethnicity from the child care sample and whole sample analyses, Table 18.2 provides predicted values for sensitivity, adjusted for all other predictors in the model, for white children and for African

American, Hispanic, and other nonwhite children who experienced low amounts of child care (defined as the 25th percentile value in our sample distribution; 7.6 hours) and who experienced high hours of care (defined as the 75th percentile value; 35.6 hours). Across the whole sample and the child care sample analyses, high hours of early child care was related to lower maternal sensitivity for the white sample but to higher maternal sensitivity for the nonwhite groups.

In addition, the whole sample analysis of maternal sensitivity contained evidence for a significant interaction of hours of early child care with time ($F[2, 1, 163] = 3.10, p < .05$). Tests of the significance of the hours coefficients at each age indicated that in the whole sample more hours of child care in the first 3 years was related to lower maternal sensitivity at age 3 (beta = $-0.09, p <$ .05) but not at subsequent ages (beta = -0.02, NS, at both ages).

Quality of Child Care

As shown in Table 18.1, early child care quality was significantly associated with maternal sensitivity, with higher-quality child care experience in the first 3 years related to greater maternal sensitivity at 36 months and subsequently through first grade. This main effect of quality, however, was qualified by a significant interaction between quality and quantity of care. Higher-quality early child care was significantly associated with greater maternal sensitivity at low hours of care but not at high hours of care. Mothers were more sensitive across observations at 36 and 54 months, and in first grade when their children experienced higher-quality care and relatively few hours of child care across the first 3 years.

Associations of Sensitivity with Family and Child Factors

Table 18.1 shows predictions of maternal sensitivity from the family and child covariates in the models. Greater sensitivity was related to more maternal education, higher income-to-needs, and white ethnicity. Interactions of the predictors with time indicated significantly less sensitivity with sons than daughters at 36 months but greater sensitivity with sons than daughters in first grade. A significant depression × time interaction indicated that maternal depressive symptoms were associated with significantly less sensitivity at 3 years, but less strongly related at subsequent ages.

Child Care and Child Positive Engagement of Mother

Table 18.3 displays results of the analyses of child engagement of mother. There were no main effects of hours, quality, or stability of child care in the first 3 years on child engagement of mother. Significant interactions of

TABLE 18.1. Results of the Repeated-Measures Regression Model Predicting Maternal Sensitivity (Sample Observed in Early Child Care [n = 895])

	$F_{main}{}^a$	F_{time}	β	β_{36}	β_{54}	β_{G1}
Site	3.62 (9, 875)***					
Child care block	5.52 (5, 875)***					
Child care hours	NS	NS	−0.02 (0.03)	−0.06	0.02	0.03
Child care no. arrangements	NS	NS	0.00 (0.02)	0.004	−0.005	0.014
Child care quality	10.8 (1, 875)**	NS	0.08 (0.02)**	0.09	0.06	0.09
Quality × hours^b	6.99 (1, 875)**	NS				
Quality @ low hours			0.14 (0.04)***	0.16	0.12	0.15
Quality @ high hours			0.02 (0.03)	0.03	−0.00	0.03
Ethnicity (white) × hours	9.11 (1, 875)**	NS				
Hours @ white			−0.06 (0.03)	−0.10	−0.06	−0.01
Hours @ nonwhite			0.13 (0.06)*	0.09	0.13	0.18
Demographics block	56.1 (2, 875)***	NS				
Maternal education	65.3 (1, 875)***	NS	0.23 (0.03)***	0.19	0.22	0.27
Income	10.1 (1, 875)**	NS	0.08 (0.03)**	0.13	0.06	0.07
Child block	23.9 (3, 875)***	4.28 (6, 875)***				
Gender	NS	8.62 (2, 875)***	0.00 (0.05)	−0.14^a	0.01^c	0.14^b
Temperament	NS	NS	−0.01 (0.02)	−0.01	0.00	−0.01
Child ethnicity (white)	69.6 (1, 875)***	4.34 (2, 875)*	0.54 (0.06)***	0.41	0.53	0.68
Family block	NS	2.54 (6, 875)*				
Maternal depression	NS	5.87 (2, 875)**	−0.03 (0.02)	−0.10^{a*}	−0.01^b	0.03^b
Partner in home	NS	NS	0.07 (0.05)	0.13	0.06	0
Separation anxiety	NS	NS	−0.01 (0.03)	−0.03	−0.01	0

Note. Coefficients with different subscripts (a, b) reflect significant changes over time in the association between that predictor and maternal sensitivity; comparisons were tested only when interaction with time was significant.

^{a}F for the effect of the predictor × time.

^{b}Maternal depressive symptoms × child care variables, income × child care variables, and child ethnicity (white vs. nonwhite) × child care variables were added to the model simultaneously; only significant interactions are listed.

*p < .05; **p < .01; ***p < .001.

TABLE 18.2. Predicted Adjusted[a] Values of Maternal Sensitivity Illustrating Significant Interactions in the Regression Models

	Maternal sensitivity			
	Whole sample hours		Sample observed in child care hours	
	Low[b]	High[b]	Low	High
Hours × ethnicity[c]				
Ethnicity				
White	0.17	0.05	0.17	0.06
African American	−0.64	−0.53	−0.68	−0.45
Hispanic	−0.24	−0.07	−0.32	−0.02
Other	−0.41	−0.37	−0.58	−0.37
Quality × hours[d]				
Quality				
Low quality[e]			−0.09	0.11
High quality[e]			−0.03	−0.00

[a]Values adjusted for all other predictors in models.
[b]Low hours = 7.6; high hours = 35.6.
[c]Predicted values from follow-up model with four-way classification of ethnicity.
[d]Predicted values from original model with two-way classification of child ethnicity.
[e]Low quality = 2.58, high quality = 3.1.

hours × child ethnicity and quality × maternal depression indicated conditions under which the amount and quality of early child care were related to child engagement of mother in mother–child interaction.

To interpret the significant ethnicity × hours interactions for child engagement, regression coefficients show (see Table 18.3) that more early child care hours predicted less child engagement of mother through first grade for white children but more positive child engagement through first grade for nonwhite children. A somewhat similar hours by child ethnicity interaction was found in analyses of the whole sample ($F[1, 1, 164] = 5.18$, $p < .05$), with evidence that hours of early child care was negatively related to child engagement of mother for white children but unrelated to child engagement for nonwhite children. For the white sample, children were more positively engaged with their mothers when they experienced few hours of early child care. For the African American and Hispanic groups (examined in the follow-up analyses), children were more positively engaged with their mothers when they experienced more hours of early child care.

The meaning of the significant quality × depression interaction from the child care sample analyses is suggested by the significant regression coefficient for the prediction of child engagement from quality of child care for mothers with high depressive symptoms and the nonsignificant coefficient for the prediction from quality for mothers with low depressive symptoms (see Table 18.3). The benefit of high-quality early child care for child

TABLE 18.3. Results of the Repeated-Measures Regression Model Predicting Child Engagement

	$F_{main}{}^a$	F_{time}	β	β_{36}	β_{54}	β_{G1}
Site	2.53 (9, 876)**					
Child care block	3.64 (5, 876)**					
Child care hours	NS	NS	−0.02 (0.03)	−0.06	0.02	0.00
Child care no. arrangements	NS	NS	0.03 (0.02)	0.01	0.00	0.07
Child care quality	NS	NS	0.04 (0.02)**	0.06	0.01	0.06
White ethnicity × hours[b]	7.46 (1, 876)**	NS				
Hours @ white			−0.06 (0.03)***	−0.09	−0.06	−0.04
Hours @ nonwhite			0.12 (0.06)	0.09	0.12	0.14
Quality × maternal depression	5.45 (1, 876)*	NS				
Quality @ low depression			0.00 (0.03)	0.03	−0.03	0.02
Quality @ high depression			0.07 (0.03)*	0.09	0.03	0.08
Demographics block	12.9 (2, 876)***					
Maternal education	10.2 (1, 876)**	NS	0.09 (0.03)**	0.04	0.10	0.14
Income	5.48 (1, 876)***	NS	0.07 (0.03)*	0.11	0.06	0.03
Child block	6.48 (3, 876)***					
Gender (male)	NS	2.25 (6, 876)*	0.01 (0.05)	−0.17[a]	0.10[b]	0.09[b]
Temperament	NS	6.49 (2, 876)***	−0.01 (0.03)	0.00	−0.02	−0.01
Child ethnicity (white)	18.7 (1, 876)***	NS	0.29 (0.07)***	0.27	0.32	0.29
Family block	3.09 (3, 876)*					
Maternal depression	5.06 (1, 876)*	3.05 (2, 876)**	−0.05 (0.02)*	−0.11[a]	0.06	0.01[b]
Partner in home	NS	NS	0.03 (0.05)	0.10	−0.02	0.02
Separation anxiety	NS	NS	−0.05 (0.03)	−0.06	−0.01	−0.07

Note. Coefficients with different subscripts (a, b) reflect significant changes over time in the association between that predictor and child engagement of mother; comparisons were tested only when the interaction with time was significant.

[a]F for interaction of predictor × time.

[b]Maternal depressive symptoms × child care variables, income × child care variables, and child ethnicity (white) × child care variables were added to the model simultaneously; only significant interactions are listed.

*$p < .05$; **$p < .01$; ***$p < .001$.

256

engagement was seen far more for children of mothers with relatively high numbers of depressive symptoms than for children of mothers with few depressive symptoms. Moreover, the more positive engagement of their mothers by children of depressed mothers when the children had experienced high-quality early child care indicates some buffering of maternal depression on children's engagement of mother. The experience of low-quality early child care adds risk for the child's engagement with mother when mothers have high depressive symptoms.

Significant predictors of child positive engagement of mother from among the covariates in the model (see Table 18.3) indicated that children were more positively engaged with their mothers when family income-to-needs ratios and maternal education were higher, children were female (but only for interactions at age 3), children were white rather than nonwhite, and mothers had fewer depressive symptoms. Predictions from maternal depressive symptoms differed over time; more depressive symptoms were related to less positive child engagement of mother only at age 3.

Follow-Up Analyses Omitting Father Care from Child Care Experience

A final set of follow-up analyses was examined to ask whether the associations between early nonmaternal child care experience and mother–child interaction through first grade would differ if *nonparental* care were the focus of interest. We omitted hours of care by father and recalculated hours of child care to represent hours of care by someone other than the child's mother or father; measures of child care quality were based on observations of nonparental child care experience. This recalculation reduced the sample observed in child care from 895 to 810. When the models were retested with father care excluded, the pattern of significant findings remained the same, with significant interactions between hours of care and child ethnicity, between quality and hours of care, and between quality of care and maternal depression (predicting child engagement). Results of these analyses are available upon request.

DISCUSSION

Very few studies have examined qualities of mother–child interaction longitudinally over several years' time spanning from preschool into the school-age years (Weinfield, Ogawa, & Egeland, 2002). Prior to the present inquiry, questions of the relation between early child care experience or maternal employment and mother–child interaction at different ages have relied primarily on cross-sectional evidence, with only a few exceptions (see Gottfried, Gottfried, & Bathurst, 1995). In this study, findings relating early child care experience to mother–child interaction in the first 3 years of life were extended to examine associations of the early child care experience to mother–child interactions from age 3 through the children's transition to school. Results deviated in several respects from those reported in the earlier years. The previously found relations between more hours of child care and lower-quality mother–child relations in the first 3 years and between higher-quality child care and greater maternal sensitivity were restricted to certain subsamples at these later ages, and a buffering effect of higher-quality care was found for effects of maternal depression on children's positive engagement of mother. These results are the first to highlight differences in relations of child care with mother–child interaction by child ethnicity, and for this reason merit replication and require further study to discern why these processes relating to the amount of child care appear to operate differently for white and nonwhite children and their mothers. Further study of the various conditions under which child care experiences relate to children's development and family processes would appear warranted.

VI

Child Care and Psychological Development

In the United States, many children are placed in nonmaternal child care during the early months of life. Frequently, these children are separated from their mothers for many hours on a daily basis, and while a small percentage experience either very high quality or very low quality of care, the care experienced by most children ranges from low to fair (see Part II). Children also are frequently moved from one child care arrangement to another or experience changes in the providers responsible for their care. Based on most developmental theories, an argument can be made that many hours in child care, poor quality of care, and instability of care are psychological stressors and, as such, may undermine emotional adjustment as well as social, cognitive, and linguistic development. Based on other theories, however, the provision of responsive and cognitively stimulating child care environments and of opportunities for interaction with peers are expected to promote young children's cognitive, language, and social development.

This section includes chapters that explore the relation between variations in children's experiences of quality of care, amount of time in care, and type of care and variations in their behavioral development, social skills, and intellectual performance over time. In each of the chapters, "effects" were assessed in terms of statistical significance (i.e., the extent to which the findings could not have been obtained by chance). In addition, in some of the chapters effects were tested using other strategies: (1) The magnitude of the effects was assessed in terms of the percent of individual differences that could be explained by child care predictors or in terms of methods that are independent of the number of children in the sample; (2) child care effects were compared to family effects—including income and maternal behaviors during interactions with the child; and (3) the stability of the results across time was examined. In some instances, consistency in the results across settings could be studied (e.g., the child care setting as compared with the home). And, in one instance, five criteria were applied to test whether child care experience actually has a causal effect on behavioral development (see Chapter 23).

The first three chapters focus exclusively on the effects of child care on the social outcomes of children. The next two chapters focus exclusively on child care effects on cognitive, language, and academic outcomes. The final three chapters in this section examine child care effects on both cognitive and social outcomes. Within each set of chapters we first present those pertaining to the children's performance when they were younger.

In Chapter 19, we report that children who had experienced higher-quality care and who were in group care had fewer provider-reported problems and were more compliant than those in lower-quality care. Those who entered care early and had experienced more hours in care, however, had higher provider-reported problems at 24 months but not at 36 months of age, though data presented in Chapters 21 and 26 reveal that the link between quantity of care and problem behavior reemerged at older ages.

Consistent, albeit modest, relations were found between child care experiences in the first 3 years of life and peer competencies (Chapter 20). Positive, responsive caregiver behavior was the feature of child care most consistently associated with positive, skilled peer interaction in child care. Children with more experience in child care settings with other children were rated by their caregivers as more negative with playmates but were observed to be more socially skillful. Children who were in child care for more hours per week were rated by their child care providers as more negative in peer play, but observations did not show the same.

The results pertaining to social outcomes at 54 months are reported in Chapters 21 and 26 (kindergarten data are also included in Chapter 21); these are generally consistent with findings from the second and third years of life. More hours in child care over the first 54 months of life predicted more caregiver-reported but not mother-reported behavior problems at 54 months (Chapter 26) but both more mother and caregiver reports of problem behavior at kindergarten (Chapter 21).

High-quality child care is a consistent predictor of global intellectual functioning, knowledge, achievement, and language skills at ages 15, 24, and 36 months (see Chapter 22). The most important feature of quality care predicting child outcomes was caregiver language stimulation. More frequent and synchronous language stimulation was linked to better cognitive and language outcomes than less stimulation. Enrollment in center-based care was also associated with more positive cognitive outcomes, controlling for quality of care.

No statistical link was found between the number of hours children spent in child care and their cognitive, achievement, or language outcomes.

The relation between child care and school readiness is examined in Chapters 24 and 26: Chapter 24 indicates that the more standards of quality met by child care centers, the better the children's readiness for school and the fewer behavior problems reported by mothers. In Chapter 26, quality of care over the first 54 months and improved quality of care over time both predicted preacademic and language skills, with better quality of care and increases in quality of care linked to better outcomes.

Results reported in Chapter 25 suggest that regulatory standards of quality are linked to school readiness outcomes through the cognitively stimulating behaviors of the child care providers. Child care settings that meet standards of quality (e.g., child–staff ratio or caregiver training) have child care providers who behave toward children in a way that supports children's psychological development. The caregivers' behavior, in turn, is linked to child's language, cognitive, and academic development. The mediated connection between the structural measures and the outcome measures assists greatly in interpreting the data from many child care studies.

Given that the results showing linkages between child care experience and the child's behavior are correlational, questions arise as to whether child care experience has a causal impact on behavioral development. In an attempt to determine the extent to which quality of care causes the outcomes measured, in Chapter 23, the research team evaluated the findings reported in this section against five criteria that support a causal interpretation. Specifically, we proposed that if child care quality affects child outcomes, (1) the association between child care quality and child outcomes should be apparent even when child and family background factors are taken into account; (2) analyses should indicate specificity of associations between child care quality and child care outcomes; (3) the quality of earlier care should be associated with child outcomes even when the quality of the concurrent care is statistically controlled; (4) associations between child care quality and child outcomes should remain when indices of the child's earlier ability are taken into account; and (5) associations between child care quality and child outcomes should be stronger if children spend more time in the care setting. Three of the five criteria were met, thus leaving the causal issue unresolved.

Because the analyses controlled for the effects of family variables, the chapters provide a comparison between the effects of the quality of the family and the quality of child care. For example, results reported in Chapter 19 showed that higher maternal sensitivity predicted more positive social behavior at 24 and 36 months and that these findings were stronger and more consistent than those pertaining to child care predictors. Consistent with these findings, Chapters 21 and 26 present findings showing that family characteristics were stronger predictors of behavior problems when children were 54 months and at kindergarten age than the number of hours they experienced in child care. In particular, greater maternal sensitivity was associated with lower ratings of problem behaviors. In Chapter 22, background variables (primarily family measures) explained more of the variance in the cognitive, language, and preacademic skill measures than the child care variables, with higher family quality predicting to better outcomes at 15, 24, and 36 months of age. In Chapter 25, quality of maternal caregiving is, once again, shown to be the strongest predictor of both cognitive and social outcomes among these children, although the importance of the quality of nonmaternal care giving is also demonstrated. The effect size for child care quality was about one-quarter of the effect size associated with parenting. In Chapter 26, the effect size for child care quality was also about one-quarter of the effect size associated with parenting. Taken together, the findings suggest the primacy of the family in the development of these children.

19

Early Child Care and Self-Control,
Compliance, and Problem Behavior
at 24 and 36 Months

NICHD EARLY CHILD CARE RESEARCH NETWORK

One of the foremost goals of socialization is the promotion of children's self-control, cooperation, and management of aggressive and antisocial impulses (Maccoby & Martin, 1983). Much research on the early childhood years highlights the role of both temperament and caregiving practices in fostering cooperation and compliance as well as noncompliance and problem behavior. A difficult and negative temperament is regarded by many as a risk factor for the development of externalizing behavior (e.g., Kochanska, 1991; Rothbart, 1986), and parenting that is based on power assertion rather than supportive guidance fosters similar behavioral tendencies (e.g., Belsky, Woodworth, & Crnic, 1996; Crockenberg & Litman, 1991; Power & Chapieski, 1986). In this chapter, we examine, in addition to the influence of parenting and early temperament, the effects of child care in the first 3 years of life on self-control, compliance, and problem behavior.

Theoretically, there are several reasons why relations between early child care and problem behavior and noncompliance might be anticipated. One possibility is that time away from parents might undermine children's responsiveness to parents' socialization efforts and, thereby, foster noncompliance and aggression. Relatedly, time spent with agemates, particularly under conditions of poor quality of care, might foster a peer orientation or the view that the way to get what you want is simply to take it. Inconsistency

From *Child Development*, 1998, Vol. 69, pp. 1145–1170. Reprinted with permission of the Society for Research in Child Development.

in rearing regimens across either multiple child care arrangements or between child care and home could also contribute to the development of problem behavior.

Since the early 1970s, investigators have repeatedly chronicled relations between early child care experience and developmental outcomes that might be considered markers of maladaptation or maladjustment (for review, see Belsky, 1988, 1990a, 1994). Much of the earliest such work was criticized for its failure to take into consideration selection effects (Phillips, McCartney, Scarr, & Howes, 1987); that is, families that rely on early child care differ in many ways from those that do not, and such differences could account for early findings.

Yet over the past decade, a number of large-sample studies that have controlled for selection effects have continued to report evidence consistent with results from the older, methodologically limited investigations (e.g., Crockenberg & Litman, 1991; Egeland & Hiester, 1995). Although this more recent body of work does not address each and every feature of child care that merits attention, it does illuminate the features of timing and/or quantity that are central to understanding the effects of child care (Baydar & Brooks-Gunn, 1991; Sternberg et al., 1991; Varin, Crugnola, Ripamonti, & Molina, 1994).

The strategy of examining care across several years rather than just one has yielded intriguingly similar results in several large U.S. studies that have controlled for selection effects (e.g., Belsky & Eggebeen, 1991; Park & Honig, 1991). However noteworthy and consistent results may appear, other investigations have failed to discern relations between early care experience and noncompliance, aggression, and problem behavior (Howes, 1988b; Macrae & Herbert-Jackson, 1976; McCartney & Rosenthal, 1991; Prodromidis, Lamb, Sternberg, Hwang, & Broberg, 1995), or have presented evidence counter to the findings just reviewed (Clarke-Stewart, Gruber, & Fitzgerald, 1994).

Many of the studies cited through this point have not included assessments of the quality of child care in their research designs. Others that do, however, show rather consistently that when quality of care is high, any adverse effects associated with early, extensive, and/or continuous care are mitigated, if not eliminated entirely (Field, 1991; Field, Masi, Goldstein, Perry, & Park, 1988; Howes & Olenick, 1986; Howes, Phillips, & Whitebook, 1992).

THE ECOLOGY OF EARLY CARE: INTERACTIONS BETWEEN CARE AND FAMILY AND CHILD FACTORS

Because it is unlikely that child care experience affects all children in exactly the same way, it is necessary to consider interactions between child care features and attributes of the child and family when seeking to identify conditions under which early care enhances and/or undermines children's socioemotional functioning (McCartney & Galanoupoulos, 1988). Available research draws attention to three kinds of interactions that might be discerned, one reflecting compensatory or protective processes, another lost resources, and a third multiple risks. Central to a compensatory or protective conceptualization is the notion that vulnerability resulting from a child characteristic (e.g., temperament) or family attribute (e.g., poverty) is not realized when a compensatory child care experience serves to mitigate risk. Although child care may serve as a protective factor for children with risk, it is possible that it functions as a risk factor for children without family and child risk. In particular, when families have many resources, especially a sensitive and skilled mother, child care might provide the child with poorer rearing experiences than would otherwise be the case (Desai, Chase-Lansdale, & Michael, 1989). Finally, interactions between child care and family or child factors can function to increase risks.

This chapter examines which, if any, child care experiences in the first years of life (e.g., quantity, quality, and stability) predict self-control, compliance, and problem behavior at 24 and 36 months of age and whether child and family factors moderate these effects. In all analyses, controls for selection effects are implemented because it is well established that children from poorer, less child-centered, and more stressed homes tend to receive lower-quality child care than do other children (Howes & Olenick, 1986; National Institute of Child Health and Human Development [NICHD] Early Child Care Research Network, 1997b; Phillips, McCartney, Scarr, & Howes, 1987). In addition to selection-effect covariates, analyses assess child care effects both prior to and following controls for additional child and family factors (i.e., gender, infant temperament, attachment security, and sensitivity of maternal care).

METHOD

Participants

Chapter 1 provides a detailed description of the recruitment process and eligible participants.

Two-year child outcome data were available for 1,085 children, and 3-year child outcome data were available for 1,041 children. Compared with nonparticipating children from the originally enrolled sample, participants came from households with a higher income-to-needs ratio (see below), M's: 2.88 versus 2.01, $p < .001$, with more educated mothers, M's: 14.4 years versus 13.2 years, $p < .001$, with two parents, 78% versus 27%, $p < .001$, who identified themselves as white, non-Hispanic, 78.51% versus 63.78%, $p < .001$, and in which mothers scored higher (i.e., better) on an aggregate measure of maternal psychological adjustment, M's, standardized: 0.59 versus − 0.52, $p < .01$.

Measures

Selection-Effect Covariates

A number of background variables were considered possible selection-effect covariates. On the basis of their associations with the dependent variables and child care predictors as well as with each other, two were selected, one economic and the other psychological.

Income-to-needs ratio, computed from maternal interview items collected at the 1-month visit, is calculated as family income divided by the appropriate poverty threshold (U.S. Department of Labor Women's Bureau, 1994) for each household size.

A composite measure of the mother's psychological adjustment was created using three scales of the Neuroticism Extraversion Openness (NEO) Personality Inventory (Costa & McCrae, 1985) obtained at 1 month along with the (reversed) average of repeated evaluations of maternal depressive symptomatology assessed at 1, 6, 15, 24, and 36 months using the Center for Epidemiologic Studies—Depression (CES-D) scale (Radloff, 1977). The three NEO scales were Neuroticism (reversed), Extraversion, and Agreeableness.

Family and Child Predictors

Family and child variables include child gender, temperament, positive qualities of maternal behavior, and infant–mother attachment security. Infant temperament was based on 55 6-point items from the Infant Temperament Questionnaire administered at 6 months (Medoff-Cooper, Carey, & McDevitt, 1993). Cronbach's alpha was .81. Higher scores reflect a more negative disposition, that is, a child seen as more intense, less positive in mood, and less adaptable to daily routines.

A global maternal behavior composite was calculated from two sources: (1) mother's behavior during videotaped interactions of mother–child interaction in the home (6, 15 months) or the laboratory (24, 36 months) under semistructured, free-play conditions and (2) mother's behavior assessed by the Home Observation for Measurement of the Environment (HOME; Caldwell & Bradley, 1984) at the 6- 15- and 36-month home visits.

The videotaped episodes of mother–child interaction from all sites were coded. A composite score of maternal sensitivity was created at each age of measurement. At 6 and 15 months it reflected the sum of three 4-point ratings: sensitivity to the child's nondistress expressions, positive regard, and intrusiveness (reversed); at 24 months a fourth rating, negative regard (reversed), was included as well; and at 36 months three different 7-point ratings were combined—supportive presence, respect for autonomy, and hostility (reversed). Intercoder reliability on the composite was .87 at 6 months, .83 at 15 months, .85 at 24 months, and .84 at 36 months. Alphas were .75, .70, .79, and .78, respectively.

Factor analyses of the items on the HOME were conducted separately for each age of assessment, and the first factor from each was retained for analysis. Variables with loadings of greater than .4 on this factor were summed at each age of measurement. The resulting positive involvement factor assessed the extent to which mother was positively responsive and affectionate to the child during the visit. At 6 months, the positive involvement factor consisted of six items (i.e., mother spontaneously vocalizes, responds verbally to child, initiates verbal interaction with home visitor, voices positive feelings for child, hugs/kisses child, watches child; alpha = .52). At 15 months, the positive involvement factor consisted of the same six high-loading items (alpha = .55), except that "praises child" replaced "watches child." At 36 months, the positive involvement factor consisted of six somewhat different items (encourages child to talk and listen, maternal voice positive in tone, talks to child two or more times, answers child's question verbally, responds to child's speech, caresses/kisses/cuddles child; alpha = .65). The composite scores from the HOME and from the video-taped interaction episodes were standardized and averaged at each time of measurement to create the mothering composite for that particular measurement occasion. At 24 months, this mothering construct was represented exclusively by maternal sensitivity in free play because the HOME was not administered at this age.

Infant–mother attachment security was assessed at 15 months using the Ainsworth and Wittig (1969) Strange Situation procedure. Videotapes of 1,201 Strange Situation assessments were coded using the standard classifications of secure (B), insecure–avoidant (A), insecure–resistant (C), disorganized (D), and unclassifiable (U). Across all coder pairs, before conferencing, agreement for the two category system (secure/ insecure) was 86% (kappa = .70) (for details, see Chapter 14).

Characteristics of Child Care

Measures of child care were obtained from two sources: (1) information on the child's age of entry into care, quantity of care, stability of care, and group-type care was obtained from mothers during face–face interviews at 6, 15, 24, and 36 months and phone calls every 3 months beginning at 3 months of age; and (2) quality of care was observed in the child care setting.

Age of entry into care was defined as the child's age in weeks when reported nonmaternal child care experiences totaled at least 10 hours per week. Nonmaternal care was defined in terms of regularly scheduled care provided by anyone other than the mother when the mother was not present. It included care by father, babysitter, relative, or neighbor and was not restricted to "formal" center-based care arrangements. (Although issue can be taken with the decision to include father care as a form of nonmaternal care, it should be noted that when analyses to be presented were carried out focusing exclusively on nonparental rather than nonmaternal care, results remained the same.) Quantity of care was the sum of all hours in all nonmaternal arrangements, scored as mean hours per week during the period 4–36 months. Children who experienced no routine nonmaternal care received a score of zero for quantity. Stability of care reflected the number of different child care arrangements the child experienced as reported by the mother. For purposes of this report, and in accord with other studies linking group care with problem behavior and noncompliance (e.g., Haskins, 1985), group-type care was operationalized in terms of children's primary nonmaternal care arrangement (the one they spent the most time in, or the more formal, institutional arrangement if time across settings was equal) at each of four ages (6, 15, 24, and 36 months). Children were considered to be in group-type care if there were at least three other (nonsibling) children in addition to the study child in the child care arrangement.

The quality of care was assessed during two half-day visits to the child's primary nonmaternal care setting at 6, 15, 24, and 36 months. Only settings in which children spent 10 or more hours per week were assessed. Visits were conducted within 2 weeks of the child's 6-month birthday and within 4 weeks of the 15-, 24-, and 36-month birthdays. The quality-of-care measures used in the present analyses were obtained by the Observational Record of the Caregiving Environment (ORCE; see Chapters 3 and 6). At each age of measurement, two composite measures of child care quality were created, one based on frequencies of behaviors, the other on qualitative ratings of behavior. The positive caregiving frequency composite represented the summed, standardized frequencies of nine categories of positive caregiving behavior. At 6 months the categories included were shared positive affect, positive physical contact, responds to infant's vocalization, asks question of infant, other talk to infant, stimulates infant's development, facilitates infant's behavior, and reads to infant (Cronbach's alpha = .89). At 15, 24, and 36 months, five additional categories were included in the composite: positive talk to child, restricts child's activity, negative talk to child, negative physical contact with child, and child unoccupied, with negatively oriented behaviors (e.g., restricts) scored in reverse (alpha = .78). Interobserver reliability estimates (Pearson correlations) at 6, 15, 24, and 36 months, respectively, for positive caregiving frequency were .98, .91, .92, .90 (videotapes), and .86, .97, .98, .98 (live).

The second composite variable at each age, positive caregiving ratings, was generated at 6, 15, and 24 months by summing five qualitative ratings made at the end of each observation cycle: Sensitivity/responsiveness to child's nondistress expressions; positive regard; stimulation of cognitive development; detachment (reversed); and flat affect (reversed). At 36 months, two additional categories, fostering exploration and intrusiveness (reversed), were added to the composite. Cronbach's alphas were .89, .88, .86, and .82 at 6, 15, 24, and 36 months, respectively. Interobserver reliability estimates (Pearson correlations) for positive caregiving ratings reliabilities were .94, .86, .81, .80 (videotapes), and .90, .89, .89, .90 (live) at each age. For the purposes of this chapter, the two composites at each age—which were highly intercorrelated (r > .64)—were themselves standardized and averaged to generate an overall index of child care quality.

Child Outcome Measures

Maternal and Caregiver Reports of Behavior Problems and Social Competence

At both 24 and 36 months, the 99-item Child Behavior Checklist–2/3 (CBCL; Achenbach, Edelbrock, & Howell, 1987) was used to assess behavior problems. In this chapter we used the two broad-band factors from factor analyses on the original standardization sample (Achenbach, 1991b), externalizing (aggressive and destructive) and internalizing (social withdrawal and depression), and two narrow-band factors, sleep problems and somatic problems. Research indicates that the CBCL–2/3 shows good test–retest reliability and concurrent and predictive validity (Achenbach et al., 1987).

Social competence and disruptive behavior were assessed with the Adaptive Social Behavior Inventory (ASBI) at 24 and 36 months (Hogan, Scott, & Bauer, 1992). Factor analysis on the original sample yielded three interpretable factors with good internal consistency and concurrent validity (Hogan et al., 1992). The express scale (13 items) taps sociability and empathy; the comply scale (10 items) measures prosocial engagement and cooperation; and the disrupt scale (7 items) assesses resistant and agonistic behavior. In the current sample the 24/36-month coefficient alphas for these scales completed by mothers were .77/.76 for express, .82/.82 for comply, and .60/.62 for disrupt, and .82/.84, .84/.87, and .70/.73 for those completed by caregivers.

Laboratory Assessments: Overview

Children were observed in a multiepisode laboratory session within 4 weeks of their second birthday and within 6 weeks of their third birthday. Four of the episodes yielded scores used in this chapter to assess self-control, compliance, and problem behavior.

The Cleanup Task (24/36 Months)

At the end of a 15-minute toy-play period that opened each laboratory session, the visit coordinator handed the mother containers for the toys and instructed her to have the child participate in picking up the toys; no other directions were given to mother. The child and mother were videotaped for the next 5 minutes or until all toys had been placed in the containers.

Videotapes were centrally coded by coders blind to child care status (and to attachment security and maternal sensitivity). The child's behavior was rated on 5-point global scales developed for this study (1 = not at all characteristic to 5 = very characteristic). Compliance and three forms of noncompliant behavior—assertive noncompliance (e.g., saying "no"), passive noncompliance (e.g., ignoring), and defiance (e.g., angry behavior and doing opposite of request)—were rated in reference to general or explicit directions from the mother. Dyadic cooperation was also rated on a single 5-point scale to capture the extent of mutuality, cooperation, reciprocity, and smoothness of interaction between mother and child. In addition, the child's negative affect during the cleanup was rated on separate 5-point scales. Reliability of the ratings was determined in terms of intraclass correlations (Winer, 1971) yielding estimates at 24/36 months of .92/.93 for compliance, .84/.79 for assertive noncompliance, .86/.86 for passive non-compliance, .82/.91 for defiance, and .91/.81 for dyadic cooperation.

Compliance with Bayley Test Examiner (24 Months)

Because there is empirical evidence suggesting that children's compliance with nonparental adults is affected by experience in child care, it was important to obtain measures of compliance outside the mother–child relationship. We standardized the administration of several items of the Bayley exam to assess compliance with the examiner at this age (blue shape board, pegboard, crayon/paper, nesting cups, stacking cubes, train of cubes): The examiner first made a request verbally without accompanying gestures ("It's time to clean up; please give me the TOY"), waited 10 seconds, and then made a second request if necessary. If the child did not comply after two requests, the examiner continued with the next item.

Two types of compliance were scored by the Bayley examiner: the child's willingness to attempt the task and the child's response to the request to give back the materials. Each child received 0 (did not comply) or 1 (complied) for each compliance request for each item; scores were summed over items to provide a total compliance score.

Resistance to Temptation (36 Months)

Approximately midway through the 2-hour laboratory session, the visit coordinator initiated the Forbidden Toy Task while the mother worked on questionnaires in a corner of the room. The task was designed to measure the child's ability to resist temptation. The task began with a brief period of play involving the child and the visit coordinator with a new and attractive toy, Ski Boat Crocs (TOMY no. 1009). The visit coordinator then initiated a waiting period by telling the child that she could play by herself during this period with toys which she had already played with during an earlier procedure but should not touch the crocodile toy until told she could do so. The toy was then placed at arm's length from the child while the visit coordinator did paperwork in a corner of the room. After 2½ minutes the visit coordinator gave the child permission to play with the Crocs and played with the child for 2 additional minutes.

Videotapes of the child's behavior during the waiting period were scored from videotapes of the procedure. Two mutually exclusive codes were used in the current analyses: active engagement time, which was scored whenever the child manipulated and played with the forbidden toy, and minimal engagement time, which was scored whenever the child made simple momentary touches of the object. These two variables correlated .11 with each other. Reliability estimates were computed based on the repeated measures formulation presented in Winer (1971), yielding estimates of .98 and .83 for active and minimal engagement, respectively.

The Three Boxes Interaction Procedure (24/36 Months)

Mother–child interaction was videotaped in a 15-minute semistructured context using three numbered boxes each containing toys (Vandell, 1979). The mother was instructed to have her child spend time with the toys in each of the boxes, beginning with Box 1 and ending with Box 3.

Of several ratings made using global 4-point scales (1 = uncharacteristic to 4 = characteristic), this chapter includes two scales considered to index active, off-task child behavior, activity level and sustained attention (labeled persistence at 36 months) and one reflecting negative mood. Intraclass correlations used to estimate interrater reliability were .69 for each of the off-task scales and .73 for the mood scale.

Child Care Observations (24/36 Months)

Child compliance and problematic behavior were also assessed in the child care setting. As part of the ORCE, several child behaviors were recorded and rated in addition to caregiver behavior.

Coded Behaviors

Children's negative interactions with peers and negative acts toward adults or peers, as well as their verbal and physical aggression to adults or peers, were recorded, all of which were composited to yield a single variable, negative social interaction (Cronbach's alpha = .65/.74 at 24/36 months). Negative behavior was defined as the involvement of the study child in an unfriendly overture from another child (video r = .90/.92, live r = .95/.96). Negative act was defined as unfriendly but not aggressive behavior directed by the study child to an adult or another child (video r = .85/.85, live r = .92/.90). Verbal aggression included name calling, threatening, or hostile teasing toward adults or children but did not include fantasy or playful aggression where the participants were clearly enjoying themselves (r = .99/.70). Physical aggression included hitting, fighting, spitting, biting, or otherwise physically threatening or attacking another child or an adult; again mock aggression, fantasy aggression, and play fighting were excluded (live r = .95/.75).

The incidence (i.e., presence/absence) of compliance with caregivers' requests and two forms of noncompliance, autonomous self-assertion and defiance, were coded each minute during the first three 10-minute epochs of each of four 44-minute observation cycles. The variable "% complies" reflected the percentage of occasions on which a child was instructed by a caregiver to do something and complied with the request or directive within 30 seconds (video $r = .83/.70$ at 24/36 months, live $r = .81/.95$ at 24/36 months). The variable "% autonomous self-assertion" reflected the percentage of times that the child responded to such caregiver directives by saying "no" or "mine" or some other emphatic but nonaggressive assertion or by refusal to cooperate (video $r = .69/.64$, live $r = .92/.91$); ignoring the caregiver was not counted as a form of autonomous self-assertion. The variable "% defies" reflected the percentage of responses to caregiver directives that involved expressions of anger or aggression by the child; intensifying an explicitly prohibited behavior was also coded as defiance, as when a caregiver told a child to put toys away but the child kept taking them from a shelf (live $r = .82/.91$).

Ratings

Several aspects of children's behavior were also rated at the end of each 44-minute observation cycle and then averaged across cycles. Negative mood reflected the extent to which the child cried, whined, yelled, or otherwise expressed discontent, anger, or hostility; lack of negative mood was expressed as contentment or positive affect (video $r = .66/.70$, live $r = .88/.80$). Sustained attention assessed the child's involvement with physical objects; higher ratings reflected greater duration of sustained, focused, undistracted interest in, attention to, and engagement with physical objects such as toys and books, whereas lower ratings reflected boredom, aimlessness, distractibility, or apathy (video $r = .65/.75$, live $r = .81/.77$). Activity level assessed how motorically active the child was, considering speed, frequency, and intensity of activity, as well as involvement in or preference for high energy and gross motor activity; high scores reflected a child high in energy and activity, whereas low ratings reflected passivity, inactivity, or lethargy (video $r = .66/.96$, live $r = .99/.99$).

RESULTS

Data on child behavioral functioning at 24 and 36 months were subjected to separate factor analyses for purposes of data reduction and then to analyses designed to assess the external validity of the composite constructs derived from the factor analyses (for details, see NICHD Early Child Care Research Network, 1998a).

Results indicated that six of the seven composite dependent variables at 24 months met our criterion as having external validity (i.e., significantly covaried with at least two of the six external correlates): cleanup defy, mother-reported problems, mother-reported social competence, three-box negative, caregiver-reported problems, child care noncomply. Five of the seven 36-month composite dependent variables met the criterion for validation: mother-reported problems, mother-reported social competence, cleanup comply, three-box neg./resist. temp., and caregiver-reported problems. Thus, a total of 11 dependent variables were included in the data set for final analysis.

Cumulative Child Care Effects

We restrict reporting of results to analyses focused exclusively on children who had some nonmaternal child care experience during their first 24 months ($n = 653$) and first 36 months ($n = 720$) and which included assessments of quality, quantity, stability, entry age, and group-type care. All the significant quantity and entry age effects that emerged in the entire-sample analyses also emerged in the child care-only analyses to be presented below.

24-Month Outcomes

To assess effects of cumulative child care (and family) experience through the first 2 years of life on child functioning at 24 months, we examined quantity, quality, stability, and type of care, as well as age of entry of 10 or more hours of care. In these analyses, independent variables pertaining to mothering and child care quality, quantity, and stability reflected the cumulative experience of the child through 24 months of age.

A series of ordinary least-squares (OLS) regression analyses was conducted to examine the explanatory power of different sets of predictor variables in accounting for variation in each of the six 24-month composite dependent variables. Multiple models were evaluated to gain insight into the effects of child care over and above the influences of selection effects and family and child variables and in interaction with these other potential sources of influence.

Model I included only the two selection-effect variables. Model II included selection variables plus the child variables (gender, temperament). Model III evaluated the extent to which child care variables (quality, quantity, entry, stability, group type) predicted—as main effects—child functioning over and above the selection and child variables. Model IV was important principally because it served as the base (or comparison) for Model V (see below). This fourth model evaluated the extent to which family factors (attachment security, mothering) predicted child functioning beyond the selection and child variables; thus, its base of comparison was also Model II. Model V tested whether child care variables added to the prediction of child outcomes over and above the selection, child, and family variables; thus, Model IV served as its base of comparison. Additional models examining the effect of two-way interactions between child care variables and child variables, among different child care variables, and between child care and family variables were also tested to evaluate compensatory process and lost-resource perspectives. Because so few significant interaction effects were detected—fewer than expected by chance alone—in both the 24- and 36-month analyses, and because the few significant interactions failed to yield results consistent with any of the interactional hypotheses outlined in the introduction, they are not discussed any further.

Table 19.1 displays the results of the first model and the subsequent four model comparisons. The table displays, in bold print, the variance explained by a particular set of variables (e.g., child, child care, and family) over and above the particular base model. Thus, with the exception of Model I, which included only the selection effects and did not have a formal base model, the numbers printed in bold represent change in variance explained (i.e., ΔR^2). Significance levels reflect the significance of the change in R^2 (rather than of the total model). Also displayed in the tables are the standardized regression coefficients (i.e., betas) of individual predictors that proved significant. These latter numbers are displayed only when the block of variables in question significantly increased the predictive power of the particular dependent variable under consideration.

As can be seen in Table 19.1, child care variables' main effects after covarying selection and child variables accounted for only a small amount of variance in the 24-month dependent variables, resulting in significant contributions ranging from 1–2.8% of the variance in the case of mother-reported problems and social competence, caregiver-reported problems, and child care noncompliance. The more hours of care the child experienced in the first 2 years, the less social competence reported by mother and the more problem behavior reported by caregiver. The lower the quality of care experienced, the more problem behavior and less social competence reported by mother, and the more problem behavior reported by caregiver. Later entry into care was associated with more problems reported by caregiver; less stable child care arrangements were associated with more problem behavior reported by mother but less noncompliance observed in care; and more time in group-type care was associated with more compliance observed in the laboratory during cleanup and less noncompliance observed in child care. In the case of two of the four dependent measures significantly predicted by the block of child care variables (mother-reported problems and social competence), this significant contribution became insignificant once family variables were controlled.

The data presented in Table 19.1 also indicate that selection-effect variables accounted for a significant proportion of the variance (1.6–15%) in mother-reported problems and social competence, three-box negative, and caregiver-reported problems. Child factors also contributed significantly to the first two of these child outcomes (2.4% and 4.0%). Family factors accounted for significant variance (0.7–7.0%) in all four outcomes. When mothers were economically and psychologically advantaged and described

TABLE 19.1. Multiple Prediction of 24-Month Child Outcomes: Main Effects—Blocks and Variables

Model	Cleanup defy	Mother-reported problems	Mother-reported social comp.	Three-box negative	Caregiver-reported problems	Child care noncomply
I. Selection	.000[a]	.150***	.111***	.016***	.027***	.002
1. Income/needs		-.09[b]	.17***			
2. Psychological adjustment		-.36***	.25***	-.12**	-.16***	
II. Child[c]	.002	.024***	.040***	Red.[d]	.002	Red.
1. Gender			.17***			
2. Temperament		.17***	-.13***			
III. Child care[e]	.005	.010**	.010*	.003	.028**	.013
1. Quantity			-.09*		.16**	
2. Entry age					.14**	
3. Quality		-.11**	.13*		-.14*	
4. Stability		.07				-.09*
5. Group type			.10*			-.13**
IV. Family[f]	.000	.010*	.07***	.059***	.022**	Red.
1. Attachment security				-.08*		
2. Mothering		-.13**	.30***	-.26***	-.17**	
V. Child care[g]	.006	.006*	.005	Red.	.020**	.012*
1. Quantity					.15**	
2. Entry age					.13*	
3. Quality					-.11*	
4. Stability						-.09*
5. Group type						-.12**

[a]Variance accounted for by block of variables.
[b]Beta.
[c]Tested *after* selection effects.
[d]Entry of this block of variables resulted in reduction of adjusted R^2.
[e]Tested *after* selection and child main effects.
[f]Tested *after* main effects of selection, child, and child care.
[g]Tested *after* selection, child, and family main effects.
*$p < .05$; **$p < .01$; ***$p < .001$.

275

their 6-month-olds as having easier temperaments, they reported fewer child behavior problems and described their children as more socially competent. Girls were characterized by mothers as more socially competent than boys. Children who experienced more positive mothering had less problem behavior according to mothers and caregivers and were observed to be more compliant with mother during cleanup in the laboratory. Finally, 2-year-olds with secure attachment histories were also more compliant during cleanup.

36-Month Outcomes

Table 19.2 displays the results of the relevant model comparisons at 36 months. Inspection of the table indicates that child care variables contributed significantly to the prediction of four of the five tested dependent variables, contributing between 0.6% and 2.8% of explained variance over and above selection and child effects. In three of these cases, child care quality was a significant contributor and in two cases group-type care: Children who had experienced higher-quality child care across their first 3 years were more cooperative and compliant with mother during cleanup; less negative in interaction with mother and more able to resist the forbidden toy; and, according to caregiver reports, exhibited fewer behavior problems in child care. Children with more group-type care experience were less negative during the three-boxes play procedure, touched the forbidden toy less often in the laboratory, and exhibited fewer problem behaviors in child care according to caregivers. For all but one of these dependent variables, the significant effect of the child care block was no longer significant once family variables were controlled (see Model V).

Beyond child care effects, the data presented in Table 19.2 indicate that selection-effect variables accounted for 0.9–12.2% of the variance in 36 month child outcomes. Mother-reported problems and social competence, along with three-box negative/resist. temp., were also predicted by child factors, with 2.6–4.3% of the variance explained. Finally, family factors contributed additional and significant variance (2.7–11.0%) to four of the five child outcomes. When families were more economically and mothers more psychologically advantaged, mothers reported fewer child behavior problems and described their children as more socially competent. Under these conditions, children were more compliant during cleanup in the laboratory, less negative during the three-boxes play procedure and able to resist temptation longer, and regarded by caregivers as having fewer behavior problems. Girls were described by mothers as more socially competent and were observed to be less negative during the three-boxes play procedure and more able to resist temptation in the laboratory. Children described by mothers as more difficult as infants were characterized as having more problems and as being less socially competent. Finally, mothers observed to provide more positive caregiving had children whom they described as

TABLE 19.2. Multiple Prediction of 36–Month Outcomes: Main Effects—Blocks and Variable

Model	Mother-reported problems	Mother-reported social comp.	Cleanup comply	Three-box neg./resist. temp.	Caregiver-reported problems
I. Selection	**.122***[a]**	**.109***	**.009****	**.048***	**.020***
1. Income/needs	-.34***	.10**[b]		-.16***	-.09*
2. Psychological adjustment		.29***	.08*	-.12*	-.10*
II. Child[c]	**.040***	**.043***	**.004**	**.026***	**.000**
1. Gender		.11***			
2. Temperament	.22***	-.20***		-.17***	
III. Child care[d]	**.006**	**.002**	**.008***	**.016***	**.028****
1. Quantity					
2. Entry age					
3. Quality			.11***	-.16**	-.15**
4. Stability					
5. Group type				-.10**	-.17***
IV. Family[e]	**.005**	**.027***	**.043***	**.110***	**.032***
1. Attachment security					
2. Mothering		.20***	.24***	-.37***	-.22***
V. Child care[f]	**.006**	**.001**	**.002**	**.001**	**.013****
1. Quantity					
2. Entry age					
3. Quality					.11***
4. Stability					
5. Group type					-.14***

[a]Variance accounted for by block of variables.
[b]Beta.
[c]Tested after selection effects.
[d]Tested after selection and child main effects.
[e]Tested after main effects of selection, child, and child care.
[f]Tested after selection, child, and family main effects.
*p <.05; **p <.01; ***p <.001.

more socially competent; who were observed to be more compliant in the laboratory during cleanup, less negative in interacting with their mothers during the three-boxes procedure, and more able to resist temptation; and whom caregivers described as having fewer behavior problems.

DISCUSSION

In the discussion that follows, we consider results pertaining to the effects of quantity, quality, entry age, stability, and group-type care, as well as inter-actions between these child care features and the quality of family care on 2- and 3-year-olds' compliance, self-control, and problem behavior.

Quantity of Care

Although 2-year-olds who spent more time in nonmaternal care were reported by their mothers to be less cooperative and by their caregivers to exhibit more behavior problems (after controlling for selection effects and child characteristics), by the time children were 3 years of age, no significant effects for amount of child care experience could be detected. In sum, we found little evidence that the amount of time children spend in non-maternal child care in the first 2 or 3 years of life is, in and of itself, system-atically related to children's self-control, compliance, or problem behavior by age 3.

Why do the results of this inquiry appear to diverge from those of prior work? Perhaps the most likely explanation concerns the age of the children studied in the current investigation. In other work early, extensive, and con-tinuous care has been related to elevated rates of aggression, noncompli-ance, and other potential indices of maladjustment when children are 4–8 years of age (Bates et al., 1994; Baydar & Brooks-Gunn, 1991; Belsky & Eggebeen, 1991; Vandell & Corasaniti, 1990). This suggests that effects of lots of time in care may take some time to materialize, at least in more pro-nounced form.

Quality of Care

Explanations offered as alternatives for the findings Belsky (1986, 1988) highlighted, linking extensive time in nonmaternal care with elevated lev-els of aggression and noncompliance during the preschool and early school years, emphasized the importance of child care quality (Fein & Fox, 1988; Phillips, McCartney, Scarr, & Howes, 1987). But this explana-tion, too, received limited support in the current investigation. All but two of the six significant effects of cumulative quality of care were reduced to nonsignificance once family variables were controlled. Nevertheless, the evidence that did emerge indicated that higher quality of observed care predicted fewer mother- and caregiver-reported problems and more mother-reported social competence at 2 years of age, and more compliance with mother and fewer caregiver-reported behavior problems at 3 years of age.

Age of Entry and Stability

With respect to two other features of child care examined in this investigation, it was once again the case that effects were quite limited. Even when family processes (attachment security, mothering) were controlled, later age of entry continued to predict more caregiver-reported behavior problems, and instability continued to predict more observed problems in the child care setting.

Group-Type Care

Recall that cumulative group experience through 24 months was associated with more cooperation with mother in the laboratory and fewer caregiver-reported behavior problems at 2 years. And more such experience through 36 months was associated with less negative interaction with mother in the laboratory and fewer caregiver-reported behavior problems at 3 years.

Child Care × Family Interactions

In light of prior studies and contemporary theorizing about the complex ecology of child development, the general absence of strong or consistent effects of child care by itself may not be surprising. After all, the compensatory-process, cumulative-risk, and lost-resource perspectives outlined in the introduction led us to anticipate findings highlighting interactions between child care and family factors more than main effects of child care. Yet in this examination of toddlers' self-control, compliance, and problem behavior, significant interactions emerged no more frequently than would be expected on the basis of chance alone, and those few that were significant failed to conform to any of interactional hypotheses guiding this inquiry.

Child and Family Effects

Although features of child care proved to be only modestly and sporadically related to self-control, compliance, and problem behavior at 2 and 3 years of age, child characteristics and family processes displayed stronger and more consistent associations.

CONCLUSION

The fact that family factors were more strongly predictive of child outcomes than were child care factors is consistent with the results of our prior examination of the effects of child care on infant–mother attachment security (NICHD Early Child Care Research Network, 1997b). Both sets of results underscore what may be the principal conclusion to be drawn from our large-scale, multisite research project. That is, what transpires in the family appears to be more important in explaining children's early social and emotional development than whether children are cared for by someone other than their mothers on a routine basis or the quality, quantity, stability, and type of care or age of entry into such care.

It must be acknowledged that family-process measures similar to those used in this inquiry have been found to reflect heritable variation, so it cannot be presumed that the discerned family effects exclusively reflect the influence of family experience (Braungart, Fulker, Plomin, & DeFries, 1992).

20

Early Child Care and Children's Peer Interaction at 24 and 36 Months

NICHD EARLY CHILD CARE RESEARCH NETWORK

Children's peer relationships are critical to their developing social compe-tence (Berndt & Ladd, 1989; Hartup. 1983, 1996). Individual differences in peer interaction appear as early as the second year (Brownell & Brown, 1992), and by early to middle childhood they predict later social compe-tence and psychological adjustment (Coie, Terry, Lenox, & Lochman, 1995; Morison & Masten, 1991). A key question, therefore, concerns the origins of individual differences in peer relations.

The evidence currently suggests that young children's developing com-petence with peers is related to their experiences with both adults and peers in their child care settings, but with a few exceptions (Howes, 1988a; Galluzzo, Matheson, Moore, & Howes, 1990), researchers have not consid-ered both amount of peer experience and quality of children's interactions with their caregivers in the same analysis. Nor have they typically included family and child characteristics when examining child care factors. The larger implication is that we do not yet have a coherent picture of which fac-tors in very young children's social environments help to shape their devel-oping peer competence. In particular, we do not know how young chil-

From *Child Development*, 2001, Vol. 72, pp. 1478–1500. Reprinted with permission of the Society for Research in Child Development.

dren's experiences with children and adults outside the family, either independently or in concert with family factors, relate to early peer skill. In this chapter we address these issues. The primary purpose of this chapter is to examine how children's experiences in child care relate to individual differences in peer social competence at 24 and 36 months, a time at which peer skills are rapidly developing. We studied three specific features of early-child care experience: (1) amount of time in child care; (2) quality of care as indexed by caregiver responsiveness and sensitivity; and (3) availability of other children in the care setting. On the basis of previous research, we expected that sensitive caregiving and amount of experience with other children would be positively associated with children's developing peer competence, but it is unclear from existing work whether the amount of nonmaternal care would be positively or negatively related to early peer competence.

METHODS

Participants

Chapter 1 describes the participants.

Sample Observed in Child Care

At 24 months, when peer behavior was first systematically assessed, 669 of the 1,364 children in the sample were observed in child care (336 boys; 333 girls). The rest either were not in regular care for at least 10 hours per week ($n = 549$) or were not observed because of refusals or scheduling problems ($n = 145$). At 36 months, 706 children were observed in child care (352 girls; 354 boys); 515 children were not in regular care, and 143 children were in child care that was not observed. In general, children observed in child care came from more educated, economically advantaged, and stable two-parent families than did children not in child care, and than children in child care who were not observed.

Sample Observed in Dyadic Peer Interaction

At 36 months, 612 preschoolers were observed in dyadic interaction with a familiar peer. Children whose parents or caregivers were able to identify a same-sex, frequent playmate close in age to the study child were observed in dyadic play. Data are missing because some children did not have same-sex regular playmates, because the peer's parents did not agree to the observation, or because of scheduling difficulties. Children who participated in the dyadic peer observation differed significantly ($p < .001$) from those who did not on income-to-needs ratio ($M = 3.76$ vs. 2.52), a measure of family economic resources (family income divided by the poverty threshold), on maternal education (M = 14.79 vs. 13.46 years), and on family structure (75.6% vs. 49.7% from two-parent families).

Procedure

Chapter 1 provides an overview of data collection.

Measures

Selection-Effect Covariates

Two measures—maternal education and maternal beliefs about the risks of maternal employment—met our criteria for selection-effect covariates, which required that they be significantly related both to outcome measures of peer competence and to child care predictors. They also tapped both family resource and maternal attitude domains, and they were relatively independent of one another.

Maternal Education was the number of years of schooling reported by the mother at the 1-month interview. The measure of *Beliefs about the Risks of Maternal Employment* was created by summing six 6-point items from the Attitudes toward Employment Questionnaire (Greenberger & Goldberg, 1989) administered at the 1-month visit (Cronbach's alpha = .88). Higher scores reflected the belief that maternal employment carried risks for children's development.

Child Factors

In addition to gender, children's cognitive competence at 24 months and language competence at 36 months were entered into the analyses, as was a measure of difficult temperament in infancy. Children's *Cognitive Competence* was assessed at 24 months using the revised Bayley Scales of Infant Development (BSID-II; Bayley, 1993) administered during a laboratory visit, yielding a single score, the Mental Development Index (see Chapter 22).

Language Competence was assessed at 36 months using the Reynell Developmental Language Scales (Reynell, 1991), administered during the laboratory visit. For the current analyses, only the expressive language subscale was used (e.g., child has one or more appropriate uses of past tense, uses complex sentences, labels or describes objects or activities, and defines words). Internal consistency exceeded .85 on this subscale.

Temperament was assessed when infants were 6 months old by completion of the 55-item Infant Temperament Questionnaire by the mothers (Medoff-Cooper, Carey, & McDevitt, 1993). A composite measure was created to index difficult temperament (Cronbach's alpha = .81).

Maternal Sensitivity

A composite measure of the mother's sensitivity during play with her child was constructed based on ratings of 15-minute videotaped episodes of mother–child play in the home at 6 and 15 months of age and in the laboratory at 24 and 36 months of age. At 6 months, mothers were asked to play with their infant for 7 minutes with any toy or object available in the home (or none at all), and then to play for 8 minutes with a standard set of toys provided by the examiners (rattles, activity center, ball, rolling toy, book, stuffed animal). At 15, 24, and 36 months, mothers and children were provided three containers of age-appropriate toys and were instructed to play with these toys as they wished (see Chapter 17).

At each age an *a priori* maternal *Sensitivity in Play* composite was constructed based on these ratings. At 6, 15, and 24 months, this was the sum of three 4-point ratings: sensitivity to nondistress (including vocal, facial, and postural expressions and communication), positive regard, and intrusiveness (reversed). The 36-month sensitivity composite was the sum of three 7-point ratings: supportive presence, respect for autonomy, and hostility (reversed). Intercoder reliability on the composite (Pearson correlations) was .87 at 6 months, .83 at 15 months, .85 at 24 months, and .84 at 36 months. Internal consistency (Cronbach's alpha) was .75, .70, .74, and .78, respectively. (See Chapter 7 for details about assessment procedures and coding.)

Child Care Factors

Three aspects of children's experiences in child care were entered into analyses.

For amount of care, average weekly hours of care was computed as the mean number of weekly hours in all nonmaternal care arrangements from 0–24 and 0–36 months of age. Children who received no nonmaternal care during a given 3-month epoch were assigned scores of "0."

Availability of other children in child care settings was determined from 5 months onward using maternal reports collected at 3-month intervals. If mothers reported that two or more other children were available in either a primary or secondary child care arrangement, then a score of 1 was recorded for the 3-month period. At 24 months, scores could range from 0 to 7, with higher scores representing more 3-month epochs with other children available in the child care setting. At 36 months, scores could range from 0 to 11.

Positive caregiving was observed and rated in the child care setting at 6, 15, 24, and 36 months for children who spent at least 10 hours per week in a regular, nonmaternal child care arrangement. Observations in child care settings were made using the Observational Record of the Caregiving Environment (ORCE; see Chapters 2 and 5 for details). For this chapter, five of the qualitative ratings were summed to index the positive quality of the primary caregiver's interaction with the study child: sensitivity/responsiveness to child's nondistress expressions; stimulation of cognitive development; positive regard; detachment (reversed); and flatness of affect (reversed). Fostering exploration and intrusiveness (reversed) were added to the 36-month composite. Higher scores on the composites represent more positive, responsive, and sensitive caregiving. Cronbach's alphas for the composites were .89, .88, .86, and .82 at 6, 15, 24, and 36 months, respectively. All scales had adequate intercoder agreement with "gold standard" videotapes master-coded by the investigators who developed the ORCE (r's = .94, .86, .81, and .80 at each age), and with live reliability partners (r's = .90, .89, .89, and .90 at each age).

Child Outcome Measures: Peer Interaction

Maternal and Caregiver Reports

Mother and caregiver reports of peer social behavior were obtained at 24 and 36 months, when all mothers and all primary caregivers in observed child care arrangements completed the Adaptive Social Behavior Inventory (ASBI; Hogan, Scott, & Bauer, 1992). For this report, two subscales representing positive and negative peer social behavior were obtained by summing the scores of items specifically related to peer interaction. *Positive Sociability* consisted of 10 items (e.g., is helpful to other children; follows rules in games; joins others' play; shares toys). *Negative/Aggressive* consisted of four items (e.g., teases others; bullies others). Cronbach's alphas for the positive sociability subscale at 24/36 months were .75/.74 for mothers' reports, and .78/.82 for caregivers' reports; for the negative/aggressive subscale alphas were .51/.57 for mothers' reports and .68/.69 for caregivers' reports. Alphas are low for the negative/aggressive subscale because the individual items are relatively low frequency at these ages, and because a child who engages in one type of aggression (e.g., bullying) may not engage in others (e.g., teasing). Because early aggression has been shown to be stable, we felt it was important to assess it even if it occurs infrequently.

Observations in Child Care

Child care observations of positive and negative social behavior were conducted as part of the ORCE, described earlier. Several aspects of the study child's behavior with peers were recorded at 24 and 36 months during four 44-minute observation cycles, by the same observers who recorded caregiver behavior. In each observation cycle, specific features of peer social behavior were recorded for their presence/absence during successive 1-minute time samples (30 seconds observe, 30 seconds record) for three 10-minute periods. After 14 minutes of additional observation and note taking, observers made qualitative ratings of the study child's social behavior over the entire 44-minute observation period. Frequencies and qualitative ratings of peer social behavior were standardized and summed to create two larger composites for substantive analyses, Positive Peer Play and Negative Peer Interaction.

Positive Peer Play represented the complexity and positive sociability of children's interactions with their peers as observed in the child care setting. It was defined as the sum of standardized scores on positive/neutral interaction with other children, proportion high level play, and positive sociability (Cronbach's alphas = .62 and .70 at 24 and 36 months, respectively). Positive/neutral interaction reflected how frequently the child engaged other children in any type of nonnegative interaction. Proportion high level play reflected how much of the child's play with peers was both complex and reciprocal. Positive sociability was the observer's rating on a 1–4 scale of the child's interest in and positive engagement with other children. Children with high scores on the composite were often engaged positively with other children and their peer play frequently included joint pretend play. Interobserver reliabilities with gold standard videotapes (conducted before data collection began) and with live reliability partners (conducted on at least four regularly spaced intervals during data collection) on the individual scores constituting the composites ranged from .89 to .96.

Negative Peer Interaction was also observed using the ORCE, and represented the proportion of peer interaction that was negative or aggressive. It was calculated as the number of observed segments in which the child was involved in negative interaction with a peer divided by the total number of segments of peer interaction. Negative interaction was defined as the child's giving or receiving an unfriendly overture and included verbal and physical aggression. Thus, children high on Negative Peer Interaction were proportionately more often engaged in unfriendly or negative interactions with other children. Interobserver reliabilities ranged from .92 to .96.

Observations in Dyadic Play

Dyadic peer play was observed at 36 months when children participated in a semistructured play session with a same-sex playmate close in age to the study child who had been identified by the child's parent or child care provider as someone the child plays with regularly (n = 612). Mean age of the familiar playmate was 39.3 months (SD = 5.0 months). These interactions were videotaped for later coding and are independent of the ORCE observations. Three measures of peer competence were derived from videotape ratings: peer skill, peer aggression, and self-assertion/control.

The dyadic play observations were carried out in a portable playroom set up in the child's regular child care arrangement or in one of the children's homes if the study child or the friend was not in child care. The playroom, constructed of heavy cardboard, was 3 feet high, 5 feet in diameter, and open at the top. This arrangement shielded the children from distractions in the surrounding environment and permitted us to standardize the children's play context. After being introduced to the playroom, the children were asked to sit down and three different toys were presented to them sequentially, in fixed order: a Magnadoodle, a Fisher-Price toy kitchen set, and a pair of flashlights, one of which was inoperable. The toys were selected to permit a range of play types and quantity, from cooperative and prosocial to solitary or negative. The experimenter set each toy one at a time on the floor between the two children, demonstrated how it worked, and then left the playroom. Children played with the Magnadoodle for 4 minutes, the kitchen set for 5 minutes, and the flashlights for 3 minutes. Children's interactions were videotaped through a curtained opening into the playroom. Children enjoyed playing in the playroom and rarely stood up or asked to leave.

The tapes were sent to a central site different from the one where mother–child interaction was coded, for scoring by coders unaware of the study children's family and child care history. Play sessions were rated for several aspects of the study child's peer social behavior using 3- or 5-point scales with higher scores representing higher skill: amount of positive interaction; clarity of verbal interaction; positive mood; cooperation; concern for peer; quality of fantasy play; complexity of social play. Each scale was rated separately for each toy, and the codes were then averaged across the three toy episodes. In addition, two nominally scaled items were later recoded into the following ordinal scales: Response to provocation: shares (originally scored yes/no for each toy episode) was recoded as 0 to 3 based on the number of toy episodes out of three in which the child tried to resolve conflict by sharing a toy when the peer had tried to take the toy from the study child; and social problem solving: property rights was recoded as 0–3 based on the number of toy episodes out of three in which the child tried to gain possession of the peer's toy by using an approach other than physical force or verbal demands (e.g., recognition of the other's ownership and negotiation). These eight scores were standardized and summed to form the composite variable, *Peer Skill* (Cronbach's alpha = .80). Children with high scores on this variable played in more positive, cooperative, complex ways, and more often resolved conflict by prosocial means.

A composite variable of *Peer Aggression* for the dyadic play session was derived by standardizing and summing the ratings for instrumental aggression, hostile aggression, and negative mood averaged over the three toy episodes (Cronbach's alpha = .74). *Self-Assertion and Control* was retained as a separate measure, to distinguish between aggression and assertion in the children's play (see Clarke-Stewart, Gruber, & Fitzgerald, 1994). Several parallel measures of the peer's behavior during the dyadic interaction were correlated with the study child's behavior to determine whether they should be controlled in substantive analyses. Correlations were low (r's = .003 to .17), so the peer's behavior was not considered further.

RESULTS

Analysis Plans for Predictive Analyses

Regression analyses examined the extent to which the measures of peer competence were related to selection, child, maternal, and child care factors, and for repeated measures whether those patterns of association changed over time. All regression models were fit simultaneously and included site as a covariate to adjust for differences among the 10 sites.

The repeated-measures regression analyses were fit using a general linear mixed-model-analysis approach (Jenrich & Schluchter, 1986; Laird & Ware, 1982). These analyses estimated a separate set of regression coefficients for each age under the assumption that there was a common covariance structure over time. For example, the analysis of maternal report of positive peer play involved one set of coefficients that described the relations between the predictors and positive peer play as measured in the first 2 years and a second set of coefficients that described the relations between the predictors and positive peer play between the second and third year.

The overall analysis plan involved testing the main effects and interactions with age for each block of predictors. First, we tested whether each block of predictors showed a different pattern of association with the outcome at 24 than at 36 months. At the same time, we tested whether each block of predictors contributed significantly to predicting a given outcome over time. Individual parameter estimates were interpreted only if block tests were significant. All continuous predictors were standardized to have a mean of 0 and standard deviation of 1 to enhance interpretation of coefficients. Thus, the main effect parameter for each predictor reflects the across-time association between that predictor and the peer outcome measure when all other predictors were at their mean values.

For the three measures of dyadic play at 36 months, which were assessed only at this age and not at 24 months, the multiple regression analyses involved the same blocks of predictors. In these analyses, we computed cumulative scores for the time-varying measures of maternal sensitivity, quantity of child care, quality of caregiving in child care, and number of times in care settings with peers available. A cumulative score was computed for each family that represented the mean of the maternal sensitivity at 6, 15, 24, and 36 months; the average hours of child care from birth through 36 months; the mean of the positive caregiving composite from 6, 15, 24, and 36 months; and the number of times in which the child had two or more peers in the child care setting. The other predictors included site, maternal education, risks of employment, gender, the 36-month Reynell receptive language score, and temperament. Again, the contribution of each block of predictors was tested, and individual predictors were interpreted only if the block test was significant.

Effect sizes were computed when either main effect or interaction tests were significant. Partial correlations were computed to provide an index of the magnitude of the observed associations for continuous variables and standardized mean differences (the difference between group means divided by the root mean squared-error) were computed for the categorical variables. All other predictors were included as covariates in these computations. Cohen (1988) recommends that $r = .10$ be regarded as a small effect size, $r = .30$ as a moderate effect size, and $r = .50$ as a large effect size when partial correlations are examined.

Longitudinal Predictions

Repeated-measures regression analyses examined the 24 and 36 month measures of maternal and caregiver report and observed play in child care. Tables 20.1 through 20.3 show results from these analyses. The first column for each outcome lists the coefficients and standard errors estimated for each 24-month predictor. The second column lists the coefficients and standard errors estimated for each 36-month predictor. The third column, labeled main effect lists the F statistic from the block test for the main effect across time for that set of predictors. Significant main-effect F's for individual predictors are also shown in this column. The final column, labeled effect × age lists the F statistic from the block test that compared the 24-month and 36-month coefficients for each predictor. This determined whether the association between predictors and the outcome changed over time.

The first columns of Table 20.1 show the results from the analysis of maternal report of positive sociability. These analyses indicate that mothers reported more positive sociability at 36 months than at 24 months, $F(1,766) = 31.16$, $p < .0001$, as can be seen by comparing the estimated intercepts for the two ages in Table 20.1. However, the associations between the selection, child, maternal, and child care blocks and maternal report of positive sociability did not change significantly from 24 to 36 months as indicated in the effects × age column. The child and maternal blocks provided the only significant associations with this outcome, with maternal reports of more positive peer play associated with more advanced cognitive/language skills, $F(1,766) = 25.89$, $p < .001$, less difficult temperament, $F(1,766) = 8.50$, $p = .004$, and greater maternal sensitivity, $F(1,766) = 6.52$, $p = .01$. Partial correlations between maternal report of positive sociability and cognitive/language skills ($r = .15$ at 24 months and $r = .18$ at 36 months), difficult infant temperament ($r = -.10$ at 24 months and $r = -.11$ at 36 months), and observed maternal sensitivity ($r = .10$ at 24 months and $r = .07$ at 36 months) indicated that these tended to be small effects.

For maternal report of negative/aggressive peer interaction (Table 20.1), mothers reported increasing levels of agonism from 24 months to 36 months, $F(1,765) = 14.16$, $p < .001$, but the patterns of association between the predictors and outcome did not differ between 24 and 36 months. The selection, child, and maternal blocks were significantly related to maternal

TABLE 20.1. Longitudinal Analysis of 24- and 36-Month Peer Social Behavior: Maternal Ratings

	Maternal ratings of positive sociability						Maternal ratings of negative/aggressive					
	24 months		36 months		Main effect F	Effect × age F	24 months		36 months		Main effect F	Effect × age F
	β	SE	β	SE			β	SE	β	SE		
Intercept	2.372	.013	2.45	.012		31.16**	1.373	.013	1.436	.014		14.16*
Site[a]					1.51						1.76	
Selection					1.59	.02					3.57*	.36
Maternal education	-.004	.014	-.006	.013			-.013	.014	-.004	.015		
Beliefs about employment risks	-.018	.013	-.018	.012			.032*	.013	.023	.013	6.13*	
Child					13.77***	.03					5.13**	.94
Gender (male = 1)	-.018	.011	-.017	.011			-.030*	.012	-.010	.013	3.94*	
Cognitive/language competence	.048***	.014	.053***	.012	25.89***		-.025	.015	-.029*	.015	5.82*	
Temperament	-.028*	.012	-.028**	.011	8.50**		.023	.012	.033*	.013	7.56**	
Maternal Sensitivity	.023	.012	.023	.012	6.52*	.00	-.021	.013	-.047*	.014	11.20***	2.04
Child care					.44	1.65					.89	1.22
Hours	.017	.014	-.013	.013			.021	.015	.010	.014		
Peer availability	-.007	.013	-.009	.010			-.011	.014	.018	.013		
Positive care	-.001	.010	.011	.011			-.003	.011	.017	.014		

Note. Beta coefficients and standard errors (*SE*) are shown for each predictor at each age. The main effect *F* corresponds to the test for each block of predictors across age, and is also shown for individual predictors when the block was significant. The effect × age *F* tested whether the association between predictors and outcome changed with age.

[a]Individual site coefficients are not reported because site was included only as a control variable.

* *p* < .05; ** *p* < .01; *** *p* < .001.

290

report of negative social behavior over time. Specifically, mothers reported higher levels of negative peer behavior when they perceived more costs associated with employment, $F(1,765) = 6.13$, $p = .014$, the child was male, $F(1,765) = 3.94$, $p = .048$, the child had lower cognitive/language skills, $F(1,765) = 5.82$, $p = .016$, when mothers had reported more difficult temperament in their infants, $F(1,765) = 7.56$, $p = .006$, and when the mother was rated as less sensitive in play with the child, $F(1,765) = 11.20$, $p = .0009$. Partial correlations between maternal report of negative/aggressive play and her report of the risks of employment ($r = .11$ at 24 months and $r = .05$ at 36 months), the child's cognitive/language skills ($r = -.07$ at 24 months and $r = -.09$ at 36 months), maternal report of difficult infant temperament ($r = .07$ at 24 months and $r = .10$ at 36 months) and observed maternal sensitivity ($r = -.05$ at 24 months and $r = -.13$ at 36 months) again indicate modest effects.

The first columns of Table 20.2 show results from the analysis of the caregiver's report of positive peer sociability. These results indicate that caregivers reported increased positive social play from 24 to 36 months, $F(1,706) = 12.87$, $p < .001$, and that the patterns of association between the selection, child, maternal, and child care predictors were similar across time. The child, maternal, and child care blocks significantly predicted caregiver ratings, with higher ratings of positive peer play related to whether the child was a girl, $F(1, 706) = 4.19$, $p = .041$, to higher cognitive/language skills, $F(1,706) = 17.20$, $p < .001$, greater maternal sensitivity, $F(1,706) = 7.54$, $p = .006$, and more positive caregiving in child care, $F(1,706) = 10.45$, $p = .001$. Again, modest effects were observed. The partial correlations between the caregiver ratings of positive social play and cognitive/language skills ($r = .11$ at 24 months and $r = .16$ at 36 months), observed maternal sensitivity ($r = .09$ at 24 and 36 months), and positive caregiving ($r = .12$ at 24 months and $r = .07$ at 36 months) were small. The standardized difference (effect size) between boys and girls was also small ($d = .08$ at 24 months, and $d = .05$ at 36 months).

For caregivers' report of negative or aggressive peer play in child care (Table 20.2) there was no reliable change from 24 to 36 months, $F(1,701) = 1.63$, $p = .20$, and the patterns of association with the selection, child, maternal, and child care predictors did not differ significantly across time. The maternal and child care blocks predicted caregiver ratings, with higher ratings of negative play related to lower maternal sensitivity, $F(1,701) = 5.50$, $p = .019$, more hours of child care, $F(1,701) = 6.96$, $p = .009$, and being in child care settings with peers available more often, $F(1,701) = 7.86$, $p = .005$. Again, modest effects were observed. The partial correlations between the caregiver ratings of negative social play and maternal sensitivity ($r = -.07$ at 24 months and $r = -.10$ at 36 months), hours of child care ($r = .11$ at 24 months and $r = .04$ at 36 months), and amount of experience with peers in child care ($r = .07$ at 24 months and $r = .10$ at 36 months) were small.

Table 20.3 shows results from the analysis of peer play observed in child care. These results indicate that observed positive social play did not

TABLE 20.2. Longitudinal Analysis of 24- and 36-Month Peer Social Behavior: Caregivers' Ratings

	Caregivers' ratings of positive sociability						Caregivers' ratings of negative/aggressive					
	24 months		36 months		Main effect F	Effect × age F	24 months		36 months		Main effect F	Effect × age F
	β	SE	β	SE			β	SE	β	SE		
Intercept	2.310	.018	2.393	.016		12.87***	1.365	.020	1.397	.018		1.63
Site[a]					2.02*	.20					1.12	
Selection					1.03						2.42	.87
Maternal education	-.017	.019	-.004	.017			-.037	.020	-.029	.019		
Beliefs about employment risks	-.013	.018	-.018	.016			.009	.019	-.019	.018		
Child												
Gender (male = 1)	-.028	.015	-.019	.014	9.11***	.32	.016	.017	.009	.016	.38	.50
Cognitive/language competence	.045*	.020	.067***	.017	4.19*		.010	.021	-.017	.019		
Temperament	-.019	.016	-.013	.015	17.20***		.007	.017	-.007	.016		
Maternal												
Sensitivity	.037*	.018	.031	.017	7.54**	.06	-.023	.019	-.041**	.018	5.50*	.48
Child care												
Hours	.011	.021	.008	.017	3.56**	.86	.060*	.023	.022	.019	7.04***	.87
Peer availability	-.011	.019	.019	.015			.043**	.020	.033	.017	6.96**	
Positive caregiving	.045**	.015	.028	.017	10.45**		-.006	.016	-.028	.019	7.86**	

Note.—Beta coefficients and standard errors (*SE*) are shown for each predictor at each age, and is also shown for individual predictors when the block was significant. The main effect *F* corresponds to the test for each block of predictors across age, and it changed with age. The effect × age *F* tested whether the association between predictors and outcome changed with age.

[a]Individual site coefficients are not reported because site was included only as a control variable.

* $p < .05$; ** $p < .01$; *** $p < .001$.

TABLE 20.3. Longitudinal Analysis of 24- and 36-Month Peer Social Behavior: Observed Peer Interaction in Child Care

	Observed positive peer play						Observed negative peer interaction					
	24 months		36 months		Main effect F	Effect × age F	24 months		36 months		Main effect F	Effect × age F
	β	SE	β	SE			β	SE	β	SE		
Intercept	−.19	.138	−.372	.133			.206	.012	.146	.008		
Site[a]					7.43***	.98					6.69***	18.65***
Selection					1.02	2.01					2.94	2.09
Maternal education	.105	.123	−.209	.124			−.017	.010	−.001	.007		
Beliefs about employment risks	−.076	.117	−.165	.112			.019	.010	.002	.007		
Child					2.59	.63					2.23	1.04
Gender (male = 1)	−.187	.103	−.048	.103			.007	.009	.012	.006		
Cognitive/language competence	.106	.138	.265*	.107			.008	.011	−.014	.007		
Temperament	−.032	.107	−.110	.105			.010	.009	.008	.006		
Maternal					5.41*	.02					.00	.46
Sensitivity	.206	.115	.185	.117			.004	.010	−.004	.007		
Child care					4.79**	1.61					3.41*	.5
Hours	−.029	.142	.225	.116			−.007	.012	−.005	.007		
Peer availability	.155	.157	.412**	.134			−.020	.013	−.000	.008		
Positive caregiving	−.168	.100	−.139	.118	7.30**		−.015	.008	−.016*	.007	8.25**	

Note. Beta coefficients and standard errors (SE) are shown for each predictor at each age. The main effect F corresponds to the test for each block of predictors across age, and is also shown for individual predictors when the block was significant. The effect × age F tested whether the association between predictors and outcome changed with age.

[a]Individual site coefficients are not reported because site was included only as a control variable.

* p < .05; ** p < .01; *** p < .001.

293

change from 24 to 36 months, $F(1,622) = 0.98$, $p = .32$; and that the patterns of association with the selection, child, maternal, and child care predictors did not change significantly across time. The maternal and child care blocks significantly predicted observed positive play, with more positive play related to greater maternal sensitivity, $F(1,662) = 5.41$, $p = .02$, and more frequent experience with peers in child care, $F(1,662) = 7.30$, $p = .007$. Again, modest effects were observed. The partial correlations between observed positive peer play and maternal sensitivity ($r = .06$ at 24 and 36 months) and experience with peers in child care ($r = .06$ at 24 months and $r = .15$ at 36 months) were small.

For negative peer play observed in child care (Table 20.3), results indicate that more negative play occurred at 24 months than at 36 months, $F(1,618) = 18.65$, $p < .001$, but the patterns of association with the selection, child, maternal, and child care predictors were similar across time. Only the child care block significantly predicted observed negative play, with more negative peer play related to less positive caregiving in child care, $F(1,618) = 8.25$, $p = .004$. Again, modest effects were observed; the partial correlations between observed negative play and positive caregiving ($r = -.09$ at 24 months and $r = -.10$ at 36 months) were small.

Dyadic Peer Play at 36 Months

The final set of analyses predicted three aspects of dyadic play with a friend, which was assessed at 36 months only, precluding longitudinal analyses. Table 20.4 shows the results. The standardized regression coefficients are reported in the first column and F tests for the contribution of each block of variables was reported in the second column. The first outcome, observed peer skill, was significantly related to the selection, child, and maternal blocks. More skilled play was observed among children who were female, who scored higher on expressive language, and whose mothers were rated as more sensitive during play with their children. Small to moderate effect sizes were observed, with the partial correlations ranging from .12 (maternal sensitivity) to .22 (language skills). The effect size for gender ($d = -.10$) was also modest. The second outcome, observed aggression, was significantly related only to the maternal block, with more peer aggression associated with less maternal sensitivity (partial $r = -.10$). The third outcome, self-assertion, was related only to the child block, with more self-assertion observed among females ($d = -.15$) and among children with higher language scores (partial $r = .15$).

DISCUSSION

Children in child care become more positive and less negative in their social play between 24 and 36 months. Regular, albeit modest, relations emerged

TABLE 20.4. Regression Analysis of Cumulative Predictions of 36-Month Peer Social Behavior: Children Observed in Dyadic Play with a Friend

| | Dyadic play at 36 months | | | | | |
| | Peer skill | | Peer aggression | | Self-assertion | |
	β	F	β	F	β	F
Site		2.15*		1.09		1.11
Selection		4.43*		.55		1.72
Maternal education	−.110*		.008		−.102	
Beliefs about employment risks	−.100*		.051		.008	
Child		10.22***		.38		7.85***
Gender (male = 1)	−.091*		−.048		−.146**	
Cognitive/language competence	.261***		−.021		.182**	
Temperament	.021		.007		.031	
Maternal		6.80**		4.72*		.92
Sensitivity	.138**		−.121*		.053	
Child care		.97		.46		.46
Hours	.005		.006		.049	
Peers availability	.038		−.055		−.014	
Positive caregiving	−.059		.009		−.031	
Total R^2		.14**		.04		.08**

For each individual predictor, standardized regression coefficients are reported.
*$p < .05$; **$p < .01$; ***$p < .001$.

between child care experiences in the first 3 years of life and individual differences in children's peer competencies. Caregiver sensitivity and responsiveness were the most consistent aspects of the child care experience associated with positive, skilled peer interactions in child care, regardless of how much time children spent in child care or how much experience they had with other children in child care. Greater experience in child care settings with other children present was also associated with more competent peer play as observed in child care, above and beyond the quality of caregiving in those settings. But caregivers rated these children as more negative in peer play. They similarly rated children as more negative in peer play who had experienced more weekly hours of care, regardless of caregiving quality, although children's observed peer play did not differ in relation to amount of child care. We have suggested that these apparent inconsistencies might be clarified by conducting more differentiated observations of peer conflict among very young children, as well as by more fully exploring how caregiver reports relate to observations of children's social behavior and how they each predict later social functioning.

Child care experiences were not associated with children's peer competence either as rated by their mothers or as observed in structured dyadic play. In contrast, both maternal sensitivity and the children's own cognitive and language competence were systematically associated with the quality and complexity of their peer play across all settings and informants. Together, these findings suggest that peer competence may be acquired differently in different contexts. In this study, our observations in the child care setting may have tapped different kinds of skills than mothers were privy to or than we observed in structured dyadic play with a friend. This, in turn, raises the possibility that children's experiences in child care may be more important for their group-based peer competencies than for the growth of dyadic peer relationships. Of course, at this report the children were quite young. As a result, their rated and observed behavior was still rudimentary and their friendships not yet well developed. Future analyses as the children develop stable friendships and regular peer-group relationships in the late preschool and early school years will permit us to consider such possibilities with greater confidence.

21

Does Amount of Time Spent in Child Care Predict Socioemotional Adjustment during the Transition to Kindergarten?

NICHD Early Child Care Research Network

Today, the majority of mothers in the United States who return to work after having a child do so before their child's first birthday. Recent figures (for 1998–1999) indicate that 58% of all women with infants under 1 year of age are in the labor force (Bureau of Labor Statistics, 2000); comparable rates in 1970 and 1985 were 27% and 46%, respectively (Kamerman, 2000). In the National Institute of Child Health and Human Development (NICHD) Study of Early Child Care, the overwhelming majority of mothers who were employed in their infants' first year returned to work and placed their child in some kind of routine nonmaternal care arrangement before the child was 6 months of age (NICHD Early Child Care Research Network, 1997c; see also Hofferth, 1996).

How does such early and extensive nonmaternal care experience affect children's development, especially their socioemotional adjustment? Despite long-standing debate regarding the effects of nonmaternal care, reviews of the relevant literature published in the late 1970s and early 1980s revealed few discernible negative associations between early child care and psychosocial adjustment (Belsky & Steinberg, 1978; Clarke-Stewart & Fein, 1983). As more evidence became available, one series of papers argued that

From *Child Development*, 2003, Vol. 74, pp. 976–1005. Reprinted with permission of the Society for Research in Child Development.

early and extensive nonmaternal care—that is, care initiated in the first year of life for more than 20–30 hours per week—was associated with elevated levels of aggression and noncompliance when children were 3–8 years of age (Belsky, 1988, 1990a, 1994; Belsky & Rovine, 1988). Considerable discussion of this interpretation of the available data by a number of scholars (Clarke-Stewart, 1988; Phillips, McCartney, Scarr, & Howes, 1987; Richters & Zahn-Waxler, 1990; Thompson, 1988) followed. Moreover, the emergence of additional evidence (e.g., Bates et al., 1994; Belsky & Eggebeen, 1991; Vandell & Corasaniti, 1990) led to the suggestion that it was lots of time in spent in care across the infancy, toddler, and preschool years (i.e., early, extensive, and continuous care) that was associated with poorer socioemotional adjustment (Belsky, 1994, 2001).

Weaknesses of the data available in the 1980s were numerous and included (1) failure to take into account preexisting family background factors that could account for the association between care use and child outcomes (Richters & Zahn-Waxler, 1990; Thompson, 1988), (2) failure to evaluate the quality of care (e.g., Belsky, 1984; Goelman & Pence, 1987; Howes, 1990; Howes & Olenick, 1986; McCartney, 1984; Phillips, 1987; Phillips, McCartney, Scarr, & Howes, 1987; Thompson, 1988), and (3) questions as to whether elevated levels of aggression and noncompliance associated with the timing and amount of nonmaternal care might reflect assertiveness and independence from adults rather than problem behavior (Clarke-Stewart, 1988).

Designed to remedy a number of the problems inherent in previously collected data, the NICHD Study of Early Child Care measured children's experiences with nonmaternal care and their developmental outcomes from birth in a diverse sample of families in 10 different locations across the United States. The NICHD data are thus well suited to address the questions concerning relations between the use of nonmaternal care and children's socioemotional development that have been much discussed over the past 15 years: (1) Does cumulative amount of time spent in nonmaternal child care across the infancy, toddler, and preschool years predict children's socioemotional adjustment after considering potentially confounding family background factors? (2) Do aspects of child care other than cumulative amount of time in nonmaternal care, especially quality of care (but also type and stability), account for detected associations? (3) Might the quality of parenting explain, at least in part, the process by which cumulative amount of time in nonmaternal care is related to children's social functioning? (4) Is there a threshold at which the effects of time in care become particularly pronounced (e.g., 20 hours per week and 30 hours per week?)? (5) To what extent does timing of child care experience, in terms of average hours of care per year across the first 4½ years, account for the detected effects of cumulative quantity of care? (6) Do detected linkages between quantity of care and socioemotional adjustment reflect high levels of problem behavior and/or actual aggressive behavior and disobedience rather than assertiveness?

METHODS

A detailed description of the study design and participants is provided in Chapter 1.

Longitudinal Modeling of Repeated Measures

As many, but not all, measures were obtained more than once, hierarchical linear modeling (HLM) techniques (Bryk & Raudenbush, 1992) were often used to generate two scores to describe *patterns of change over time* from measurements of the same construct obtained by the same method on multiple occasions. One measure, the maximum-likelihood estimate of the intercept, reflects the predicted *mean* of the repeated measurements of a particular construct at the mean of the included assessment ages (i.e., 6, 15, 24, 36, and 54 months). Age was mean centered, so intercepts reflect the predicted mean for the individual's growth curve at the average age (27 months). The second measure, the individual's slope, estimates *the linear change* in the construct across the multiple measurement occasions. Positive slope values reflect degree of increase in the variable over time, whereas negative slope values reflect degree of decrease in the variable over time.

Child Care Characteristics

Nonmaternal child care was defined as regular care by anyone other than the mother—including care by fathers, relatives, and nannies (whether in home or out of the home); family-day-care providers, and centers—that was routinely scheduled for at least 10 hours per week. Several features of individual children's care experiences measured from birth through 54 months figure importantly in this report.

Quantity

Cumulative amount of time in nonmaternal care through the first 4½ years of life was determined from telephone interviews with mothers at 3- or 4-month intervals about the number of hours and the types of care used during the prior 3–4 months. Two indices were used in the analyses: the average number of hours per week that nonmaternal care was used from ages at the mean age between 3 months through 4½ years (i.e., HLM intercept) and the linear rate of change (i.e., HLM slope) of hours per week over time.

Quality

Quality was defined by the caregiver–child interaction and stimulation experienced by the target child in the child care setting. Quality was assessed during two half-day visits scheduled within a 2-week interval at 6, 15, 24, and 36 months and one half-day visit at 54 months. At each visit, observers completed two 44-minute cycles of the Observational Record of the Caregiving Environment (ORCE) during which they first coded the frequency of specific caregiver behaviors and then rated the quality of the caregiving. Positive caregiving composites were calculated for each age level observed by averaging these ratings. (See Chapters 2 and 6 for details.) For this report, two cumulative indices of positive caregiving were formed by means of HLM analyses: average quality of nonmaternal care at the mean age (i.e., HLM intercept) and linear rate of change over time in quality of nonmaternal care (i.e., HLM slope). (For further details on the ORCE, see Chapters 3 and 6.)

Type

For each of 16 epochs (3-month intervals from birth to 36 months and 4-month intervals after 36 months), the child's primary care arrangement was classified as a center, a child care home (any home-based care outside the child's own home except grandparent care), in-home care (by any caregiver in the child's own home except father or grandparent), grandparent care, or father care. Information was available on each setting with respect to the number of children present other than the target child. Epochs in which children were in less than 10 hours per week of nonmaternal care were coded as exclusive maternal care. Two indicators of type of care are used in this report. "Center care" reflects the proportion of epochs in which the child received care in a center. "Peer-group exposure" reflects the proportion of epochs in which a child was in any child care setting in which there were at least two other children in addition to him/herself.

Instability

For each of 12 3-month epochs from birth to 36 months, a count was made of the number of times the mother reported that the child started a new child care arrangement, or one that had previously stopped and then started again. Because of a few extreme scores, this variable was truncated at the 95th percentile. Children who received no nonmaternal care received scores of 0. Thus, low scores reflected more stable arrangements and high scores less stable ones.

Maternal, Child, and Family Characteristics

The following maternal, child, and family characteristics were included in the analyses as controls for selection effects: maternal education in years, the mean family's income-to-needs ratio (family income divided by the poverty threshold for its household size as determined by the U.S. Census), partner status (the proportion of 3–4-month epochs during which mother reported living with a partner/husband), child sex, infant temperament (see below), ethnic group (non-Hispanic African American, non-Hispanic European American, Hispanic, or other), and maternal depressive symptoms (the intercept or predicted mean and linear slope over 4 years) as measured by the Center for Epidemiological Studies—Depression (CES-D) scale (Radloff, 1977). The mother reported the family income and household size at 6-, 15-, 24-, 36-, and 54-month assessments.

Infant temperament was measured by means of 55 6-point items from the Infant Temperament Questionnaire completed by mothers at 6 months (Medoff-Cooper, Carey, & McDevitt, 1993). Cronbach's alpha was .81.

In addition, a composite measure of maternal sensitivity, based on evaluations of observed maternal behavior at 6, 15, 24, 36, and 54 months (see Chapter 17) , served as a potential explanatory factor, rather than control variable, in the analyses to be reported.

Child Adjustment at 4½ Years and Kindergarten

The child outcomes examined in this study are mother-, caregiver- and teacher-report measures of social competence and problem behavior and child–teacher relationship conflict obtained when children were 54 months of age and/or in kindergarten. In addition, at 54 months, children were observed in a dyadic interaction with a friend and their peer interactions in child care settings were also observed.

Social Competence

Mothers completed the Social Skills Questionnaire from the Social Skills Rating System (SSRS; Gresham & Elliott, 1990; Chapter 24) for their children at both times of measurement. Teachers completed the instrument when children were in kindergarten. For children who were in child care at least 7½ hours per week at age 54 months ($n = 833$), caregivers completed a slightly modified version of the California Preschool Social Competency Scale (Levine, Elzey, & Lewis, 1969; Chapter 24).

Behavior Problems

Mothers, caregivers, and teachers completed appropriate versions of the Child Behavior Checklist (CBCL; Achenbach, 1991a; Chapter 24), a widely used measure of behavior problems. The score for the externalizing subscale served as the dependent variable in the primary analysis. Externalizing is defined as problem behavior of the "acting out" variety and includes, but is not restricted to, behaviors involving disobedience and defiance of adult requests/commands/instructions/directives (e.g., defiant, uncooperative, disobedient at school, talks out of turn, and fails to carry out assigned task), aggression (e.g., hits others, destroys others' things, and gets in many fights), and assertiveness/emotion dysregulation (e.g., argues a lot, screams a lot, has temper tantrums, and demands/wants attention). Raw scores were converted into standard *T*-scores, based on normative data for children 4–11 years of age. In secondary analyses designed to address the question of whether quantity of child care was related to aggression and disobedience or just assertiveness, three composite measures were created by summing select items from the CBCL. An assertiveness subscale was based on items such as bragging/boasting, talks too much, argues a lot, and demands attention. A disobedience subscale was based on items such as defiant–talks back to staff, disrupts classroom discipline, temper tantrums, lying/cheating, and fails to carry out assigned tasks. The aggression subscale was based on items such as cruelty to others, destroys own things, gets in many fights, attacks others, hits others, and is explosive/unpredictable.

Teacher–Child Conflict

At 54 months and at kindergarten, child care providers and teachers completed the Student–Teacher Relationship Scale (STRS; Pianta, 2001). The STRS is a widely used indicator of a teacher's perceptions of the quality of their relationship with a specific child and one specific scale, Conflict, appears to be a particularly informative indicator (e.g., Birch & Ladd, 1997; Hamre & Pianta, 2001). In the present sample, caregivers completed the STRS at 54 months for the children in child care and kindergarten teachers completed the STRS in the late fall of kindergarten. Coefficient alphas for the conflict scale were .86 at 54 months and .90 at kindergarten.

Dyadic Peer Interaction

At 54 months, study children were videotaped while they interacted with a peer during three structured play episodes and trained observers coded 10 ratings of social behavior for each episode (see Chapter 20 for details). Two composite indicators of the quality of interactions with the peer were computed for each child. Negative interaction was computed as the sum of ratings on "contributes to negative interaction," "aggression," and "negative mood." Positive interaction was computed as the sum of "contributes to positive interaction," "prosocial behavior," and "positive mood."

Behavior in Child Care

As part of the ORCE child care observation at 54 months, the interactions of the study child with peers in the child care setting were recorded during each of the observation periods (see Chapters 1 and 5). Two composites were derived from time-sampled codes of the child's behavior. The child care positive composite was computed as the sum of three separate codes: cooperative play, boisterous play, and other positive or neutral interaction. The child care negative composite was computed as the sum of four separate codes: physical aggression, verbal aggression, negative behavior toward peer, and other negative nonaggressive acts. The negative interaction composite was highly skewed and had limited nonzero values, and so was dichotomized as 0 if below the median (2) and 1 otherwise.

Table 21.1 presents the mean, standard deviation, and ranges of all variables. Overall, mothers, caregivers, and teachers rated the sample well within the normal range on all standardized measures. The mean CBCL externalizing *T*-scores were approximately 50 at both time points according to mothers and teachers, with 50 being the mean for the norming population. Very few children scored in the clinical range defined as a *T*-score of 65 or above and about 16% of the same scored in the at-risk range of a *T*-score at or above 60 (one standard deviation above the mean). The SSRS social competence mean scores range from 99 to 103, again falling close to the expected population mean of 100. Further details about all data collection procedures are documented in the manuals of operation of the study (*http://public.rti.org/secc/*).

RESULTS

Statistical analyses were undertaken to answer a series of questions posed in the introduction and some additional ones that emerged in the course of the data analysis. Fourteen outcomes were evaluated and we used the consistency of findings across the multiple indicators of social functioning as the criterion for determining when an effect was detected. Rather than relying on a single regression analysis that would include in a single prediction model all the explanatory variables considered in this inquiry, we chose to analyze the data in a series of interrelated steps (i.e., nested regression models) so that we could address distinctive and logically ordered questions in a lawful sequence.

Effects of Quantity Controlling for Background Factors

To evaluate the relation between time in nonmaternal child care and socioemotional adjustment, an initial multiple regression model (i.e., Model 1, or the base model) was run. The covariates included in the base model to control for background factors were site (represented by nine dummy-coded variables), child gender (male), child ethnicity (African American non-Hispanic, Hispanic, other), 6-month difficult temperament, maternal education at enrollment, average income-to-needs ratio across the period 6–54 months, and average maternal depression (i.e., HLM intercept) and linear change over time in maternal depression (i.e., HLM slope) across the same period. As analyses revealed that significant interactions between family and child care factors, and among child care factors, were detected at a rate no greater than chance, no interaction effects are presented.

TABLE 21.1. Descriptive Statistics on All Analytic Variables

Variable	M	SD	Minimum	Maximum	n
Quantity of child care (hours)					
Mean hours per week (3–54 mo)	26.98	15.43	−0.53	61.57	982
Linear change/slope (3–54 mo)	0.173	0.314	−1.102	1.189	982
Mean child care hours 3–6 mo	21.0	18.0	0	62.5	982
Mean child care hours 7–12 mo	23.7	18.5	0	80	980
Mean child care hours 13–24 mo	26.0	16.7	0	65.8	982
Mean child care hours 25–36 mo	26.8	17.0	0	68.8	982
Mean child care hours 37–54 mo	32.7	15.8	0	92.3	982
Child and family characteristics					
Gender (1 = male)	50.4%				982
Ethnicity					
Black	11%				982
Hispanic	6%				982
Other	4%				982
Mother's education	14.50	2.44	7.00	21.00	982
income-to-needs (6–54 mo)	3.82	2.82	0.22	27.36	982
Child temperament at 6 mo	3.16	.40	1.54	4.44	982
Depression mean (HLM intercept: 6–54 mo)	9.21	5.44	1.39	31.69	982
Depression linear slope (6–54 mo)	0.19	0.66	−2.84	4.05	982
Parenting mean (HLM intercept: 6–54 mo)	.06	.61	−2.85	1.27	982
Parenting linear slope (6–54 mo)	−.01	.07	−0.32	.20	982
Other child care experiences					
Center care: Proportion time	0.24	0.28	0.00	1.00	982
Quality mean (HLM intercept: 6–54 mo)	2.82	0.23	2.07	3.44	982
Peer-group exposure: Proportion time	0.57	0.30	0.00	1.00	982
Instability (3–34 mo): number of changes	3.27	2.62	0.00	18.00	982
Child social functioning					
Mother ratings: 54 mo					
Social competence	98.72	13.30	53.00	130.00	935
Externalizing problems	51.61	9.35	30.00	82.00	940
Caregiver ratings: 54 mo					
Social competence	104.79	13.53	46.14	135.00	725
Externalizing problems	50.12	9.54	35.00	87.00	689
Conflict	18.77	6.64	12.00	49.00	691
Observations: 54 mo					
Dyadic play positive	.06	2.46	−8.43	7.86	698
Dyadic play negative (> median)	.41	.49	0.00	1.00	694
Child care positive (log)[a]	2.33	.99	0.00	4.03	838
Child care negative (> median)	.51	.50	0.00	1.00	838
Mother ratings: kindergarten					
Social competence	102.85	14.69	56.00	130.00	938
Externalizing problems	50.01	9.72	30.00	81.00	940
Teacher ratings					
Social competence	103.48	14.08	49.00	130.00	893
Externalizing problems	49.90	8.95	39.00	89.00	903
Conflict	10.71	5.43	7.00	34.00	905

(continued)

TABLE 21.1. *(continued)*

Variable	M	SD	Minimum	Maximum	n
Child behavior problems					
Mother ratings: 54 mo					
Aggression items	1.32	1.93	0	12	931
Disobedience items	2.92	2.10	0	14	934
Assertive items	3.66	2.06	0	10	936
Caregiver ratings: 54 mo					
Aggression items	1.25	2.39	0	14	593
Disobedience items	1.87	2.63	0	14	676
Assertive items	.40	.63	0	2	698
Mother ratings: Kindergarten					
Aggression items	1.15	1.78	0	13	924
Disobedience items	2.69	2.16	0	13	925
Assertive items	3.35	2.06	0	10	926
Teacher ratings: 54 mo					
Aggression items	.69	1.79	0	16	891
Disobedience items	1.80	2.90	0	20	880
Assertive items	1.40	2.09	0	10	894

[a]Log transformation.

The effects of the two quantity-of-care predictors in the base model are detailed under three separate columns in Table 21.2, each labeled "Model 1: Base." The first such column (i.e., fourth column of table) indicates whether the two quantity variables, when considered together, significantly predicted a particular outcome (i.e., "pooled"). Inspection of the relevant data show that the two quantity variables significantly predicted three of the nine 54-month outcomes—caregiver reported social competence, externalizing problems, and conflict—and three of the five kindergarten outcomes: mother-reported externalizing problems and teacher-reported externalizing problems and conflict. The second column labeled "Model 1: Base" (i.e., seventh column in the table) presents the effect of the individual quantity predictor, mean hours per week of care, net of all other factors in the base model; and the third column labeled "Model 1: Base" (i.e., tenth column) presents the same information for the second quantity predictor, linear-change-over-time-in-hours-per-week-in-nonmaternal care.

Inspection of the relevant data indicates that children who averaged more time in nonmaternal child care across their first 54 months of life scored lower on caregiver-rated social competence and higher on caregiver-rated externalizing problems and teacher–child conflict at 54 months, and were observed to engage in more negative dyadic play at this age. More time spent in child care also predicted, at kindergarten age, more mother- and teacher-reported externalizing problems and more teacher–child conflict. Further, when hours spent in child care increased (vs. decreased) over time, children were rated by caregivers at age 4½ years as being less socially com-

TABLE 21.2. Effects of Quantity of Care (Mean Hours per Week, Linear Change over Time) in Model 1 (Base: Covariates Only), Model 2 (Plus Additional Child Care Predictors), and Model 3 (Plus Maternal Sensitivity)

	N	Stat.[d]	Pooled tests[a]			Hours of care per week[b]			Linear change over time in hours/week		
			Model 1: Base	Model 2: Adds child care	Model 3: Adds parenting	Model 1: Base	Model 2: Adds child care	Model 3: Adds parenting	Model 1: Base	Model 2: Adds child care	Model 3: Adds parenting
54 Months[c]											
M social competence	935	β		*	*	-.05	-.09**	-.07*	-.04	-.04	-.03
CG social competence	725	β	***	***	***	-.13***	-.15***	-.13**	-.12**	-.12**	-.10**
M externalizing problems	940	β				.06	.05	.04	-.01	-.01	-.01
CG externalizing problems	689	β	***	***	***	.25***	.23***	.22***	.08*	.07*	.07
CG conflict	691	β	***	***	***	.22***	.20***	.18***	.07	.06	.05
Dyadic play (positive)	698	β				.01	-.04	-.03	-.02	-.03	-.02
Child care (positive)	838	β				.02	-.01	.01	.07*	.06	.07
Dyadic play (negative)	694	OR				1.01*	1.01*	1.01	1.42	1.43	1.41
Child care (negative)	838	OR				1.01	1.01	1.01	0.92	0.86	0.85
Kindergarten[c]											
M social competence	938	β		*		-.03	-.06	-.04	-.04	-.04	-.03
T social competence	893	β				-.05	-.04	-.02	.02	.02	.03
M externalizing problems	940	β	*			.09**	.08*	.08*	.01	.00	-.00
T externalizing problems	903	β	***	**	**	.14***	.11**	.10**	-.03	-.05	-.05
T conflict	905	β	***	*	*	.13***	.09*	.09*	-.02	-.03	-.04

[a]Two degrees of freedom tests of no effect on intercept (mean) or slope (linear change).
[b]Base model with factors for site, gender, ethnicity, mother's education, maternal depression (intercept, slope) 6–54 months average income-to-needs, 6 months temperament. Model 2 adds child care factors: average quality of care, proportion of center care, proportion of peer-group exposure, instability of care. Model 3 adds parenting factors: mean (i.e., HLM intercept) and linear change (i.e., HLM slope) from 6–54 months.
[c]M, mother; CG, caregiver; T, teacher.
[d]β, Beta; OR, odds ratio.
*$p < .05$; **$p < .01$; ***$p < .001$.

petent and as showing more externalizing problems but were observed to engage in more positive behavior during the child care observations. Change in time spent in child care proved unrelated to kindergarten outcomes, however.

Alternative Explanation: Other Features of Child Care

As part of a series of nested regression analyses, a second model (i.e., Model 2) was run to determine whether effects of quantity of care just described would remain significant—or even emerge for the first time (i.e., suppression effects)—when four other features of child care were taken into consideration by adding them to the base model: average quality of child care, proportion of time spent in center care, proportion of peer-group exposure, and instability of care. To the extent that effects of quantity of care remain significant with these other variables included, this would indicate that effects of quantity were not exclusively a function of other features of child care purposefully excluded from the base model. Inspection of the fifth column in Table 21.2, which reports the significance of the two quantity-of-child care predictors combined when additional child care factors are added to the base model, indicates that in only one of six cases did a previously significant pooled effect of quantity prove insignificant in Model 2 (i.e., maternal report of externalizing problems in kindergarten: from $p < .05$ to $p > .05$) and that two previously insignificant pooled effects of quantity of care proved significant once other features of child care experience were taken into consideration (i.e., mother-reported social competence at 54 months and in kindergarten: from $p > .05$ to $p < .01$ and $.05$, respectively).

Inspection of the second column labeled "Model 2" in Table 21.2 (i.e., eighth column of table) shows that all significant effects of hours of care per week (i.e., HLM intercept) detected in Model 1 remained significant when the four additional child care variables were added to the prediction model; and that in the case of mother-rated social competence, a previously insignificant effect of hours per week in care proved significant, indicating that more time in care predicted less mother-reported social competence at 54 months. Nevertheless, comparison of parameter estimates from Model 1 and Model 2 shows that effects of hours per week were modestly smaller in the model including additional child care predictors than in the base model in the case of five of the original seven significant effects (e.g., T externalizing) and in one case larger (i.e., caregiver social competence). The largest changes in regression coefficients for hours per week emerged in the case of kindergarten teacher's report of externalizing problems and conflict.

Inspection of the third column labeled "Model 2" in Table 21.2 (i.e., 11th column of table) shows that in one of three cases a previously significant effect (in Model 1) of linear change over time in hours per week of child care became insignificant when additional features of child care were taken into consideration (i.e., positive child care). In sum, even though inclusion of four additional features of child care in the prediction model attenuated some of the originally detected effects of quantity of child care, in the main, effects of quantity remained significant even with indicators of child care quality, type, and instability taken into consideration.

Alternative Explanation: Maternal Sensitivity

As the third step in the series of nested regression analyses, Model 2 was itself modified by adding two additional predictors reflecting average maternal sensitivity (i.e., HLM intercept) and linear change in maternal sensitivity (i.e., HLM slope) so that effects of quantity of child care could be reexamined after controlling for patterns of parenting that prior work on this sample showed were themselves predicted by quantity of care (NICHD Early Child Care Network, 1999a). Although small reductions of the hours coefficients were observed for selected outcomes, of the pooled effects of the two quantity-of-care predictors in Model 3, all but one (i.e., six of seven) of these combined effects remained significant when the two maternal sensitivity predictors were added to Model 2. Consideration of specific parameter estimates from Models 2 and 3 indicates that seven of eight significant effects of hours of care per week (i.e., HLM intercept) and one of two significant effects of linear change over time in hours per week (i.e., HLM slope) remained significant when maternal sensitivity predictors were added to the prediction model. By and large, then, the previously detected effects for quantity of care remained significant when the alternative predictor of maternal sensitivity was added to the model.

At the same time, it should be noted that even children experiencing the greatest amount of nonmaternal care do not score, on average, in (or even near) the at-risk range on externalizing problems (i.e., ≥ 60). Further the absolute differences between the adjusted means for the groups with the lowest and highest amounts of care are in all cases less than one-half of the sample standard deviation (see Table 21.1).

Effect Sizes

In order to evaluate the explanatory power of each predictor included in Model 3 and, in so doing, illuminate the absolute and relative power of quantity of care to predict socioemotional adjustment, effect-size estimates were calculated for all predictors in Model 3 for those 7 (of 14) developmental outcomes found to be related to quantity of care. Two effect-size estimates were calculated for each predictor for each outcome, one more conservative and one quite liberal. The former took the form of a partial correlation representing the relation between each predictor in Model 3 and each outcome after controlling for all other predictors in the model. The latter took the form of a structural coefficient, reflecting the ratio of the correlation between the intercept from hours of care growth curve and the outcome divided by the multiple correlation from Model 3 (Courville & Thompson, 2001). Thus, the structural coefficient reflects the relative predictive power of each predictor included in the analysis model without adjusting for shared variance among the predictors. Structural coefficients reflect the attenuated zero-order correlations under the assumption that all unmeasured variance would show the same linear association as the measured variance. These coefficients are interpreted within the context of a given model by identifying the coefficients that are largest as the best unconditional predictors if the overall model provides significant prediction of the outcome. Examination of both the structural coefficients and partial correlations provide information about both the degree that predictor is associated with the outcome and provides unique prediction. Table 21.3 presents these effect-size statistics for the four relevant 54-month outcomes and Table 21.4 for the three relevant kindergarten outcomes.

Considering first the 54-month data, significant quantity-of-care effects range from small, as evident in the partial correlation of .08 ($p < .05$) linking average hours of care per week with mother-reported social competence, to rather substantial, as in the case of the structural coefficient of .64 ($p < .001$) linking the same quantity variable with caregiver-reported conflict. Certainly as noteworthy, though, is that quantity of care, especially average hours per week, is typically a stronger predictor of the child outcomes than are the other four features of child care included in Model 3. Of importance, nevertheless, is that higher quality of care significantly predicts greater mother- and caregiver-rated social competence and lower levels of caregiver-rated behavior problems and conflict, though only when the more liberal effect-size estimates are considered (i.e., no significant partial correlations); that a greater proportion of time spent in center-based care predicts more caregiver-reported behavior problems and conflict; that greater peer-group exposure predicts less social competence and greater conflict reported by caregivers; and that instability of care is generally unrelated to the outcomes under consideration.

Not to be missed in this description of child care effect sizes is the fact that several background factors treated as covariates in the nested regression analyses proved to be stronger predictors of some or several outcomes than any child care factor. This is especially true of the social class indicators of maternal education and family income-to-needs (averaged across 6–54 months) and to some limited extent of maternal depression (averaged across 6–54 months; see mother-reported social competence) and child gender. With the exception of maternal report of social competence, the maternal report measure of difficult temperament proved to be an insignificant predictor. It is maternal sensitivity, especially average sensitivity over time, that proves to be the most consistent and generally strongest predictor of all outcomes displayed, with greater sensitivity predicting greater caregiver- and mother-reported social competence and less caregiver-reported behavior problems and conflict.

TABLE 21.3. Summary of Predictors of Select Month 54 Outcomes: Conservative (r_p) and Liberal (r/R) Effect Sizes

	Mother-reported social competence		Caregiver-reported social competence		Caregiver-reported problems		Caregiver reported conflict	
	r_p	r/R	r_p	r/R	r_p	r/R	r_p	r/R
Covariate predictors								
Child gender = Male	.16***	.36***	-.15***	-.36***	-.03	-.05	.01	.06
Child ethnicity = Black	.02	-.27***	.04	-.26***	-.02	.22*	.02	.22
Child ethnicity = Hispanic	-.02	-.14	.01	-.11	-.03	.04	.02	.17
Child ethnicity = Other	-.01	-.09	-.01	-.01	.02	.03	-.00	-.05
Mother's education	-.02	.39***	.06	.49***	-.06	-.42***	-.00	-.18
Average income/needs (6–54 mo)	.00	.33***	-.02	.36***	.02	-.24***	.03	-.09
Difficult temperament (6 mo)	-.17***	-.52***	-.04	-.15	.04	.13	.05	.09
Mother's depression (average)	-.14***	-.63***	-.03	-.33***	.03	.32	.03	.28*
Mother's depression (slope)	-.01	-.00	-.04	-.08	.03	.06	.07	.20
Child care predictors								
Quantity: mean hours/week	-.08*	-.05	-.12**	-.24***	.20***	.56***	.16***	.64***
Quantity: linear change/slope	-.04	-.14	-.11*	-.37***	.08*	.25**	.05	.21
Quality mean	-.02	.16*	.00	.30***	-.01	-.32***	-.02	-.37**
Center proportion	.04	.04	.03	-.08	.06	.40***	.07	.49***
Instability (3–34 mo)	.08*	.15	.00	.01	-.05	.01	.01	.10
Peer-group exposure: proportion	-.06	-.15	-.08*	-.21***	.01	.14	.07	.28*
Parenting								
Maternal sensitivity: mean	.16***	.67***	.16***	.72***	-.13***	-.61***	-.09*	-.46***
Maternal sensitivity: linear change over time	.04	.21**	.05	.21*	-.13***	-.32***	-.07	-.26*
R^2		.18***		.16***		.17***		.11***

*$p < .05$; **$p < .01$; ***$p < .001$.

TABLE 21.4. Summary of Predictors of Select Kindergarten Outcomes: Conservative (r_p) and Liberal (r/R) Effect Sizes

	Mother-reported problems		Teacher-reported problems		Teacher-reported conflict	
	r_p	r/R	r_p	r/R	r_p	r/R
Covariate predictors						
Child gender = Male	-.05	-.11	.00	.05	.12***	.37***
Child ethnicity = Black	-.06	.15	.06	.39***	.09*	.43***
Child ethnicity = Hispanic	-.04	.02	-.00	.03	-.02	-.06
Child ethnicity = Other	-.05	-.08	-.02	-.04	-.01	-.00
Mother's education	-.00	-.41***	.02	-.29***	.01	-.24*
Average income/needs (6–54 mo)	-.01	-.36***	.00	-.22*	.00	-.17
Difficult temperament (6 mo)	.03	.24**	-.04	.06	-.05	-.02
Mother's depression (mean)	.24***	.80***	.04	.35***	.00	.22*
Mother's depression (linear change)	.08*	.23*	-.06	-.10	-.04	-.03
Child care predictors						
Quantity: Mean hours/week	.07*	.16*	.08*	.36***	.08*	.37***
Quantity: Linear change over time	.00	.09	-.06	-.00	-.03	.03
Quality	.01	-.16	-.04	-.39***	.01	-.26**
Center proportion	.02	.11	.08*	.40***	.10**	.45***
Instability (3–34 mo)	-.01	.01	.02	.08	-.03	-.00
Peer-group exposure: proportion	-.00	.06	.02	.21	-.01	.12
Parenting						
Maternal sensitivity: Mean	-.09**	-.56***	-.12**	-.63***	-.09**	-.55***
Maternal sensitivity: Linear change over time	-.13***	-.43***	-.16***	-.39***	-.14***	-.39***
R^2		.17***		.14***		.12***

*$p < .05$; **$p < .01$; ***$p < .001$.

311

Somewhat similar trends emerge when kindergarten outcomes are examined. Effect sizes of quantity of care tend to be smaller relative to those considered at 54 months, which is generally true of the explanatory power of other child care and non–child care predictors as well. In the case of average quantity of care across the first 54 months of life, significant associations range from a small partial correlation of .07 ($p < .05$) linking this quantity indicator with mother-reported problems to a moderate structure coefficient of .37 ($p < .001$) linking the same predictor with teacher-reported conflict. Even though this average hours of care per week is more consistently related to the kindergarten outcomes in question than any other child care predictor, worth noting is that in several cases other child care variables prove to be stronger predictors of particular outcomes. Specifically, more time spent in centers predicts more teacher-reported problems and conflict; and lower quality of child care predicts more teacher-reported problems and conflict (but only stronger than quantity in the former case). Neither instability of care nor peer-group exposure significantly predicts the three kindergarten outcomes under consideration.

Once again, though, maternal education, family income-to-needs, and maternal depression consistently predict the kindergarten outcomes, though only sometimes more strongly than child care variables. Finally, it is maternal sensitivity which once more most consistently and, rather often, most strongly predicts the kindergarten outcomes, with change in maternal sensitivity over time (i.e., slope) becoming a more consistent predictor than was evident in Table 21.2. Not only is greater sensitivity predictive of less negative socioemotional adjustment in kindergarten, then, but increases in sensitivity over time also predict lower levels of mother- and teacher-reported behavior problems and less teacher–child conflict.

Identifying Threshold Effects

There have been repeated suggestions in the literature that potentially negative effects of time spent in child care emerge after some threshold of hours is crossed (e.g., 20 hours per week: Belsky & Rovine, 1988; 30 hours per week: Vandell & Corasiniti, 1990). Because there is no consensus in the literature regarding specific a priori cutoffs for hours per week in care, we conducted piecewise regression in hopes of identifying thresholds. This analytic technique is designed to identify points at which the relationship between independent variable (i.e., quantity of care) and dependent variable (i.e., child outcomes) changes over the scale of the independent variable (Willett, Singer, & Martin 1998). As it turned out, no threshold effects proved detectable.

Timing of Child Care

In addressing the issue of quantity of care as a function of timing or child age, this naturalistic study confronted an ecological challenge in that hours per week in care was more rather than less stable across the first 4½ years of life. Indeed, the cross-age correlation in average hours per week in care ranged from a high of .77 ($p < .001$) across the first and second year to a low of .50 ($p < .001$) for years 1–4. In fact, the part–whole correlation between average hours of care in any one year and average hours of care across the first 54 months ranged from .95 ($p < .001$) for year 2 (as well as year 3) to .66 ($p < .001$) for year 5. In view of this circumstance, two strategies were adopted in an attempt to illuminate timing effects in predicting each of the outcomes found to be related to average hours per week of nonmaternal care across the first 54 months of life (i.e., Model 3). First, Model 3 was rerun several times in order to predict each dependent variable, replacing the variable mean hours of care per week across the first 54 months with a quantity-of-care variable reflecting different periods of time (i.e., an alternative prediction approach). Thus, in one model, average hours of care from 3–54 months was replaced with a variable reflecting average hours of care for the period 3–6 months. In a second—*and separate*—model, the quantity-of-care predictor was average hours of care across the period 3–12 months; in a third, average hours of care for the period 3–24 months; in a fourth, average hours of care for the period 3–36 months; and in a fifth, average hours of care for the period 3–54 months.

With the second strategy four different quantity-of-care variables were included as predictors in the *same* regression equation (along with co-variates, other child care variables, and maternal sensitivity), each reflecting a distinct and nonoverlapping developmental period: 3–6 months, 7–12 months, 13–24 months, 25–36 months, and 37–54 months (i.e., a unique prediction approach). In this model, then, the *unique* predictive power of amount of care experience in each developmental period (i.e., not shared with any other developmental period) is tested.

Results show that, as quantity of care across lengthier periods of time is considered, the predictive power of average hours per week of non-maternal care tends to increase, usually ever so slightly, except in the case of teacher-reported externalizing problems and conflict, where prediction remains virtually unchanged from the period 3–6 months to the period 3–54 months. With the exception of predicting teacher-reported externalizing problems in kindergarten, amount of nonmaternal care neither in the period 3–6 months nor in the first year makes a significant unique prediction once time in care during other age periods is taken into consideration. The same is true across all outcomes for the second year of life and for most outcomes for the third year of life and for the period 37–54 months. Note, however, that more time in nonmaternal care during the third year of life uniquely predicts greater caregiver-reported externalizing problems and conflict at 54 months (but not in kindergarten), and that more time in care for the period 37–54 months uniquely predicts less caregiver-reported social competence at 54 months. These results may reflect the results found for the effect of hours slope reported in Table 21.2.

Predicting Higher Levels of Problem Behavior

Having found in the first set of analyses presented in Table 21.2 that more time in nonmaternal child care through 54 months of age predicted more problem behavior, as reported consistently by teachers at both 54 months and kindergarten, but by mothers only at kindergarten age, we sought to determine whether children who experienced more hours of child care were more likely to evince levels of problems considered high by certain *a priori* standards. It is important to note that we were not able to examine the criteria for identifying *clinical* levels of problems (i.e., scores above 2 standard deviations above the mean at any time or above 1.5 standard deviations according to two informants) because too few children in our sample met those criteria ($n < 50$ in the largest group and < 20 in other groupings). Instead, we used a recommended "risk" cutoff score of 1 standard deviation above the mean (e.g., $t \geq 60$). This corresponds to scoring at or above the 84th percentile. Achenbach (1991a) recommended that children in this range could be, but not necessarily should be, referred for further evaluation for clinical-level problems.

Logistic regression analyses examined whether children classified in the four quantity-of-care groups reflecting limited, moderate, high, and very high levels of child care across their first 4½ years of life care differed in the proportions of children scoring in that "at-risk" range of t 60. The full model covariates were included in these analyses, along with the four child care hours groups. Descriptive results indicate that the proportion of children scoring in the at-risk range tended to increase as amount of time in care increased, relative to the proportion of children in the at-risk range who experienced lower amounts of nonmaternal care. At the same time, the overwhelming majority of children did not score in the at-risk range, even when considering those experiencing the most child care.

Aggression and Disobedience or Assertiveness?

When data such as those emerging from this inquiry have been reported in the past linking amount and/or timing of child care with problem behavior, the suggestion has been advanced that assertiveness may be confused with aggressive and disobedient behavior by raters (Clarke-Stewart, 1989). In order to address this issue, items on the externalizing-problem behavior scale were sorted to create three subscales, one reflecting aggression (e.g., cruelty to others, destroys own things, gets in many fights, threatens others, and hits others), one reflecting disobedience/noncompliance (e.g., defiant, uncooperative, fails to carry out assigned tasks, has temper tantrums, and disrupts class discipline), and a third reflecting assertiveness (e.g., bragging/ boasting, talks too much, demands/wants attention, and argues a lot). Internal consistency reliability (i.e., coefficient alpha) for these three subscales for mothers (54 months, kindergarten), caregivers (54 months), and teachers (kindergarten) ranged from .67 (54 months, mother-rated assertiveness) to .85 (54 months, kindergarten teacher-rated aggression). The resulting scale scores were then subjected to a Poisson regression that included all the predictors from Model 3 (i.e., covariates, multiple child care predictors, maternal sensitivity).

The more time children spent in nonmaternal care across their first 4½ years, the more mothers, caregivers and teachers characterized them as assertive at 54 months and in kindergarten, and the more caregivers at 54 months and teachers in kindergarten characterized them as aggressive and disobedient. It would seem, then, that more time in care across the first 4½ years, though not change in hours of care per week over time, is predictive of more aggression and disobedience, according to caregiver and teacher reports.

CONCLUSION

The results of the present study advance understanding of potential effects of amount of time spent in early child care in showing, most significantly, that the more time children spend in any of a variety of nonmaternal care arrangements across the first 4½ years of life, the more externalizing problems and conflict with adults they manifest at 54 months of age and in kindergarten, as reported by mothers, caregivers, and/or teachers; that these effects remain, for the most part, even when quality, type, and instability of child care are controlled, as well as maternal sensitivity and other family background factors; that the magnitude of quantity-of-care effects are limited, though typically greater than those of other features of child care, though not of maternal sensitivity and family socioeconomic status; that there is no apparent threshold for quantity effects; that in most cases that effects of quantity of care are of a cumulative nature or that effects of time spent in nonmaternal care in the earliest months and years of life are contingent upon amount of care experienced subsequently; and that more time in care not only predicts problem behavior measured on a continuous scale but at-risk (though not clinical) levels of problem behavior, as well as assertiveness, disobedience, and aggression. It should be noted that these correlational findings also imply that lower levels of problems were associated with less time in child care.

Even though the effects of time spent in nonmaternal care were statistically significant, effect sizes associated with them were, for the most part, limited (Cohen, 1988). When it comes to interpreting effect sizes, it is important to remember that Cohen offered conventions to guide power analysis, not as a metric with which to dismiss statistically significant findings. Evaluations of the practical importance of research findings that are modest in magnitude are not straightforward, because effect-size estimates are affected by measurement, design, and method (McCartney &

Rosenthal, 2000). In the health domain, small effects are taken seriously. Consider the fact that the effect of aspirin on reducing heart attack is statistically very small (r^2 = .001, with corresponding r = .034; Rosenthal, 1994) and yet the findings have influenced medical practice.

In advancing the aforementioned conclusions, we acknowledge that despite the inclusion of controls for selection effects, it remains possible that the detected relations between time in care and problem behavior could reflect effects of children's behavior on utilization of nonmaternal care. Conceivably, children who are more aggressive and disobedient than others could be placed in child care at younger ages and for longer periods of time; and children who are shy and nonaggressive may be less likely to be placed in child care, particularly with large groups of children. Seemingly inconsistent with this analysis, however, is the fact that effects of time in care remained even when mother-reported difficult temperament at age 6 months was taken into consideration and were evident when just time in care in the first 6 months of life was used to predict socioemotional adjustment. Nevertheless, the correlational nature of our longitudinal data does not permit an unambiguous determination of causal direction.

This observation highlights the need for future work focused on mechanisms or processes of influence, especially as most quantity effects remained significant, even if somewhat attenuated, when maternal sensitivity and other features of child care were controlled. In addition to future work focused on family interaction processes, including parenting, children's physiological stress reactivity may also be worthy of investigation (Booth, Carver, & Granger, 2000; Stansbury & Gunnar, 1994). The reason is that relations have been detected between separation from mother and children's threshold for cortisol production as well as the size of the cortisol increase in response to a stressor (Gunnar, Mangelsdorf, Larsen, & Herstgaard, 1998). In fact, recent research indicates that long days in child care are associated with elevated levels of cortisol among 3- and 4-year-olds (Dettling, Gunnar, & Donzella, 1999; Tout, de Hann, Kipp Campbell, & Gunnar, 1998). Additional research on social processes taking place within child care environments also merits consideration.

When set in a larger context, the results summarized earlier regarding amount of time spent in child care may have implications for school readiness and the transition to school (Pianta & Cox, 1999). National surveys of kindergarten teachers reveal the emphasis they place on the importance of social and emotional competencies—following directions, getting along with peers, cooperation with adults, and other markers of self-regulation—in determining the degree to which a child is succeeding in making an adjustment to kindergarten (Rimm-Kaufman, Pianta, & Cox, 2000). In light of these views, there is reason to wonder whether amount of time in child care will prove related to children's adjustment as they progress in elementary school (and beyond). Despite the fact that there remains healthy debate about the size and meaningfulness of virtually all child care effects (Scarr,

1998), it must be remembered that more and more children are spending more and more time at younger and younger ages in nonmaternal care arrangements in the United States. Even small effects, when experienced by many children, may have broad-scale implications for larger policy discussions (Fabes, Martin, Hanish, & Updergraff, 2000; Jeffrey, 1989). Indeed, the detected effects may have no implications for how any individual child should be cared for or how any individual family function but could have implications at broader levels concerning how classrooms, communities, and even societies operate.

22

The Relation
of Child Care to Cognitive
and Language Development

NICHD EARLY CHILD CARE RESEARCH NETWORK

Experiences in the first year or two of life are particularly formative, establishing the fundamentals of language and cognitive functioning. For example, one hallmark of language, vocabulary development, begins in the first 2 years of life, before children enter preschool. The relationship between language input from caregivers and children's early vocabulary acquisition is well documented (for reviews, see Adamson, 1995; Messer, 1994). Moreover, the first 2 years mark an important period of brain development during which the density of short-range synaptic connections reaches its peak. These connections are formed on the basis of available input from the environment (Elman et al., 1996). Hence, verbal and cognitive stimulation by caregivers in the first 2 years may have a pronounced impact on later language and cognitive competence. This leads us to ask how the quality, type, and amount of care relate to cognitive and language outcomes in the first 2 or 3 years of life.

QUALITY OF CARE

Quality of care has typically been indexed by process features of adult–child interaction that represent good caregiving, whether provided by a parent or someone else. These features include sensitivity and responsiveness to the

From *Child Development*, 2000, Vol. 71, pp. 960–980. Reprinted with permission of the Society for Research in Child Development.

child's needs and signals, positive affect, frequent verbal and social interaction, and cognitive stimulation (e.g., Friedman & Cocking, 1986; Hart & Risley, 1995). In naturalistic investigations, high-quality care during the infant and toddler years is generally associated with better cognitive functioning, complex play, and language development when both are measured at the same age (e.g., Burchinal, Roberts, Nabors, & Bryant, 1996; Howes, Smith, & Galinsky, 1995; McCartney, 1984; Phillips, McCartney, & Scarr, 1987). Although this finding is consistent across studies, there is some question about how to interpret these results. Some argue that although most of the effects are statistically significant, they are trivial in magnitude (Lamb, 1997), suggesting the need to determine effect sizes, particularly in studies with large samples. Others, like Scarr (1998), have asserted that even if there are effects of quality, they do not endure into later childhood and are therefore not sufficiently important to justify large public investments in high-quality care. Evidence for durability of effects is mixed (e.g., Broberg, Wessels, Lamb, & Hwang, 1997; Chin-Quee & Scarr, 1994; Rosenthal, 1994).

The effects of child care quality have also been studied experimentally in investigations of planned early interventions for economically disadvantaged children or for those at risk for developmental problems. The findings here are very consistent. Intensive, high-quality interventions begun in infancy have a positive effect on measures of intelligence and on school achievement throughout childhood and adolescence (e.g., Burchinal, Campbell, Bryant, Wasik, & Ramey, 1997; Lamb, 1997; McLoyd, 1997; Ramey & Ramey, 1998). Furthermore, early gains are associated with language ability in early childhood (Feagans, Fendt, & Farran, 1995; Roberts, Rabinowitch, Bryant, & Burchinal, 1989). Such programs not only enhance intellectual functioning but contribute to infants' responsiveness to their environments, which may further enable children to elicit stimulation from a range of environments (Burchinal et al., 1997). Although some of these effects dissipate during the early school years, the impact of some high-quality infant and preschool programs on school performance and educational attainment continue into middle childhood, adolescence, and, in some instances, adulthood (e.g., Campbell & Ramey, 1994; Currie & Thomas, 1995; Luster & McAdoo, 1995; McLoyd, 1997).

TYPE OF CARE

Despite the fact that most infants and very young children are cared for in child care homes (Hofferth, 1996), most research has been conducted in child care centers. Child care centers are more likely than child care home settings to have a planned curriculum and trained caregivers—features that might enhance cognitive development. On the other hand, the centers attended by children in the present study at age 6 months had higher child–

adult ratios and lower levels of positive caregiving than did children in child care homes or those in relative care or in in-home care (National Institute of Child Health and Human Development [NICHD] Early Child Care Research Network, 1996). In general, children from low-income families with experience in center-based infant and toddler care have more advanced language development and perform better on measures of intelligence and achievement than do children in child care homes, but the differences may be a function of program quality or family characteristics (Broberg et al., 1997; Caughy, DiPietro, & Strobino, 1994).

TIMING AND AMOUNT OF CARE

One major debate about the effects of infant child care revolves around the possibility that early entry into extensive amounts of nonmaternal care is harmful to infant development, regardless of the quality of the care, because it disrupts the parent–child bond (e.g. Barglow, Vaughn, & Molitor, 1987). Because socioemotional and cognitive/linguistic development are believed to be intimately linked in infancy and beyond (e.g. Kopp, 1997; Lazarus, 1991; Lewis & Michalson, 1983), the disruption of the parent–child relationship due to extensive child care and its impact on socioemotional development raises the possibility that there will be secondary or mediated negative effects of early and extensive child care on cognitive development (e.g., van IJzendoorn, Dijkstra, & Bus, 1995).

Another concern related to extensive child care is that in settings with more than one child, adults spend less time with any given child, thereby reducing the amount of language and cognitive stimulation. Less overall stimulation might impede development, as was shown in a study comparing language stimulation and language outcomes in singletons and twins of the same age (Tomasello, Mantle, & Kruger, 1986).

Most reviews of the literature have concluded that the evidence is mixed about whether the timing and amount of infant child care has positive, negative, or no relation to intellectual and language development (Ackerman-Ross & Khanna, 1989; Clarke-Stewart, 1986; Hayes, Palmer, & Zaslow, 1990; Lamb, 1997).

VARIATIONS IN RELATIONS OF CARE TO OUTCOMES FOR CHILDREN OF DIFFERENT ENVIRONMENTS

The relation between infant care and intellectual development appears to depend partly on the family's income and environment. Positive relations of infant care to intellectual development and achievement have been found more consistently for children from low-income families than for children from more advantaged families (Caughy et al., 1994; Lamb, 1997). This pattern is consistent with the "compensatory education" notion that children from home environments with limited opportunities for cognitive stimulation will obtain more benefits from high-quality care than will children from more advantaged family environments. However, some recent studies with preschool age children failed to find evidence for compensatory child care effects under conditions of lower parent education (Stipek, Feiler, Daniels, & Milburn, 1995), poverty, or developmental risk due to gender (Burchinal, Peisner-Feinberg, Bryant, & Clifford, 2000).

The mirror image of the "compensatory education" hypothesis, known as the "lost resources" hypothesis, has also been advanced. It has been suggested that for affluent children, child care environments often provide less optimal stimulation, structure, and support than their family environments (Desai, Chase-Lansdale, & Michael, 1989). Consequently, the prediction is that the cognitive and language outcomes for these children would be less optimal than if they were not in child care.

Finally, there are reasons to expect ethnic differences in the relations between child care and development, even when the confound of ethnic group with income is taken into account. For minority children, family environment may be different than those for majority culture children (Garcia Coll et al., 1996). One problem in testing these and other hypotheses about the role of child care in children's development is the confound between child care experiences and other features of children's lives. Hence, in studies about the effects of child care on child development, child and family attributes must be either experimentally or statistically controlled in order to detect the unique contribution of child care.

PURPOSES OF THIS RESEARCH

Five questions were addressed in this research. First, does the cumulative quality, type, and amount of child care predict children's cognitive and language skills during the first 3 years of life? Second, assuming some effects of cumulative quality, type, and amount of care on outcome, what are the magnitudes of these effects? Third, how do children raised almost exclusively by their mothers compare with children who have experienced different levels of quality of child care? Fourth, does child care in the first year or two of life have lasting associations with cognitive and language development at subsequent ages? Fifth, are the relations of child care to cognitive and language outcomes different for children from different income levels, home environments, genders, or ethnic groups?

METHOD

Participants

For a detailed description of the recruitment procedure and of the sample itself, see Chapter 1. All the analyses about the effects of child care parameters on cognitive and language outcomes are based on data from children who were observed in child care and for whom we had complete data on predictor variables and data on at least one outcome variable (NS = 595 at 6 months, 595 at 15 months, 739 at 24 months, 856 at 36 months). The same analyses (but not including observed quality of care as a variable) were run on data from all the children participating in the study. On variables other than quality of care, these analyses yielded results that shadowed the ones we obtained for the more restricted sample of children observed in child care. Consequently, this chapter focuses on the children observed in child care.

Any child who was spending 10 or more hours per week in non-maternal care at 6, 15, 24, or 36 months was eligible for a child care observation. Of those eligible, 78.6% were observed at 6 months, 77.4% at 15 months, 85.8% at 24 months, and 90.3% at 36 months. The families in the observed sample had higher incomes and provided more stimulating home environments than in the nonobserved sample; the mothers had more education, had higher Peabody Picture Vocabulary Test (PPVT) scores, and were rated as more stimulating in interactions with the child; and the observed children experienced more hours of child care and were more likely to be in a child care center or a child care home than to be in less formal child care (all differences were significant at $p < .05$).

The sample observed in child care includes a full range of families with diversity in ethnicity, maternal education level, income, and family structure. In addition, the children were placed in diverse child care arrangements. The children who were observed in care entered child care at mean age of 4.3 months (SD = 5.3). The mean age for entry into extensive child care, (i.e., for at least 30 hours per week) was 7.2 months (SD = 8.1). By 6 months of age, 61% of the children were in child care for at least 30 hours a week, and by 12 months of age, the comparable figure is 69%. Children who entered care early also experienced a higher quantity of care during the first 3 years of life. The correlation between entry into care for any amount of time and quantity of care was moderate (r = –.49). The correlation between entry into care for a minimum of 30 hours per week and quantity of care was high (r = –.63).

Procedures

Mothers and children were visited in their homes when the children were 1, 6, 15, 24, and 36 months old; the primary child care environment was observed at 6, 15, 24, and 36 months of age; and children and their mothers were seen in the laboratory at 15, 24, and 36 months. At each assessment point, mothers responded to standardized interview questions about family demographics and other domains of family life not dealt with in this report. The families were telephoned at 3-month intervals between assessment points to update information about child care and family characteristics. All data collectors were highly trained and certified on data collection procedures. The performance of data collectors was monitored centrally to ensure uniform, high-quality data collection across the 10 sites.

Measures

Demographic, maternal, child, family environment, child care characteristics were selected as predictors of cognitive outcomes and language outcomes. As many of the predictor measures were collected longitudinally, cumulative scores were computed as the mean of that family's scores up to and including the age at which the dependent variable was assessed.

Maternal and Family Characteristics

Maternal vocabulary was assessed by the Peabody Picture Vocabulary Test–Revised (PPVT-R; Dunn & Dunn, 1981), administered to the mothers when children were 36 months old. Family income was defined as an income-to-need ratio, computed as reported family income (exclusive of Aid to Families with Dependent Children) divided by the federal poverty threshold for that family size for the year. Consequently, a ratio of 1 is the federal poverty threshold.

Two measures of the family environment included: the total Home Observation for Measurement of the Environment (HOME) score and the amount of maternal cognitive stimulation in a videotaped observation. The HOME (Caldwell & Bradley, 1984) was coded live to assess the overall quality of the physical and social resources available to the child in the family context. (For further details of the HOME, see Chapter 8.)

A more targeted measure of maternal cognitive stimulation was obtained from a semistructured mother–child interaction procedure conducted and videotaped at the family's home at 6 and 15 months and in the laboratory at 24 and 36 months of age. At 6 months mothers were instructed to play with their children using toys in two containers. Some of the toys were provided by the experimenter, and others were the child's toys that were selected by the mother. At 15, 24, and 36 months, toys were provided by the experimenter and were placed in three containers (Vandell, 1979). Maternal stimulation of cognitive development was rated for the number and quality of activities presumed to enhance perceptual, cognitive, linguistic, and physical development on a 4-point scale at 6, 15, and 24 months and on a 7-point scale at 36 months. Low scores indicate that mothers made little or no attempt to stimulate or teach the child, were totally uninvolved, or provided stimulation that was very poorly matched to the child's developmental level or interest. High scores indicate that mothers consistently provided age-appropriate cognitive stimulation that was likely to lead to a higher level of mastery, understanding, or sophistication. Intercoder reliability was .81 at 6 months, .69 at 15 months, .72 at 24 months, and .78 at 36 months.

Child Care

Three dimensions of nonmaternal care were included in the analyses. These were observed quality, type, and quantity of care.

Quality of Care. Measures of child care quality were coded live using the Observational Record of the Caregiving Environment (ORCE; Chapter 3).

Positive Caregiving Rating. A positive caregiving rating composite was created by summing the ratings for five scales: sensitivity to nondistress, stimulation of cognitive development, positive regard, detachment (reversed), and flatness of affect (reversed). At 36 months, two additional scales were included: fostering exploration and intrusiveness (reversed). The composites had good internal consistency (Cronbach's alphas = .89 at 6 months, .88 at 15 months, .87 at 24 months, and .83 at 36 months).

Frequency of Language Stimulation. Because of the centrality of language stimulation to cognitive and language development, a subset of observed caregiving behaviors was identified as constituting language stimulation: asks questions of child, responds to child's vocalizations, and other (nonnegative) talk to child. Frequencies of each behavior were standardized and then summed to create composite scores at 15, 24, and 36 months. The internal consistency of these composites was high (Cronbach's alphas = .88, .92, and .90 at 15, 24, and 36 months, respectively). This score was not computed at 6 months. At each age, frequency of language stimulation was positively correlated with positive caregiving ratings (correlations ranged from .58 to .71, p's < .001).

Type of Care. The primary care arrangement of each child was classified at each of the four child care assessments as one of three types: (1) child care center; (2) child care home (care in someone else's home by a nonrelative or relative other than the child's grandparents); or (3) grandparent or in-home care (care in the child's home, including care by father). For the purpose of data analysis, two variables of type of care were created. The first consisted of the number of times a child was observed in center care (numbers could be between 0 and 4). The second consisted of the number of times a child was observed in child care homes (numbers could be between 0 and 4).

Quantity of Care. This construct was defined as the average number of hours per week of regular, nonmaternal care the child received up to the age point that was the focus of each analysis. Quantity of care was calculated on the basis of information obtained every 3 months by telephone or face-to-face interviews.

Cognitive and Language Outcomes

Cognitive performance was measured at 15 and 24 months using the Bayley Scales of Infant Development (BSID; Bayley, 1969, 1993) and at 36 months using the school readiness subtest of the Bracken Scale of Basic Concepts (Bracken, 1984). Language measures were the MacArthur Communicative Development Inventory (CDI) at 15 and 24 months (Fenson et al., 1994) and the Reynell Developmental Language Scales (RDLS) at 36 months (Reynell, 1991). At 15 months, the Bayley Mental Development Index (MDI) was modestly to moderately correlated with the CDI vocabulary comprehended ($r = .30$) and vocabulary expressed ($r = .45$) scores. The two CDI scores were more highly correlated ($r = .57$). At 24 months, the MDI was moderately correlated with the CDI vocabulary comprehended ($r = .49$) and sentence complexity ($r = .50$) scores. The two CDI scores were more highly correlated ($r = .68$). At 36 months, the Bracken school readiness score was modestly to moderately correlated with the Reynell expressive vocabulary ($r = .35$) and receptive vocabulary ($r = .65$) scores. The two Reynell scores were moderately correlated ($r = .52$).

Cognitive Measures. The original version of the Bayley (1969) was administered at 15 months. It assesses sensory perceptual acuity and discriminations; memory, learning, and problem solving; early verbal communication; and the ability to form generalizations and classifications. The extensively revised Bayley (BSID-II; Bayley, 1993) was administered at 24 months. The revision covers the age range of birth to 42 months, reducing the kind of ceiling level problems for 24-month-olds that might have occurred with the original scale. The correlation between the 15-month BSID scores and the 24-month BSID-II scores is $r = .49$

The Bracken school readiness composite consists of 51 items grouped into five categories: knowledge of color, letter identification, number/counting, comparisons, and shape recognition (Bracken, 1984). The score analyzed was the percentile rank. The correlation between the Bracken scores and the 15-month BSID scores is $r = .27$ and between the Bracken scores and the 24-month BSID-II scores is $r = .50$.

Language Measures. Age-appropriate versions of the MacArthur CDI were used (Fenson et al., 1994). The infant version of the CDI, administered when the children were 15 months, is a vocabulary checklist. Mothers check each word that the child understands (vocabulary comprehension) and produces (vocabulary production). Percentile scores for each scale were calculated. The toddler version of the CDI, administered when the children were 24 months, includes a vocabulary production checklist and a section designed to assess syntactic and morphological development as well as nominal/pronominal style. Two percentile scores were generated: vocabulary production and sentence complexity. The correlation between the 15-

month and the 24-month percentile scores of vocabulary produced was r = .56. The correlation between the vocabulary produced percentile score and the 24-month sentence complexity percentile score was r = .42. Cronbach's alphas for the three vocabulary scales (infant comprehension, infant production, and toddler production) were .95, .96 and .96, respectively. In earlier reports, test–retest reliability was presented as .87 and .95 for comprehension and production, respectively (Fenson et al., 1994).

The RDLS (Reynell, 1991) was administered at 36 months of age during the laboratory session. Composed of two 67-item scales, the scale assesses verbal comprehension and expressive language. The correlation between the 15-month CDI and the RDLS verbal comprehension scores is r = .12. The correlation between the 15-month CDI vocabulary produced percentile scores and the RDLS expressive language percent score is r = . 14. The correlation between the 24-month CDI vocabulary produced percentile score and the RDLS expressive language percent score is r = .31. Alphas were .93 for verbal comprehension and .86 for expressive language.

RESULTS

Hierarchical Regressions

Does the cumulative quality, type, and amount of child care predict children's cognitive and language skills during the first 3 years of life? Cumulative quality was defined as the average quality rating up to and including the age being considered for the analysis. Cumulative-type ratings were calculated for center care and for care in child care homes. Each child received a score representing the number of assessment periods up to and including the age under consideration in which the type of care observed was in a child care center and a second score representing the number of assessment periods in which care was observed in a child care home. Cumulative quantity of care was the average number of hours of care per week that the child had received up to and including the age being analyzed. Hierarchical regressions were used to examine the association between child care experience, cognitive development, and language development. Two models were fit. Both models included controls for site, maternal PPVT, gender, HOME total, and maternal stimulation as background variables. In Model 1, quality (positive caregiving rating), type (proportion of times observed in center and child care homes), and amount (average hours of care per week) were the child care variables tested. If the variance accounted for by the child care block of variables was significant, we examined the coefficients associated with each child care variable. If the global measure of child care quality was significant in these analyses, a second model was tested adding frequency of language stimulation to determine whether this aspect of the child care environment mediated the association between global positive caregiving and a child outcome. This measure was selected because it is correlated with the positive caregiving rating and it represents a moment-to-moment index of caregivers' talk to the child. Evidence of mediation was obtained when the positive caregiving rating was significantly related to outcomes in Model 1 but markedly less related in Model 2 (Baron & Kenny, 1986).

Table 22.1 displays the results of these analyses. The child care block accounted for a small but significant amount of variance in all outcomes at each age (1.3–3.6%). When the variance accounted for by child care was calculated as a proportion of the total variance explained by all predictors, it ranged from .042 to .735.

Quality of Care

Both indices of the quality of child care were positively related to most of the language and cognitive outcomes. According to Model 1, children who experienced more positive caregiving scored higher on both language measures at 15 months, the Bayley MDI and CDI sentence complexity at 24 months, and school readiness and both language measures at 36 months.

According to Model 2, cumulative observed language stimulation would be the significant predictor for all measures at ages 15 and 24 months and for the RDLS expressive language score at 36 months. A comparison of Models 1 and 2 suggests that language stimulation accounted for the relations of the more global indicator of child care quality (positive caregiving) to cognitive and language scores, at least at 15 and 24 months, and to the expressive language score at 36 months.

Type of Care

The type of child care was related to children's competence, especially at 24 and 36 months (see Table 22.1). The more times children were observed in child care centers (the maximum possible were four times, when the children were 6, 15, 24, and/or 36 months of age), the better they performed on all cognitive and language assessments taken at 24 and 36 and the higher were their CDI expressive vocabulary scores at 15 months (Table 22.1, Model 2). The more time children were observed in child care homes, the higher were their 24-month Bayley scores and 36-month verbal comprehension scores.

Amount of Care

The cumulative number of hours in child care did not contribute to the prediction of children's cognitive or language development in any analysis. As shown in Table 22.1, there were no significant relations between average hours/week of child care and children's cognitive and language performance.

TABLE 22.1. Standardized Regression Coefficients and Adjusted R^2's for Cumulative Child Care Variables as Predictors of Cognitive and Language Scores at 15, 24, and 36 Months for Children Observed in Child Care

	BSID: 15-month MDI		CDI: 15-month Vocab. Prod.		CDI: 15-month Vocab. Comp.	
	Model 1	Model 2	Model 1	Model 2	Model 1	Model 2
Background variables						
Maternal PPVT-R	.16*	.17*	.01	.02	−.04	−.03
income-to-needs ratio	.06	.05	−.02	−.03	−.04	−.04
Gender (male)	−.13*	−.13*	.12*	.12*	.07	.07
HOME total	.10*	.09	.17*	.14*	.09	.07
Maternal stimulation	.04	.03	.03	.02	.09	.08
Adjusted R^2 for background variables	.129*	.129*	.037*	.036*	.013*	.013*
Child care						
Average hours/week	−.01	−.03	.03	.00	−.01	−.03
No. times center care	.04	.07	.06	.11*	.03	.06
No. times child care home	.06	.08	−.02	.02	−.10	−.07
Positive caregiving rating	.08	−.02	.12*	−.01	.15*	.05
Language stimulation	—	.17*	—	.25*	—	.18*
Adjusted R^2 for child care	.000	.013*	.005	.032*	.024*	.036*

	BSID-II: 24-month MDI		CDI: 24-month Vocab. Prod.		CDI: 24-month Sentence Complex.	
	Model 1	Model 2	Model 1	Model 2	Model 1	Model 2
Background variables						
Maternal PPVT-R	.17*	.17*	.04	.04	.11*	.10*
Income-to-needs ratio	.11*	.10*	.03	.02	.05	.04
Gender (male)	−.15*	−.15*	.04	.04	−.21*	−.21*
HOME total	.12*	.11*	.15*	.14*	.08	.07
Maternal stimulation	.15*	.15*	.08	.06	.04	.03
Adjusted R^2 for background variables	.268*	.269*	.053*	.053*	.109*	.110*
Child care						
Average hours/week	−.00	−.02	−.04	−.06	−.04	−.05
No. times center care	.17*	.20*	.06	.10*	.07	.10*
No. times child care home	.08*	.10*	.01	.04	.03	.06
Positive caregiving rating	.16*	.08	.07	−.07	.12*	.02
Language stimulation	—	.14*	—	.23*	—	.16*
Adjusted R^2 for child care	.025*	.032*	.001	.023*	.007*	.016*

(continued)

TABLE 22.1. *(continued)*

	Bracken: 36-month School Readiness		Reynell: 36-month Express. Lang.		Reynell: 36-month Verbal Comp.	
	Model 1	Model 2	Model 1	Model 2	Model 1	Model 2
Background variables						
Maternal PPVT-R	.16*	.15*	.10*	.10*	.24	.24
income-to-needs ratio	.14*	.14*	−.01	−.01	.12*	.12*
Gender (male)	−.16*	−.16*	−.13	−.12	−.16*	−.16*
HOME total	.22*	.21*	.22*	.21*	.16*	.16*
Maternal stimulation	.10*	.09*	.09*	.09*	.16*	.16*
Adjusted R^2 for background variables	.316*	.316*	.164*	.164*	.387*	.388*
Child care						
Average hours/week	−.02	−.03	.03	.02	−.02	−.03
No. times center care	.12*	.14*	.09*	.12*	.14*	.16*
No. times child care home	.04	.05	.05	.07	.08*	.09*
Positive caregiving rating	.12*	.07	.10*	.03	.15*	.12*
Language stimulation	—	.08	—	.12*	—	.06
Adjusted R^2 for child care	.012*	.014*	.008*	.014*	.021*	.021*

Note. Regression coefficients are from the full model. The adjusted R^2s are reported from the hierarchical model as the contribution of that block as it enters the model.
*$p < .05$.

Magnitude of Differences Associated with Child Care

The second and third questions posed in this research were the magnitude of the effects associated with child care and how children raised almost exclusively by their mothers compare with children who experienced different various levels of quality of care. Answers to these questions were derived from two analyses of covariance (ANCOVA) that compared the cognitive and language performance of children for groups of children. The first analysis compared children who were observed in different levels of quality of care with one another and with children who received exclusive maternal care during the first 3 years of life. This ANCOVA included the same control variables and the measures of child care types and amount that were used in the cumulative regressions. The child care quality measure was transformed for these analyses. Four groups differing in levels of quality of care were created by performing a quartile split on whichever cumulative quality measure was the best predictor of child outcomes at a given age. This was frequency of language stimulation at 15 and 24 months and positive caregiving at 36 months. A fifth group was added, consisting of children who received less than 10 hours/week of child care from birth through the assessment age of the dependent variable. Effect sizes were computed as pairwise comparisons of the means from the five-level "group" factor divided by the pooled standard deviation as estimated by the root mean squared error under that analysis model. The estimated means for each group appear in Table 22.2. The second analysis compared the cognitive and language performance of children who were observed in different levels of quality of care with one another and with children who received exclusive maternal care during the first 3 years of life. The second ANCOVA compared children who were and were not observed in center care and included the same control variables and the measures of child care quality and amount that were used in the cumulative regressions.

Child Care Quality and Type: Effect Sizes

The largest discrepancy in quality was the top (High) vs. the bottom (Low) quartile. Two effect sizes were greater than .40. The effect size for the 36-month RDLS verbal comprehension battery was .48 and for the 24-month MDI it was .43. Four were between .30 and .39; two were between .20 and .29; the lowest was .18 for 36-month RDLS expressive language battery. All but one fell between "small" (.20) and "medium" (.50) according to Cohen's (1988) guidelines.

Comparisons of Quartile 1 (Low) with 3 (Medium High) and of 2 (Medium Low) with 4 (High) each represent groups separated by two steps. Effect sizes were greater than .30 for three comparisons, between .20 and .29 for nine comparisons, and less than .20 for the remaining six comparisons. Most of the comparisons of adjacent quartiles yielded effect sizes less than .20.

Comparisons of children observed in center care with those not observed in center care show only four effect sizes ranging between Cohen's "small" and "medium" levels. The effect size for the 24-month BSID-II was .43, for the 36-month Bracken it was .28, for the RDLS expressive language, it was .21 and for the RDLS verbal comprehension measure it was .38.

Exclusive Maternal Care

In these ANCOVA, children observed in the different levels of child care quality were also compared with children who were in the exclusive care of their mothers for their first 3 years. The overall difference among the five groups was tested first. Pairwise comparisons were tested only when the overall effect of group was significant. Table 22.2 shows the results of these analyses with adjusted means for each group.

For the most part children in full-time maternal care had scores that were similar to those of children in child care (see Table 22.2). The only exceptions were 24-month language scores (CDI vocabulary production and sentence complexity) and 36-month verbal comprehension. Children in

TABLE 22.2. Adjusted Means for Children in Exclusive Maternal Care and Children Observed in Four Levels of Quality of Care

	15 months			24 months				36 months	
	Bayley MDI	CDI Vocab. Prod.	CDI Vocab. Comp.	Rev. Bayley MDI	CDI Vocab. Prod.	CDI Sentence Complex.	Bracken School Readiness	Reynell Express. Lang.	Reynell Verbal Comp.
n	891	771	771	925	856	856	985	983	1008
R^2									
Total	.16***	.08***	.08***	.32***	.10***	.15***	.35***	.21***	.41***
Group	.005	.006	.011	.012**	.018**	.015**	.011**	.003	.012***
Adjusted means									
Low quality	107.3	35.4	35.6	90.5^a	41.4^a	37.8^a	38.6^a	42.3	41.7^a
Low/average quality	107.9	36.1	40.0	$91.5^{a,b}$	$43.5^{a,b}$	$39.3^{a,b}$	$39.5^{a,b}$	45.2	46.9^b
High/average quality	109.8	39.9	45.2	$93.6^{b,c}$	$48.3^{b,c}$	$43.9^{b,c}$	$43.4^{b,c}$	46.1	47.1^b
High quality	110.0	42.4	45.0	95.6^c	50.1^c	45.6^c	47.2^c	46.7	52.7^c
Exclusive maternal care	110.7	38.5	41.2	$93.5^{a,b,c}$	37.2^a	36.0^a	$43.6^{a,b,c}$	45.6	$50.9^{b,c}$
Range of cell sizes	$140 < n < 245$			$155 < n < 200$				$135 < n < 225$	

Note. Means adjusted for maternal PPVT-R, income-to-needs ratio, child gender, HOME total, and maternal stimulation. Within a column of adjusted means, values with the same superscript are not significantly different from each other.
*$p < .05$; **$p < .01$; ***$p < .001$.

331

exclusive maternal care performed less well than did children in medium-high- and high-quality care on the former, and they performed better than children in low-quality care on the latter.

Developmental Patterns

The fourth question concerned whether child care in the first year or two of life would have lasting associations with cognitive and language development at subsequent ages. Some theoretical positions (cf. Lamb, 1997) predict that experiences very early in life may have a particularly strong relation to subsequent cognitive and language development. Because there is some stability in children's care situations, it is also possible that apparently cumulative relationships are, in fact, primarily a function of current features of child care. Therefore, a set of analyses was performed to determine whether earlier child care experiences predicted child outcomes independently of concurrent care. The child care indices were divided into measures collected at the same age as the outcome measure (concurrent measures) and measures collected prior to that assessment point (lagged measures). Hierarchical regressions were computed to test the relations of concurrent child care characteristics to child outcomes (Model 3). In Model 4, lagged child care measures were entered to determine whether they made additional contributions to explained variance that was independent of children's current child care experiences. Table 22.3 shows the results.

Quality

At 24 months, language stimulation in the concurrent child care setting was positively related to all three outcome variables—Bayley MDI, vocabulary production, and sentence complexity. The amount of language stimulation received at 15 months predicted additional variance in children's scores on the two language measures.

At 36 months, concurrent positive caregiving predicted the RDLS verbal comprehension score but not expressive language or school readiness. The amount of language stimulation in earlier child care experiences, however, was positively related to both the RDLS expressive language and the RDLS verbal comprehension scores.

Type of Care

At age 24 months, children who were currently cared for in child care centers and child care homes performed better on all outcomes than did children in other forms of care. By 36 months, children who were currently in child care centers performed better than children in other types of care, but being in a child care home at age 3 was not related to performance.

TABLE 22.3. Relations of Concurrent and Lagged Child Care Variables to Cognitive and Language Scores at 24 and 36 Months

		BSID-II: 24-month MDI		CDI: 24-month Vocab. Prod.		CDI: 24-month Verbal Comp.	
		Model 3	Model 4	Model 3	Model 4	Model 3	Model 4
Background variables	R^2	.25***	.25***	.05***	.05***	.10***	.10***
Concurrent child care	ΔR^2	***	***	***	***	***	*
Average hours/week	β	−.02	−.01	−.07	−.07	−.05	−.02
No. times in center		**.29**	**.22**	**.22**	**.23**	**.17**	.13
No. times in home		**.15**	**.13**	**.15**	**.24**	**.15**	**.20**
Positive caregiving		.04	.05	−.09	−.10	−.03	−.04
Language stimulation		**.24**	**.20**	**.36**	**.29**	**.26**	**.18**
Lagged child care	ΔR^2		NS		*		*
Average hours/week	β				.01		.06
No. times in center					.05		.09
No. times in child care home					−.12		−.08
Positive caregiving					.02		.05
Language stimulation					**.16**		**.15**
Total R^2		.31***	.31***	.11***	.13***	.14***	.15***

		Bracken: 36-month School Readiness		Reynell: 36-month Express. Lang.		Reynell: 36-month Verbal Comp.	
		Model 3	Model 4	Model 3	Model 4	Model 3	Model 4
Background variables	R^2	.29***	.29***	.16***	.16***	.36***	.36***
Concurrent child care	ΔR^2	**	**	*	NS	***	***
Average hours/week	β	.00	.01	−.07	−.07	.01	.01
No. times in center		**.16**	**.15**	**.13**	.10	**.15**	**.13**
No. times in home		.03	−.03	.07	.02	.02	−.08
Positive caregiving		.07	.05	.05	.05	**.09**	**.09**
Language stimulation		.08	.08	−.02	−.09	−.03	**−.11**
Lagged child care	ΔR^2		NS		**		***
Average hours/week	β				−.02		−.03
No. times in center					.10		.08
No. times in child care home					**.12**		**.19**
Positive caregiving					.03		.02
Language stimulation					**.18**		**.21**
Total R^2		.31***	.31***	.16***	.18***	.38***	.41***

Note. R^2: *p <.05; **p < .01; ***p < .001.
Significant coefficients are **bolded** and underlined.

Children who had been in child care homes during the first 2 years of their lives, however, performed better at age 3 than did children whose earlier experience had been in other types of care.

Variations in Relations of Child Care to Outcomes for Children from Different Environments

The fifth question was whether the relations of child care to cognitive and language outcomes are different for children from different income levels, ethnic groups, home environments, or genders.

To address this question, the hierarchical regression analyses shown in Table 22.1 were modified slightly, and interaction terms were added. Family income and HOME were each categorized into three groups. Ethnicity was entered as a dichotomous variable: white, non-Hispanic or not white, non-Hispanic. Gender was dichotomous.

Interactions of these four variables with each characteristic of child care were tested. These analyses did not suggest that the relations of child care quality, type, or amount to cognitive and language outcomes differed by family income, home environment, gender, or ethnic group.

DISCUSSION

Results indicate that quality of child care was a reasonably consistent predictor of children's cognitive and language performance. One measure of quality consisting of ratings of responsive, sensitive caregiving was related to cognitive and language outcomes throughout the first 3 years of life. The other more specific measure of frequency of language stimulation appears to be a particularly important component of such caregiving, especially during the first 2 years of life. This finding is consistent with theoretical predictions as well as with earlier cross-sectional studies pinpointing the importance of linguistic stimulation in child care for children's language development (McCartney, 1984; Melhuish, Mooney, Hennesey, & Martin, 1992). By identifying a specific feature of the child care environment that appears to facilitate language and cognitive development, this study extends findings from the current literature.

Although child care quality was a consistent predictor of cognitive and language outcomes, quality, and the other child care predictors accounted for only between 1.3% and 3.6% of the variance. Although this proportion of variance seems relatively small, the effect-size analyses indicated that the differences between scores of children in the highest and lowest quartiles of quality generally ranged from .18 to .48. Differences in performance of these magnitudes are nontrivial and could have importance for subsequent language and cognitive development. In fact, Cohen (1988) suggests that these magnitudes are to be expected in naturalistic studies that are "noisy" because of the many factors that influence the conditions and behaviors observed.

These results represent the unique variance predicted by child care parameters after controlling for selection, family, and child variables. The child's gender and the selection and family variables, taken together, accounted for a higher proportion of the variance than did the child care variables for the cognitive measures in most of the analyses. It should be noted, however, that limiting the discussion of child care contributions to the unique variance associated with child care may provide a conservative estimate because of the substantial proportion of variance shared by family and child care settings. More advantaged families tend to select higher quality child care, and child care quality may influence the quality of the parent–child relationship and the home environment (Clark, Hyde, Essex, & Klein, 1997; Lamb, 1997; NICHD Early Child Care Research Network, 1997c, 1997d; Weinraub, Jaeger, & Hoffman, 1988). On the other hand, as in any naturalistic study, there is always the possibility that unmeasured variables associated with child care quality could inflate the estimate of child care effects. For children in child care, the observed association between caregivers' language stimulation to the child and the child's language development leaves open the question of the direction of effect. Is children's cognitive and language development influenced by language stimulation, or do children who are more linguistically advanced elicit more language stimulation from their child care providers? The naturalistic design of the study does not permit one-way causal inferences. Whereas some of the observed association may be due to children's elicitation of language stimulation from caregivers, these findings are consistent with prior research showing that cognitive and language stimulation is associated with cognitive and language gains (Friedman & Cocking, 1986; Hart & Risley, 1995; Hoff-Ginsberg, 1991; Tomasello & Farrar, 1986). In this study, the longer children were in centers, beginning at age 6 months, the better they performed on cognitive and language measures, when the positive caregiving ratings and frequency of caregiver–child verbal interactions were comparable to quality in child care home settings. Center care appears to provide some advantages over child care homes for cognitive and language development, perhaps because children in centers are typically exposed to a more diverse array of language models, a richer language environment, and greater opportunities to encounter developmentally stimulating materials and events than are children in less formal settings. Children in centers are also more apt than those in child care homes to be exposed to same-age peers, and the group setting may make more demands on children to use language to meet their needs. The prospective, longitudinal design of the present study indicated that sensitive and responsive caregiving is important throughout the age period studied and that language stimulation during the child's first 2 years is particularly important for subsequent language functioning. Earlier research led to the expectation that the associations between child care and developmental outcomes might be different for children from different home environments. Child care might compensate for limited resources and opportunities for learning at home, and, conversely, it might provide a less optimal environment than advantaged homes that offer rich and stimulating environments. Like the studies by Burchinal and colleagues (2000) and Stipek and colleagues (1995), our analyses did not provide support for these expectations.

23

Does Quality of Child Care Affect Child Outcomes at Age 4½?

NICHD EARLY CHILD CARE RESEARCH NETWORK

Developmental research consistently links higher-quality child care with children's well-being, developing skills, and subsequent adjustment (Lamb, 1998; Love, Schochet, & Meckstroth, 1996; Scarr & Eisenberg, 1993; Smith, 1998; Vandell & Wolfe, 2000). But the utility of this evidence is weakened by the fact that it is based largely on correlational studies of child care that do not provide causal evidence linking child care quality to children's development. To the extent that pertinent causal evidence exists, it derives from experimental evaluations of relatively high-quality early intervention programs (see Barnett, 1995; Campbell, Pungello, Miller-Johnson, Burchinal, & Ramey, 2001; Currie, 2000; Shonkoff & Meisels, 2000; Shonkoff & Phillips, 2000; Yoshikawa, 1994, 1995). Both short- and longer-term effects of such programs have been documented for children's early learning, cognitive and language development, progress through school and eventual attainments, social skills, and the reduction of conduct problems and subsequent delinquency. The extent to which the quality of care provided by early intervention programs overlaps with the range of quality provided by child care programs is unknown but probably quite limited.

This chapter takes a first step toward moving from the correlational literature on child care to questions that bear on causal relations between child care quality and children's development. In the philosophy of science,

From *Developmental Psychology*, 2003, Vol. 39. pp. 451–469. Copyright 2003 by the American Psychological Association. Reprinted by permission.

the issue of providing empirical proof of causality remains somewhat controversial. The gold standard is clearly experimentation, but experimental designs are not without their fallibilities. Using data from the nonexperimental, longitudinal National Institute of Child Health and Human Development (NICHD) Study of Early Child Care, we examined a series of propositions that, if satisfied, would suggest that relations found between child care environments and development are causal. These propositions address issues of selection into child care, the specificity and developmental sequencing of associations between child care quality and child outcomes, and dose–response relations between quality and outcomes.

• *Proposition 1:* If child care quality affects child outcomes, associations between child care quality and child outcomes should be apparent even when child and family background factors are taken into account.
• *Proposition 2:* If child care quality affects child outcomes, analyses should indicate specificity of associations between child care quality and child outcomes: The quality of cognitive and language aspects of care should be related to cognitive and language outcomes; the quality of social aspects of care should be related to social outcomes; and the emotional quality of care should be related to emotional outcomes and attention regulation.
• *Proposition 3:* If child care quality affects child outcomes, the quality of earlier care should be associated with child outcomes even when the quality of concurrent care is statistically controlled.
• *Proposition 4:* If child care quality affects child outcomes, associations between quality of care and child outcomes should remain when indices of the child's earlier ability are taken into account.
• *Proposition 5:* If child care quality affects child outcomes, associations between child care quality and child outcomes should be stronger if children spend more time in the care setting; that is, there should be a dose–response relation between (the quantity of) child care quality and outcomes.

In this chapter we explore these propositions bearing on the causal nature of relations between child care quality and children's development. The propositions trace the historical course of advances in this field as researchers came to impose more controls—for selection, for concurrent care, for earlier child abilities—in their analyses and probed the interactions among independent variables in their predictions of child outcomes. As we move through the propositions, evidentiary standards get more strict. Finding support for only the first few propositions would not be as convincing as finding support for all them or finding support for the final two. Finding support for all the propositions would still not prove that child care quality affects child outcomes, but such results would greatly strengthen this argument. On the other hand, failing to find support for the propositions would not prove that child care quality does not affect child outcomes, only that evidence of causal links was not provided by this particular study.

METHOD

Participants

Chapter 1 provides a detailed description of the study design and participants. At 4½ years, 1,083 children and their parents were still enrolled in the study. Mothers had an average of 14.4 years of education, and 16.5% were single. Average family income was 3.6 times the poverty threshold; 79% of the infants were non-Hispanic European Americans. The participants differed in the following ways from the 281 children who were recruited but were lost during follow-up: Mothers of participants had significantly ($p < .05$) more education ($M = 14.4$ years vs. 13.6 years) and higher family incomes (income–poverty ratio: $M = 3.6$ vs. 3.2) and were more likely to have a husband or partner in the household (85% vs. 76%). The children were less likely to be African American (11% vs. 19%). The children included in this report consisted of all those who were assessed at 54 months and were in child care at 6 months ($n = 689$), 15 months ($n = 762$), 24 months ($n = 799$), 36 months ($n = 844$), or 54 months ($n = 1,075$). For a variety of reasons—caregiver or parent refusal, inability to schedule child care visits within the 2-month assessment windows—it was not possible to observe all eligible children. Participation rates were highest for in-home caregivers (92%) and centers (91%), somewhat lower for fathers (83%) and grandparents (79%), and lowest for child care homes (75%). Mothers in the observed sample had higher levels of education than mothers in the nonobserved sample (see Chapter 1).

Child Care Measures

Quantity

Quantity of care was measured as (1) the average hours per week in any nonmaternal care from 3 to 54 months (used as a control variable; alpha = .94) and (2) the average hours per week in observed nonmaternal care (used to test Proposition 5; alpha = .92).

Type

Types of care arrangements were classified as child care center, child care home (any home-based care outside the child's own home except grandparent care), in-home care (any care in the child's own home except by fathers or grandparents), grandparent care, and father care. On the basis of these reports, two variables were created: the proportion of 3–4-month intervals from 3 to 54 months of age (16 epochs in all) in which the child received care in a center and the proportion of epochs in which the child was in a child care home.

Quality

Observational assessments of children's experiences in care were obtained in the primary nonmaternal care arrangements of children who were in care for the required number of hours per week. Five assessments were possible for each child (at 6, 15, 24, and 36 months and at 4½ years), but because not all children were in care at all five ages and because not all children could be assessed even if they were in care owing to scheduling problems and refusals, children had differing numbers of assessments. At least one assessment was obtained for 985 children, and at least two assessments were obtained for 779 children. Assessments were conducted during two half-day visits scheduled within 2-week intervals at 6, 15, 24, and 36 months and during one half-day visit at 4½ years. At each visit, observers completed two 44-minute cycles of the Observational Record of the Caregiving Environment (ORCE) (see Chapters 3 and 6 for further details).

The following measures of child care quality were analyzed for this chapter:

1. *Overall rating of positive caregiving quality*: At 6, 15, and 24 months, caregiving quality ratings were the mean of five 4-point subscales (Caregiver's Sensitivity to Child's Nondistress Signals, Stimulation of Child's Development, Positive Regard Toward Child, Detachment [reflected], and Flatness of Affect [reflected]). Cronbach's alphas for the composite ranged from .87 to .89. At 36 months, these five scales plus two additional subscales, Fosters Child's Exploration and Intrusiveness (reflected), were included in the composite (alpha = .83). At 4½ years, the positive caregiving composite was the mean of 4-point ratings of caregivers' sensitivity, stimulation of cognitive development, intrusiveness (reflected), and detachment (reflected) (alpha = .72).

2. *Language stimulation* was a composite variable based on the number of 30-second observation intervals in which a caregiver responded to the child's vocalization or question, read aloud to the child, asked a question, directed other talk to the child, or stimulated the child's cognitive development (at 6 and 15 months) or taught the child an academic skill (at 24, 36, and 54 months). Standardized Cronbach's alphas were .78 at 6 months, .82 at 15 months, .78 at 24 months, .75 at 36 months, and .68 at 54 months.

3. *Watching TV* consisted of the number of intervals in which the child was watching TV (at 6, 15, 24, 36, and 54 months).

4. *Positive physical contact* was the number of intervals in which the child had positive physical contact with the caregiver (at 6, 15, 24, and 36 months).

5. *Positive talk* consisted of the number of intervals in which a caregiver spoke positively to the child—giving praise, encouragement, or affection (at 15, 24, 36, and 54 months).

6. *Positive interaction with other children*, measured at 15, 24, and 36 months, was the number of intervals in which the study child experienced positive or neutral interaction with another child. It was divided into three categories: none, a little (less than the 75th percentile), and a lot (greater than the 75th percentile).

7. *Stimulating physical materials*: At the end of the second observation visit, observers evaluated the quality of the physical learning environment at ages 6 to 36 months using the Assessment Profile for Early Childhood Programs (Abbott-Shim & Sibley, 1987) and at 54 months using an adaptation of this checklist developed for the NICHD study. Scores reflected the number, variety, and organization of stimulating materials accessible to the child (standardized Cronbach's alphas were .60 [for centers]/.62 [for homes] at 6 months. 67/.67 at 15 months. 76/.77 at 24 months. 80/.78 at 36 months, and .75 at 54 months).

All but one of the variables reflecting these different aspects of child care quality (variables 2 through 7) were significantly related to the overall rating of positive caregiving quality (variable 1) at levels ranging from $r = -.16$ ($p < .001$) for watching TV to $r = .61$ ($p < .001$) for language stimulation. The only specific aspect of care that was not related to overall quality was the child's positive interactions with other children.

Family Background and Child Characteristics (Control) Variables

Family Background.

Family background variables were as follows:

1. The *geographical location* (study site) in which the family resided.
2. *Mother's education*.
3. *Family income-to-needs ratio*: the family income divided by the poverty threshold for a household of that size, averaged across assessments from 1 to 54 months (alpha = .94).
4. *Mother's partner status*: the proportion of the assessment periods (data were collected every 3 months in the first 3 years of life and every 4 months thereafter) during which the mother lived with a husband or partner (alpha = .90).
5. *Child's ethnicity* in non-Hispanic African American, non-Hispanic European American, Hispanic, or other ethnic group.
6. *Maternal depression* (Center for Epidemiologic Studies—Depression scale; Radloff, 1977), with scores averaged across assessments from 1 to 54 months (alpha = .83).

7. *Parenting quality*: composite scores based on (a) maternal behavior ratings and (b) scores on the Home Observation for Measurement of the Environment (HOME; Caldwell & Bradley, 1984). The maternal ratings were based on videotaped mother–child play with toys. At 6, 15, and 24 months, the rating scales included were Maternal Sensitivity, Positive Regard for the Child, and Intrusiveness; at 36 and 54 months, the scales were Supportive Presence, Respect for the Child's Autonomy, and Hostility. (For more details, see Chapter 18.) The HOME was administered at 6, 15, 36, and 54 months (alpha = .78–.87). To create the composite variable of parenting quality, we standardized and combined mean scores from the maternal behavior ratings and total scores from the HOME inventory and averaged them across age (alpha = .89). (For more details on the composite parenting measure, see Chapters 19 and 24.)

Child Characteristics

Child characteristics measured were as follows:

1. *Gender.*
2. *Earlier cognitive ability* measured at 36 months with the Bracken Basic Concept Scale school readiness composite (Bracken, 1984).
3. *Earlier language ability* measured at 36 months with the Reynell Developmental Language Scale (Reynell, 1991), which consists of two subscales, expressive vocabulary and language comprehension.
4. *Earlier attention* measured by the average duration of bouts of attention at 36 months in a solitary, free-play situation with toys in the laboratory.
5. *Earlier social competence* consisted of scores on the Adaptive Social Behavior Inventory (ASBI; Hogan, Scott, & Bauer, 1992) completed by mothers and caregivers at 36 months. Two subscales, expressive behavior and compliant behavior, were summed to indicate social competence (alpha = .76 and .82, respectively; r = .49).
6. *Earlier behavior problems* consisted of scores on the Child Behavior Checklist–2/3 (CBCL-2/3; Achenbach, Edelbrock, & Howell, 1987), which was completed by mothers and caregivers at 36 months.

Child Outcomes at 4½ Years

Cognition and Language

Four measures of children's cognition were collected that were based on the Woodcock–Johnson Achievement and Cognitive Batteries (WJ-R; Woodcock & Johnson, 1989, 1990). These measures consisted of children's standardized scores on four subtests: Letter–Word Identification (skill at identifying letter forms and words), Applied Problems (skill at analyzing and solving practical problems in mathematics), Incomplete Words (ability to name incomplete words after hearing a recorded word that has one or more missing phonemes), and Short-Term Memory (the ability to remember and repeat simple words, phrases, and sentences). The child's language ability was assessed with the Preschool Language Scale (PLS-3; Zimmerman, Steiner, & Pond, 1979). This individually administered, standardized test assesses vocabulary, morphology, syntax, and integrative thinking, which are grouped into two subscales, Language Comprehension (what children understand) and Expressive Vocabulary (what children say). Intercorrelations among these measures of cognitive ability ranged from .36 ($p < .001$) between Letter–Word Identification and Incomplete Words to .68 ($p < .001$) between Language Comprehension and Expressive Vocabulary (average $r = .49$, $p < .001$). Although these measures of children's cognitive and language abilities were highly intercorrelated, we kept them separate in the analyses because of our interest in links between specific aspects of care and specific aspects of cognitive and language development.

Attention

Attention was measured with the Continuous Performance Task (CPT; Rosvold, Mirsky, Sarason, Bransome, & Beck, 1956), which was administered to each child individually. Dot-matrix pictures of 10 familiar objects (e.g., butterfly, fish, and flower) were generated by a computer and presented on a 2-inch-square screen. The child was asked to press the button "as fast as you can" each time a target stimulus (a chair) appeared. *Errors of omission* consisted of failing to press the button; *errors of commission* consisted of pressing the button for nontarget stimuli. Children who had fewer errors of omission had greater ability to sustain attention; children with more errors of commission were more impulsive. Children's performance on the CPT has high construct validity as a measure of attention, and measures of sustained attention and impulsivity have adequate test–retest reliability (r's = .65 to .74; Halperin, Sharma, Greenblatt, & Schwartz, 1991).

Social Behavior

There were three measures of children's social behavior: social competence assessed by mothers and caregivers and observed social competence in an interaction with a friend. Social competence was assessed by mothers with the Social Skills Questionnaire from the Social Skills Rating System (Gresham & Elliott, 1990). This instrument is composed of 38 items, each rated on a 3-point scale reflecting how often the child exhibited each behavior. Items are grouped into four areas: cooperation, assertion, responsibility, and self-control. The total score is the sum of all 38 items, with higher scores reflecting higher levels of perceived social competence. Caregivers (n = 833) were given the California Preschool Social Competency Scale (Levine, Elzey, & Lewis, 1969), a 30-item instrument assessing behaviors especially relevant in child care settings (e.g., safe use of equipment, calling others by name, greeting a new child, and initiating group activities). Four items were added to index specific features of peer play ("cooperation," "following rules in games," "empathy," and "aggression"). Items were rated on 4-point scales. Total social competency was the sum of the 34 items, with higher scores denoting greater social competence (alpha = .88).

Observed Social Competence

Observed social competence was assessed from videotaped interactions of the child playing with a friend in a portable playhouse set up at the child care facility or at the child's or friend's home. The observation lasted 15 minutes and was divided into three 5-minute sessions, each with a different toy or set of toys. The observed social competence composite consisted of the following ratings, averaged across the three sessions: (1) child's contribution to coordinated positive interaction, prosocial behavior (more frequent turn taking, turn offering, and sharing), and positive mood and (2) (inversely coded) child's contribution to negative interaction, aggression, and negative mood (interrater agreement: Pearson $r = .78$, analysis of variance estimate = .87; Cronbach's alpha = .73).

Emotional Well-Being

Behavior problems were evaluated by both mothers and caregivers, using age-appropriate versions of the CBCL (Achenbach, 1991a). Total problem raw scores (sums) were converted into standard T-scores based on normative data for children of the same age.

Statistical Analyses

The primary analyses were multiple regression analyses predicting each child outcome measure from each measure of child care quality averaged across assessments made at 6, 15, 24, 36, and 54 months and controlling for site, child's gender and ethnicity, mother's education and partner status, mother's depression, quality of parenting, and family income. Hours of child care and type of child care were also controlled. Additional analyses of subgroups were used to follow up specific research propositions.

RESULTS

Descriptive Statistics

Children were least likely to be in a center at 6 months ($n = 88$) and most likely to be in a center at 54 months ($n = 589$). The provision of care by fathers and grandmothers was relatively consistent across time ($ns = 147–188$ for fathers and 98–125 for grandmothers). Provision of care in child care homes was consistent over the first 3 years (ns = 217–262) but less frequent at 54 months (n = 131). Overall, the least common arrangement was a caregiver in the child's own home (ns = 65–96). On average, children who were in observable care spent 34 hours per week in the observed arrangement from 6 to 36 months and 27 hours per week at 54 months.

To provide a baseline background for the analyses of the five propositions, we first computed regression coefficients predicting child outcome measures at 54 months from the overall quality of care rating averaged over assessments from 6 to 54 months without any covariates included. These analyses, summarized in the first four columns of Table 23.1, revealed significant associations between quality of care and all but one of the child measures (mother-reported behavior problems). The 12 significant associations were moderate in size (Cohen, 1988), with effect sizes ranging from .29 to .55 and correlation coefficients from .12 to .23 (see Table 23.1). To place these associations in context, it is useful to compare them with another set of correlations. Table 23.2 shows the comparable correlations between child outcomes and the quality of parenting (maternal behavior ratings and HOME scores). The effect sizes for these associations ranged from .28 to .99; correlation coefficients ranged from .17 to .54.

These initial analyses thus established a baseline showing that quality of care was related to child outcomes. Associations were generally not as large as those with family care, but uniformly significant associations between overall ratings of child care quality and a broad range of child ability measures pointed to the possibility that higher quality care could be causally related to better child outcomes and laid the groundwork for more stringent analyses controlling for selection factors.

Proposition 1: Associations between Child Outcomes and Quality of Care Will Be Significant with Selection Factors Controlled

In the first analyses of the proposition, we used this extensive set of child, family, and child care covariates in a series of regression analyses to predict child measures, investigating the unique contribution of child care quality to these child outcomes at 54 months. Results of these regression analyses are presented in the second four columns of Table 23.1. These analyses revealed that controlling for selection and child care factors reduced the number of significant associations with child care quality from 12 to 8. Nevertheless, the average rating of quality care from 6 to 54 months was significantly and positively associated with all measures of child cognition assessed at 54 months. Specifically, children in higher-quality care performed better on the six intercorrelated measures of cognitive development—letter–word identification, applied problems, incomplete words, short-term memory, language comprehension, and expressive vocabulary—than did children in lower-quality care. Also, quality was related to one of the two measures of attention (children in higher-quality care were less impulsive) and one of the

TABLE 23.1. Associations between Child Outcomes and Average Quality of Care from 6 to 54 Months

	Measures of child care quality							
	Overall quality of caregiving,[a] 6–54 mo (n = 658–936)				Overall quality of caregiving,[b] 6–54 mo (n = 695–950)			
Child outcome	β	SE	Effect size[c]	r	β	SE	Effect size[c]	Partial r
Cognition and language								
MANOVA F	8.60***				2.19*			
Letter–word identification	5.68***	1.15	0.44	.19***	2.21*	1.07	0.19	.07*
Applied problems	7.82***	1.33	0.52	.20***	2.49*	1.20	0.21	.07*
Incomplete words	4.43***	1.2	0.33	.14***	2.52*	1.11	0.21	.08*
Short-term memory	6.69***	1.58	0.37	.17***	3.37*	1.52	0.20	.07*
Language comprehension	10.31***	1.69	0.54	.22***	3.00*	1.44	0.19	.07*
Expressive vocabulary	10.16***	1.63	0.55	.23***	4.47*	1.43	0.29	.10*
Attention								
Omission errors	-2.14**	0.66	0.29	-.12**	-1.1	0.66	0.15	-.06
Commission errors	-7.55***	1.71	0.39	-.16***	-3.98*	1.75	0.21	-.08*
Social and emotional								
Competence, Cg	6.61***	1.21	0.50	.20***	3.91**	1.29	0.31	.11**
Competence, M	3.94***	1.15	0.30	.12***	1.7	1.11	0.14	.05
Observation with friend	.23**	0.07	0.30	.12**	0.11	0.08	0.15	.05
Behavior problems, Cg	-3.98***	0.94	0.40	-.16***	-1.04	1.01	0.11	-.04
Behavior problems, M	-1.44	0.81	0.15	-.06	-0.25	0.79	0.03	-.01

Note. MANOVA, multivariate analysis of variance; M, mother; Cg, caregiver.
[a]With no covariates.
[b]Controlling for site, child gender, child ethnicity, mother education, partner status, parenting quality, maternal depression, family income, child care hours, and child care type.
[c]Obtained regression coefficient divided by the root mean square error for that model.
*$p < .05$; **$p < .01$; ***$p < .001$.

three measures of social competence (children in higher-quality care were more socially competent according to their caregivers). In this analysis, with a stringent set of controls, significant associations between overall ratings of child care quality and child outcome measures were consistent with the proposition that higher-quality care is causally related to better cognition, less impulsivity, and greater social competence in child care. The size of these significant associations were at the low end of the moderate range, ranging from .19 to .31, and partial correlation coefficients ranged from .07 to .11.

In the second set of analyses, we looked for interactions between the quality of care children received in child care settings and the quality of parenting they received at home, in order to determine whether associations

Measures of child care quality											
Language stimulation,[b] 6–54 mo (n = 695–950)		Watching TV,[b] 6–54 mo (n = 695–950)		Stimulating physical materials,[b] 6–54 mo (n = 695–942)		Positive interaction with other children,[b] 15–54 mo (n = 695–939)		Positive physical contact,[b] 6–36 mo (n = 554–797)		Positive caregiver talk,[b] 15–54 mo (n = 695–939)	
β	SE	β	SE	β	SE	β	SE	β	SE	β	SE
2.21*		3.04**		3.16**		1.93		0.46		0.81	
2.27**	0.85	0.05	0.64	0.23	1.12	−0.71	0.53	−0.05	0.58	0.5	0.55
2.86**	0.95	−2.13**	0.71	1.99	1.25	0.48	0.59	−0.43	0.64	0.07	0.61
1.65	0.89	−0.2	0.66	1.82	1.17	0.40	0.56	0.13	0.60	1.06	0.57
2.84*	1.22	−1.57	0.91	5.40***	1.58	0.20	0.76	0.74	0.83	0.13	0.78
2.40*	1.15	−2.34**	0.85	5.17***	1.50	1.51*	0.72	−0.59	0.78	−0.05	0.73
2.36*	1.15	−2.68**	0.85	2.85	1.50	1.54*	0.72	0.11	0.78	−0.08	0.73
−0.59	0.52	0.09	0.41	−1.21	0.69	−0.27	0.34	−0.21	0.36	−0.01	0.34
−0.59	1.40	−0.27	1.1	−4.41*	1.85	−0.47	0.91	−0.12	0.96	1.33	0.90
0.07	1.08	−0.93	0.81	2.65	1.40	1.28	0.68	0.50	0.77	−0.08	0.65
1.13	0.89	−0.26	0.66	0.07	1.17	0.63	0.57	0.60	0.59	−0.48	0.56
0.06	0.06	0.05	0.06	0.04	0.09	−0.02	0.04	0.05	0.05	0.01	0.04
1.63*	0.82	1.31	0.72	−0.35	1.10	−1.55*	0.52	−0.22	0.60	0.19	0.49
0.51	0.63	−0.04	0.47	−0.47	0.83	−0.85*	0.4	0.51	0.43	0.71	0.39

between child care quality and child outcomes were evident only for children who had advantages at home. If associations between child care and outcomes appeared only for children who received higher-quality care at home, this would cast doubt on the interpretation that child care (alone) was leading to differences in children's performance. We divided the children into four groups depending on whether they were above or below the median on the quality of child care they received and above or below the median on the quality of parenting they received, averaged over time, and we tested for interactions between parenting and overall quality of care in predicting child outcomes. There were significant main effects for both parenting quality and overall care quality, but none of the interactions was significant. Taken together, the results of this first set of analyses are consis-

TABLE 23.2. Associations between Child Outcomes and Average Quality of Parenting from 6 to 54 Months

Child outcome	Overall quality of parenting[a]				
	β	SE	Effect size[b]	r	n
Cognition and language					
MANOVA F	72.6***				
Letter–word identification	8.71***	0.67	.73	.42***	801
Applied problems	11.32***	0.75	.84	.47***	801
Incomplete words	6.88**	0.72	.53	.32***	801
Short-term memory	10.38***	0.94	.62	.36***	801
Language comprehension	16.51***	0.91	.99	.54***	801
Expressive vocabulary	14.70***	0.91	.90	.50***	801
Attention					
Omission errors	−2.85***	0.41	.39	−.24***	783
Commission errors	−6.21***	1.07	.33	−.20***	783
Social behavior					
Competence, caregiver	5.81***	0.72	.45	.28***	731
Competence, mother	5.87***	0.68	.46	.22***	816
Observation with friend	.21***	0.05	.28	.17***	658
Emotional well-being					
Behavior problems, caregiver	−3.42***	0.56	.35	.29***	695
Behavior problems, mother	−2.69***	0.49	.29	−.19***	820

Note. MANOVA, multivariate analysis of variance.
[a]With no covariates.
[b]Obtained regression coefficient divided by the root mean squared error for that model.
**$p < .01$; ***$p < .001$.

tent with the first proposition that quality of care influences child performance, independent of family factors, particularly in the cognitive domain.

Proposition 2: There Will Be Domain-Specific Associations between Child Outcomes and Quality of Care

To investigate the second proposition, we first determined that the four sets of child outcomes (cognition and language, attention, social behavior, and emotional well-being) and the three sets of child care variables (cognitive–language environment, social environment, and emotional environment) were not so highly correlated across domains that it would be impossible to detect specificity. The mean correlation between the sets of variables was only .18 (see Table 23.3). Then we examined the associations between child outcomes and specific measures of care quality from 6 to 54 months, using regression analyses controlling for the set of covariates in the previous analysis; these associations are shown in the remaining columns of Table 23.1.

TABLE 23.3. Intercorrelations among Variables

Child outcome variable	1	2	3	4	5	6	7	8	9	10	11	12	13
Cognition and language													
1. Letter-word	—						-.24	-.16	.22	.15	-.13	-.11	-.05
2. Applied problems	.56	—					-.33	-.26	.28	.17	.16	-.15	-.05
3. Incomplete words	.36	.43	—				-.20	-.14	.18	.12	.17	-.09	-.07
4. Short-term memory	.39	.48	.55	—			-.21	-.12	.21	.22	.13	-.10	-.11
5. Language comprehension	.49	.65	.41	.50	—		-.28	-.27	.34	.21	.19	-.19	-.13
6. Expressive vocabulary	.42	.57	.42	.51	.68	—	-.30	-.28	.30	.20	.18	-.18	-.12
Attention													
7. Omission errors							—	.22	-.19	-.12	-.15	.12	.10
8. Commission errors								—	-.15	-.06	-.09	.15	.11
Social behavior													
9. Competence, caregiver									—	.22	.12	-.46	-.24
10. Competence, mother										—	.08	-.18	-.30
11. Observation with friend											—	-.09	.05
Emotional well-being													
12. Behavior problems, caregiver												—	.24
13. Behavior problems, mother													—

Quality of care variable (6–54 months)	1	2	3	4	5	6
Cognitive environment						
1. Language stimulation	—					
2. Watching TV	-.08	—				
3. Stimulating materials	.23	-.17	—			
Social environment						
4. Positive interaction	-.26	-.17	-.03	—		
Emotional environment						
5. Positive physical contact	.34	.16	.01	-.18	—	
6. Positive caregiver talk	.52	-.12	.17	-.05	.14	—

Note. ns = 610–824.

349

Some specificity of associations did appear in these regression analyses—but only in the cognitive domain. Most clearly, greater language stimulation by the caregiver was related significantly to higher scores on five of the six measures of cognition—specifically, letter–word identification, applied problem solving, language comprehension, expressive vocabulary, and short-term memory. There was no indication that language input was more highly predictive of children's language ability than of other aspects of their cognition (e.g., solving math problems)—presumably because the cognitive measures were so highly intercorrelated. The only cognitive measure that was not significantly related to language stimulation was auditory processing. In contrast to these associations with cognitive outcomes, language stimulation was not significantly related to outcomes in the social–emotional domain. The specific link between language input and cognition is consistent with the proposition that quality of care influences cognitive performance.

The amount of time children spent watching TV while they were in the child care setting was also considered to reflect lower-quality cognitive input, because when children are watching TV, they are not receiving stimulation from their caregivers or instructional materials. As expected, children who watched more TV received lower scores on three measures of cognitive ability—applied problems, language comprehension, and expressive vocabulary. These associations, too, are reasonable and expectable if child care quality affects children's cognitive performance.

The physical environment of the care setting is a particularly important dimension for analysis because it is unlikely that children directly cause variations in this index of quality of care. Children with advanced language skills may elicit more language stimulation from their caregivers, and brighter children may choose to watch less TV, but it is unlikely that children with higher cognitive abilities would cause their caregiver to provide a better physical environment. (At most, the link would be indirect if parents of more cognitively advanced children selected child care settings that had more stimulating physical environments.) However, like language stimulation and TV watching, the nature of the physical environment was found to be associated with child cognitive outcomes. Children in settings with more stimulating, varied, and well-organized materials (including materials to stimulate math, movement, music, language, art, and play) received higher scores on tests of language comprehension and short-term memory. It was also expected that access to more stimulating physical materials would lead to better letter–word identification (language materials) and applied problem solving (math materials). However, these links were not found. Thus, the evidence from this analysis offered consistent but somewhat limited support for the proposition that child care quality promotes child performance.

We expected that the social quality of care—having more positive interaction with peers in the care setting—would be related to social outcomes, not cognitive outcomes. If interaction with other children is causally linked to improved child development, one would expect that children with more

such experience would be rated and observed to be more socially competent with their peers. However, our analyses showed that simply having
more positive experience with other children was not related to any of the
measures of social competence (ratings by mother or caregiver or observation of the child with a friend). Instead, experience with other children was
related to children's language ability and behavior problems. Children who
had experienced a lot of positive or neutral interaction with other children
in the child care setting had better language skills (expressive vocabulary
and comprehension) and fewer behavior problems (according to their
mothers and caregivers). These associations, although not predicted, are
reasonable: Children would be able to interact better with peers if they
could communicate better and were neither withdrawn nor aggressive.
However, these associations do not support the proposition that quality of care—as indexed by participation in more frequent, positive peer
interaction—leads to better social skills.

We expected that the emotional quality of care—caregivers' positive
physical contact and positive talk with the child—would not be strongly
related to child outcomes in the cognitive domain; these outcomes require
direct input in the form of stimulation and instruction. However, we did
expect that emotional support would be related to higher levels of emotional well-being and attention regulation in the children. The results of the
regression analyses were not consistent with this prediction. Caregivers'
emotional support was not related to any of the child outcomes measured,
including the two measures of the child's behavior problems and the two
measures of attention/impulsivity. Taken together, these analyses of associations between specific aspects of child care quality and child outcomes in
the same domains give substantial support to the proposition that child care
quality affects children's cognitive performance. There was no evidence of a
link between social–emotional aspects of child care quality and social–
emotional and attentional outcomes—as these constructs were assessed in
this study.

Proposition 3: Associations between Child Outcomes and Quality of Earlier Care Will Be Significant with Quality of Concurrent Care Controlled

For the third proposition, we analyzed whether the quality of earlier care
(from 6 to 36 months) was associated with child outcomes at 54 months
even with the quality of concurrent care (at 54 months) statistically controlled. The purpose of these analyses was to reduce the possibility that the
associations obtained in the preceding analyses, in which prior and concurrent care were combined, were child effects on quality rather than quality
effects on children.

Before conducting these analyses, we computed the association between quality of early care (6–36 months) and quality of concurrent care (54

months). We did so because if quality of care was strongly consistent over time, partialing out concurrent care would leave little residual to be correlated with child outcomes, and looking only at the unique variance of early care would underestimate the true causal variance. The correlation between early and concurrent care was only .09 ($p < .05$).

Table 23.4 presents the results of regression analyses predicting child outcomes from quality of earlier care with quality of concurrent care controlled and the results of regression analyses predicting child outcomes from quality of concurrent care with quality of earlier care controlled. The set of child, family, and child care covariates was controlled in all these analyses.

These analyses showed that even with the quality of contemporaneous care controlled, some features of children's cognitive performance were related to some features of earlier care. Specifically, children did better on letter–word identification, applied problems, language comprehension, and short-term memory if they had been in child care of higher overall quality;

TABLE 23.4. Associations between Child Outcomes and Quality of Early Care (at 6–36 Months) and Contemporaneous Care (at 54 Months)

	Measures of child care quality							
	Overall quality of caregiving				Language stimulation			
	6–36 mo.		54 mo.		6–36 mo.		54 mo.	
Child outcome	β	SE	β	SE	β	SE	β	SE
Cognition and language								
Letter–word identification	2.59*	1.22	1.17	0.86	1.44	0.90	0.22	0.75
Applied problems	2.82*	1.36	1.4	0.96	2.55*	1.00	−0.01	0.83
Incomplete words	1.97	1.30	1.08	0.91	1.74	0.96	0.35	0.80
Short-term memory	4.36*	1.71	−0.10	1.2	2.32	1.26	0.49	1.05
Language comprehension	3.39*	1.65	1.37	1.16	2.89*	1.21	−0.96	1.01
Expressive vocabulary	2.46	1.64	2.00	1.15	2.70*	1.2	−0.43	1.00
Attention								
Omission errors	−0.83	0.76	−0.82	0.54	−0.49	0.56	0.53	0.47
Commission errors	−1.05	1.84	−3.02*	1.32	−1.23	1.36	1.5	1.15
Social and emotional								
Competence ratings, Cg	1.44	1.38	2.86**	0.99	−0.58	1.04	−0.69	0.84
Competence ratings, M	1.33	1.25	2.10*	0.89	−0.10	0.92	1.52*	0.76
Observation with friend	0.07	0.09	0.17**	0.06	0.04	0.07	0.07	0.06
Behavior problems, Cg	0.02	1.11	−0.72	0.80	1.06	0.81	1.31*	0.66
Behavior problems, M	0.28	0.91	0.21	0.65	−0.01	0.67	1.19*	0.56

Note. Ns = 523–667. M, mother; Cg, caregiver. 54-month analyses control for 6–36-month quality variables; 6–36-month analyses control for 54-month quality variables; all analyses control for site, child gender, child ethnicity, mother education, partner status, parenting quality, maternal depression, family income, child care hours, and child care type.
*$p < .05$; **$p < .01$.

they did better on tests of applied problems, language comprehension, and expressive vocabulary if they received more language stimulation and watched less TV at earlier ages. Among the cognitive outcomes, only auditory processing (incomplete words) was unrelated to any index of the quality of earlier care; among the measures of cognitively stimulating care, only a stimulating physical environment at earlier ages was unrelated to child outcomes. The results of these analyses, therefore, are quite consistent with the proposition that children's cognitive development is influenced by child care quality.

In contrast, children's social–emotional behavior and attention were related to concurrent care but were not related to earlier care with quality of concurrent care controlled. The only link between social behavior and earlier care was that children who watched more TV in their care arrangement from 6 to 36 months were more competent with a friend at 54 months. Taken together, the results of these analyses are consistent with a

Measures of child care quality															
Watching TV				Stimulating physical materials				Positive interaction with other children				Positive caregiver talk			
6–36 mo.		54 mo.		6–36 mo.		54 mo.		15–36 mo.		54 mo.		15–36 mo.		54 mo.	
β	SE	β	SE	β	SE	β	SE	β	SE	β	SE	β	SE	β	SE
−0.12	0.69	0	0.48	0.86	1.35	−0.58	0.92	−.47	0.69	0.04	0.49	0.36	0.65	0.4	0.47
−1.76*	0.76	0.42	0.53	0.91	1.02	0.99	1.03	−.37	0.77	0.97	0.54	0.61	0.72	0.02	0.52
0.39	0.73	0.12	0.51	1.54	1.43	0.36	0.98	0.89	0.73	−0.92	0.51	1.08	0.68	0.33	0.49
−1.09	0.96	−0.48	0.67	2.4	1.88	0.96	1.29	0.51	0.97	−0.38	0.68	0.51	0.91	0.4	0.66
−1.82*	0.92	−0.18	0.64	2.83	1.80	2.98*	1.24	0.57	0.93	1.33*	0.66	−.81	0.88	−.20	0.63
−2.11*	0.91	0.13	0.64	1.23	1.80	1.83	1.23	0.7	0.92	1.09	0.65	0.14	0.87	−.02	0.63
0.4	0.45	−0.08	0.29	−0.80	0.84	−0.18	0.58	−.15	0.43	−0.52	0.30	0.18	0.40	−.06	0.30
−0.20	1.08	1.94**	0.69	−0.93	2.05	0.19	1.41	−.05	1.05	−1.66*	0.74	−.41	0.97	1.66*	0.73
−0.22	0.84	0.56	0.52	2.50	1.57	1.23	1.06	1.20	0.83	0.79	0.54	−.88	0.74	−.20	0.52
−0.12	0.70	0.14	0.47	−0.37	1.40	0.57	0.96	.37	0.71	−0.28	0.49	−.46	0.63	.23	0.47
0.12*	0.05	−0.03	0.04	−0.02	0.10	−0.03	0.07	−.02	0.05	−0.01	0.04	.00	0.05	.01	0.03
0.65	0.64	0.33	0.48	−0.88	1.26	1.24	0.84	−.59	0.65	−0.58	0.43	.29	0.56	.31	0.41
0.22	0.51	−0.41	0.34	−0.23	1.01	−0.36	0.69	−.33	0.52	−0.74*	0.36	.04	0.47	.58	0.35

causal argument linking quality of care with cognitive ability but not with social behavior or attention.

Proposition 4: Quality of Care Will Be Related to Child Outcomes Even When the Child's Earlier Abilities Are Taken into Account

To investigate the fourth proposition, we first analyzed the associations between overall quality of care and child outcomes at 54 months while controlling for matched child abilities assessed at 36 months. (The measure of attention at 36 months was not significantly associated with attention at 54 months [rs with omission errors and commission errors = .00], so the attention variables were not included in this analysis.) Table 23.5 presents the matched 36-month measures and the results of these analyses. As the table indicates, only 2 of the 10 child outcomes at 54 months were significantly related to child care quality after controlling for earlier ability: A higher level of quality was related to more advanced expressive vocabulary (controlling for expressive language at 36 months) and greater social competence reported by the mother at 54 months (controlling for mother-reported social competence at 36 months), and F ratios for changes in predictability when quality of care was added to the regression equations for these two variables were significant. These results provide limited evidence for a causal link between child care quality and child outcomes; they are consistent with a causal link between child care quality and cognitive outcomes only for expressive language.

In a subsequent set of analyses, we examined associations between changes in children's cognitive abilities between 36 and 54 months and changes in child care quality between 36 and 54 months. The difference between child care quality at 36 months and child care quality at 54 months was calculated, and two groups were created: children whose child care quality between 36 and 54 months had improved substantially (the top quartile of the change-in-quality distribution; $n = 102$) and children whose child care quality had declined substantially (the bottom quartile; $n = 97$). In each case, these changes substantially exceeded 1 standard deviation (for the improved-quality group, the standard deviation for quality at 36–54 months was .34, and the mean change score was .88; for the diminished-quality group, the standard deviation for quality at 36–54 months was .42, and the mean change score was .67).

We proposed that if high quality causes improved scores and low quality leads to lower scores, children whose care had substantially improved in quality should show improvement in their abilities between 36 and 54 months and vice versa. For this analysis, we selected only children who had been in their 54-month care arrangement for at least 6 months in order to ensure sufficient time for children to experience either the "benefit" or the "harm" of that care arrangement. Among the 10 associations that were

TABLE 23.5. Associations between Child Outcomes and Quality of Care at 54 Months with Earlier Child Abilities Controlled

Child outcome	Earlier ability measure	Association with earlier ability		Association with overall quality rating		F of change for quality	n
		β	SE	β	SE		
Cognition and language							
Letter–word identification	Bracken	0.27***	0.02	0.38	0.69	0.31	771
Applied problems	Bracken	0.25***	0.02	0.94	1.32	1.32	770
Incomplete words	Bracken	0.11***	0.02	0.77	0.85	0.82	767
Short-term memory	Reynell	0.66***	0.05	-0.65	1.01	0.41	779
Language comprehension	Reynell	0.73***	0.04	1.15	0.87	1.78	788
Expressive vocabulary	Reynell	0.42***	0.04	2.52*	0.99	6.53*	764
Social and emotional							
Competence, Cg	Competence, Cg	0.24*	0.09	1.88	1.16	2.62	410
Competence, M	Competence, M	1.24***	0.08	1.67*	0.71	5.56*	783
Behavior problems, Cg	Behavior problems, Cg	0.07*	0.03	-0.05	0.89	0.00	397
Behavior problems, M	Behavior problems, M	0.35***	0.02	-0.34	0.46	0.53	786

Note. Site, child gender, child ethnicity, mother education, partner status, parenting quality, maternal depression, family income, child care hours, and child care type were controlled. Bracken, Bracken Basic Concept Scale; Reynell, Reynell Developmental Language Scale; M, mother; Cg, caregiver.
* p = <.05; *** p < .001.

355

tested in these analyses, only 1 was significant. Children whose child care quality improved substantially gained more in their auditory processing (incomplete words) than did children whose child care quality had declined (Ms = 56.2 vs. 48.7), $F(1, 185)$ = 3.81, $p < .05$. Thus these analyses of changes in children's abilities over time failed to provide much support for a causal link between child care quality and child outcomes.

In these first two sets of analyses, we investigated direct effects of child care on child outcomes. It is possible, however, that although these analyses revealed few direct effects, there may be indirect effects of child care quality mediated through children's earlier abilities or through the quality of parenting. Structural equation modeling (SEM) analyses allowed us to explore indirect effects of care quality. We conducted SEM analyses that included the following variables: (1) child care quality from 6 to 36 months, (2) child care quality at 54 months, (3) parenting quality from 6 to 36 months, (4) parenting quality at 54 months, (5) child outcomes at 36 months, and (6) child outcomes at 54 months. We allowed child care quality and parenting quality from 6 to 36 months to be correlated, estimated direct paths between pairs of variables, and tested two indirect paths: (1) child care quality from 6 to 36 months → child outcomes at 36 months → child outcomes at 54 months and (2) child care quality from 6 to 36 months → parenting quality at 54 months → child outcomes at 54 months. Good fit was obtained for all models (Bollen scores were very near 1, which indicates a good fit; the lowest Bollen score was .98, and all others were ≥ .99). These analyses revealed no significant indirect paths to child outcomes at 54 months through parenting quality. However, significant indirect paths from quality of care at 6–36 months through child abilities at 36 months to child outcomes at 54 months were found for all cognitive outcomes.

Proposition 5: There Will Be a Dose-Response Relation between Quality of Care and Child Outcomes

Finally, to test the last proposition, we analyzed statistical interactions between the quality of care and the amount of time the child spent in the observed care arrangement in predicting child outcomes, controlling for the same set of covariates that had been used in earlier analyses, to determine whether associations between child care quality and child outcomes would be stronger if children spent more time in the care setting. We did this in a number of ways. In each analysis, we focused on child care at a single age, rather than using cumulative child care from 6 to 54 months, so that we could link the observations of quality with the "dose" of the particular care setting and caregiver observed. Combining across ages would have made direct links between amount and quality of care impossible.

In five separate sets of analyses of dose–response relations between child care quality and child outcomes, no significant interactions in the expected direction emerged. The results of these analyses fail to support the proposition that more exposure to high-quality care at 36 or 54 months of age causes improved performance and that more exposure to low-quality care is detrimental to development.

Given the possibility that failure to detect dose–response relations with respect to quality of care could be a function of the nonlinear nature of the dose–response relation, we carried out curvilinear analyses predicting 54-month outcomes from quality + hours + (hours × hours) + (quality × hours) + (quality × hours × hours) + covariates. These provided no evidence of a nonlinear dose–response relation; all quadratic terms were clearly non-significant.

DISCUSSION

Over the past three decades, a large body of research has accumulated demonstrating that the quality of child care predicts children's performance on cognitive and social assessments. Findings in the present study are consistent with the results reported in that research literature and extend them in a new direction. In this study, we were able to include a comprehensive assortment of child care arrangements; a wide array of child outcomes; a large and diverse geographical sample, and a longitudinal set of child, family, and child care assessments. We used these methodological advantages to explore five propositions about causal links between child care quality and child outcomes. Three of the propositions received substantial support; two received minimal or no support. When support occurred, it pertained principally to cognitive outcomes and appeared primarily for the less stringent propositions. Therefore, in this naturalistic study of child care quality in the typical range, evidence that child care quality was causally related to child outcomes was seriously limited. For now, the message to be drawn from our analyses is that although there may be a causal link between child care quality and child outcomes, the evidence for it is mixed and the "effect," if any, is not large (approximately 0.2).

24

Child Outcomes When Child Care Center Classes Meet Recommended Standards for Quality

NICHD Early Child Care Research Network

This chapter focuses on a single basic question: Do children perform better in terms of cognition, language, and social competence when they receive child care that meets professional standards for quality? Although all 50 states regulate child care centers, there is considerable variability in the stringency of regulated standards. A number of professional organizations have provided child care recommendations in an effort to set national standards to safeguard the well-being of children. The American Public Health Association and the American Academy of Pediatrics joined forces in 1992 to formulate a comprehensive set of standards, resulting in the publication of a comprehensive and detailed manual for child care workers. The view of health reflected in the standards is broader than a biomedical model (Ford & Lerner, 1992). From a systems theory perspective, child care is seen as an environment that provides opportunities for sensitive caregiving, nutrition, safety, and learning. Data are needed with which to evaluate the effectiveness of these standards in regard to children's development.

The National Institute of Child Health and Human Development

From *American Journal of Public Health*, 1999, Vol. 89, pp. 1072–1077. Reprinted with permission from the American Public Health Association.

(NICHD) Study of Early Child Care provided an opportunity to examine the consequences for children when centers meet recommended standards in child care. We predicted that children enrolled in child care center classes that met more professionally recommended standards would perform better on measures of cognition, language, and social competence than children enrolled in classes that met fewer of these standards.

METHODS

Participants

Chapter 1 provides a detailed description of the study participants.

Measures

Child Care Variables

Children were observed in their child care centers at 6, 15, 24, and 36 months of age using the Observational Record of the Caregiving Environment (see Chapter 5). Child–staff ratios were recorded by child care observers at the beginning and end of each observation cycle, and subsequently the average child–staff ratio across cycles was calculated. All adults were counted (qualified staff included caregivers, assistant caregivers, and aides who worked in classes at least 10 hours per week). Group size was calculated as the average number of children younger than 13 years across all observation cycles. Caregivers' formal training was scored from the interview to reflect training in child development or early childhood education in one of the following categories: none (scored as 0), high school courses (1), vocational/technical school courses (2), college courses (3), or college degree (4). Caregivers' education was scored as a six-level variable (1 = less than high school graduation, 6 = advanced degree).

To create an index of the extent to which a class met the standards recommended by experts, we used child–staff ratio, group size, and training requirements published by the American Public Health Association and the American Academy of Pediatrics (1992). We selected these standards because they were specific, recent, and issued by two important professional organizations. The standards were as follows: child–staff ratios of 3:1 at 6 and 15 months, 4:1 at 24 months, and 7:1 at 36 months of age; group sizes of 6 at 6 and 15 months, 8 at 24 months, and 14 at 36 months of age; and formal, post-high school training (including certification or a college degree) in child development, early childhood education, or a related field at all four ages. Because higher education has been shown to be a predictor of better practice in numerous studies (Berk, 1985; Howes, 1997;

Whitebook, Howes, & Phillips, 1990), we supplemented the preceding standards with an additional one: caregiver general education that included at least some college. Each class observed received a score of 0 or 1 on each of the four features of child care to signify whether it met the recommended standard; classes also received a total score for the number of recommended standards they met (0–4).

Family Variables

Five family variables were included as potential covariates: (1) ratio of income to needs, calculated as total family income divided by poverty threshold for family size, averaged over the four assessment points (6, 15, 24, and 36 months of age), (2) maternal education, (3) concurrent single-parent status, (4) child gender, and (5) maternal sensitivity, as assessed by mother–child interaction ratings made during semistructured play (see Chapter 19).

Child Outcome Variables

At 24 months of age, the Mental Development Index (MDI; Bayley, 1993) was administered to assess children's overall cognitive development. At 36 months of age, 51 items constituting the school readiness composite (colors, letter identification, numbers/counting, comparisons, and shapes) of the Bracken Basic Concept Scales were administered (Bracken, 1984), and total scores were converted to percentiles. The Reynell Developmental Language Scales, which consist of two 67-item instruments measuring language comprehension and expressive language, were also administered at 36 months of age (Reynell, 1991), and total scores were converted to standard scores (mean = 100, SD = 15). Prior to the beginning of data collection, testers were trained and certified in regard to all of these measures at a central location.

Mothers' reports of their children's problem behavior and positive social behavior were obtained at both 24 and 36 months of age via two instruments: the Child Behavior Checklist (CBCL; Achenbach, Edelbrock, & Howell, 1987), on which mothers rated how characteristic each of the 99 listed behaviors was of their child over the previous 2 months (0 = not true, 1 = sometimes true, 2 = very true), and the Adaptive Social Behavior Inventory (ASBI; Hogan, Scott, & Bauer, 1992), on which mothers rated 30 descriptions of the child's behavior via 3-point scales representing frequency of occurrence (1 = rarely, 2 = sometimes, 3 = always). Four scales from the CBCL (externalizing, internalizing, sleep problems, and somatic problems) and the disruptive behavior scale of the ASBI were standardized (mean = 0, SD = 1) and summed as a composite index of mother-reported behavior problems. The two remaining subscales from the ASBI (expressive and comply) were standardized and summed as mother-reported positive social behavior.

RESULTS

To determine the representativeness of the nine study states with respect to the four child care standards, we used existing state-level data for the 50 states and the District of Columbia on mandated child–staff ratios, group sizes, caregiver formal training, and caregiver education at 9 and 30 months, the two ages for which data were available (Azure, 1996; Azure & Eldred, 1997). Four t tests were conducted comparing ratio and group size between the 9 study states and the remaining 41 states and the District of Columbia at both ages. Two chi-squared tests were performed comparing the proportion of states meeting American Public Health Association standards for caregiver education and training in the nine study states versus the remaining states. All tests were nonsignificant; thus, there is no evidence of bias in the selection of the nine states.

Descriptive statistics for the four features in the observed centers show that at the three youngest ages, the average observed child–staff ratio exceeded the recommended level by 1 child per adult; specifically, the average observed child–staff ratios were 4:1 (vs. the recommended 3:1) at 6 and 15 months and 5:1 (vs. 4:1) at 24 months of age. At 36 months of age, the observed child–staff ratio was equivalent to the recommended ratio (7:1). The average observed group size also exceeded the recommended level at 6 and 15 months (8 children vs. the recommendation of 6) and at 24 months of age (11 children vs. 8), whereas, at 36 months, it approximately met the recommended standard (observed group size: 13; recommended maximum group size: 14). The average observed levels of caregiver formal training and education approximated the levels we set as guidelines in our analyses at all four ages. The majority of caregivers had some formal, post–high school training in child development or early childhood education and at least some college education.

The total number of recommended standards met increased as the children became older. Only 10–12% of the classes observed met all four standards at 6, 15, and 24 months, whereas 34% of the classes met all four at 36 months of age. Nearly 20% of the classes failed to meet any of the recommended standards at the two youngest ages, while only 3% of the classes failed to meet any at the oldest age.

Five family variables (ratio of income to needs, maternal education, single-parent status, child gender, and maternal sensitivity) known to relate to both families' child care selection and children's development were examined for possible inclusion in analyses as covariates. At 24 months of age, two of the five family variables were associated with the number of recommended standards met by child care centers: income-to-needs ratio $F(4,158) = 2.91$, $p < .03$ and maternal education $F(4,158) = 6.84$, $p < .001$. Predictably, these variables were lowest in centers that met no standards.

At 36 months of age, only maternal sensitivity was associated with number of standards met $F(4, 245) = 3.47$, $p < .01$; this variable also was lowest in centers that met no standards. Because maternal education and ratio of income to needs were highly correlated at both 24 and 36 months of age, we decided to include only one of these variables as a covariate. We selected income-to-needs ratio because it was less correlated with maternal sensitivity and thereby provided a more independent control. (Analyses were also rerun with maternal education as a covariate; a similar pattern of results was obtained.) When we conducted separate multivariate analyses of covariance (MANCOVAs) (for each of the four features) to compare children in classes that met a given standard with children in classes that did not, results indicated that concurrent child outcomes differed significantly as a function of the standards for child–staff ratio at 24 months $F(3,157) = 3.61$, $p = .015$, caregiver education at 36 months $F(5,242) = 4.94$, $p = .0002$, and caregiver training at 36 months of age $F(5,242) = 3.74$, $p = .003$. Meeting the recommended ratio standard was associated with fewer behavior problems and more cooperative behaviors at 24 months of age. Meeting standards for caregiver education and training was associated with higher school readiness and language comprehension scores and fewer behavior problems at 36 months of age.

In the next step, we examined the associations between the number of standards classes met and child outcomes. The multivariate test of the linear trend was not significant at 24 months of age; however, one of the three univariate tests was significant. Fewer behavior problems were reported for children in classes that met more standards. At 36 months of age, the multivariate test of the linear trend was significant $F(5, 239) = 3.26$, $p = .007$, and the univariate linear contrasts were significant for three of the five outcomes. Children in classes that met more recommended standards displayed higher school readiness and language comprehension scores and fewer behavior problems.

Effect sizes were computed as the average change in an outcome associated with a 1-point increase in the number of standards met, divided by the estimated standard deviation (under the analysis model). Average change was estimated from the group means based on the assumption that number of standards and outcome measures were linearly related. These analyses indicated that increasing the number of standards met by 1 was associated with modest amounts of change: decreases on the behavior problems composite of 0.53 points at 24 months of age (effect size: 0.16) and 0.84 points at 36 months of age (effect size: 0.24) and increases of 4.40 percentile points on the 36-month school readiness score (effect size: 0.20) and 2.41 points on the language comprehension standard score (effect size: 0.19).

In a set of *post hoc* analyses, we examined contrasts for possible thresholds in the linear trends. All were significant: zero or one versus two to four standards met $F(5,239) = 3.62$, $p = .004$, zero to two versus three or four standards met $F(5,239) = 4.08$, $p = .004$, and zero to three versus four standards met $F(5,239) = 4.23$, $p = .001$. Because all contrasts were significant, there did not appear to be any threshold; instead, analyses at 36 months of age consistently indicated that when children attended classes that met more standards, their cognitive, language, and social development was better than when they attended classes meeting fewer standards.

The analyses described thus far focused on the concurrent effects of child care standards on child outcomes (i.e., both measured at the same point in time). In a final set of analyses, lagged effects were examined. For the 87 children in center-based care at both 15 and 24 months of age, 24-month outcomes were predicted from the number of standards met at 15 months of age; for the 127 children in center-based care at both 24 and 36 months of age, 36-month outcomes were predicted by number of standards met at 24 months of age. In neither case were there significant lagged effects. Note that the associations between number of standards met at consecutive ages were moderate (rs = .35 between 15 and 24 months and rs = .34 between 24 and 36 months of age).

DISCUSSION

This chapter began with the question whether children have better outcomes when they attend centers where classes meet more professional standards for child–staff ratio, group size, caregiver training, and caregiver education. The answer to this question depends on a child's age, the outcome, and the specific child care standard. Outcomes were better when children attended classes that met the recommended child–staff ratio at 24 months and the recommended levels of caregiver training and education at 36 months. Furthermore, the more standards met, the better the outcomes in terms of school readiness, language comprehension, and behavior problems at 36 months. These results complement previous findings from the NICHD Study of Early Child Care showing significant associations between observed child care quality (i.e., caregiver behavior with children) and children's cognitive, language, and social outcomes (see Chapters 19 and 20).

These relations between child care standards and children's development raise important issues for policymakers. The concurrent analyses suggest that the failure of many states to impose stringent standards and the failure of many centers to meet such standards may undermine children's development. If so, these findings support a policy of more stringent child care regulation, including adoption of national standards. Some, however, might question the return on investment that might result from the added cost of raising standards, because the lagged analyses, which admittedly lacked the statistical power of the concurrent analyses, failed to reveal significant effects. Clearly, more work in this important area is needed.

25

—

Child Care Structure →
Process → Outcome
Direct and Indirect Effects of Child Care Quality
on Young Children's Development

NICHD EARLY CHILD CARE RESEARCH NETWORK

One of the most robust findings in the early-childhood literature is that good child care quality is associated with a variety of positive outcomes for young children. Specifically, children in higher-quality child care programs perform better on measures of social, language, and cognitive development when compared with other children (Clarke-Stewart & Allhusen, 2002; Lamb, 1998). Quality is typically measured by both process features, such as caregiving quality, and structural features, such as child–staff ratio. By definition, process variables are assumed to have a direct impact on children's development, whereas structural variables are assumed to have an indirect impact via process quality (see Friedman & Amadeo, 1999).

Studies have documented three types of associations: those between structural and process features of child care quality, those between structural features of child care quality and child outcomes, and those between process features of child care quality and child outcomes. In no investigation to date, however, have these three associations been brought together in a single analytic model. Of particular interest is the often assumed but never tested mediated path from structural features of child care quality through process features to child outcomes. The purpose of the present study was to test this mediated path using structural equation modeling (SEM).

From *Psychological Science*, 2002, Vol. 13, pp. 199–206. Reprinted by permission of Blackwell Publishing.

Figure 25.1 presents a general child care model that has guided researchers. Note that as with child care, there are two kinds of family variables: structural (e.g., mothers' education) and process (e.g., maternal caregiving). These two family variables are each linked to both structural and process child care quality, as well as to child outcomes; the link is direct for family process and indirect for family structure. Structural child care quality is directly linked to process child care quality. Finally, process child care quality is linked to child outcomes. We predicted that the mediated path (in **boldface** in Figure 25.1), from structure to process to outcome, would be significant; further, we predicted that this mediated path would not be accounted for entirely by family influences. In the study discussed in this chapter, we focused on child care at age 54 months, a time at which the greatest proportion of children are in care, and we included all types of child care, from center-based care to home care to relative care.

METHOD

Overview of the Study Design

Children were followed from birth through 54 months. Mothers were interviewed in person when their infants were 1 month old. Measures of the family environment and measures of primary child care settings were obtained when the children were 6, 15, 24, 36, and 54 months old. The 54-month child-outcome data used in this chapter were obtained from parents' ratings, caregivers' ratings, and laboratory assessments. All the data collectors were trained and certified on data collection procedures. Their performance was monitored centrally to ensure uniform, high-quality data across sites.

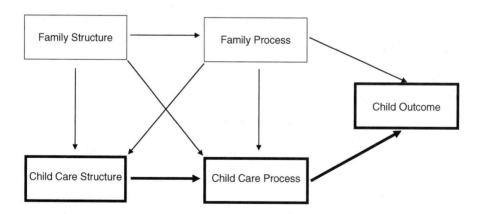

FIGURE 25.1. A generalized child care effects model. The mediated path tested in the current study is shown in boldface.

Participants

Chapter 3 provides a detailed description of the study design and participants.

Measures

Process Measures of Child Care Quality

The Observational Record of the Caregiving Environment (ORCE) was developed to assess characteristics of child care quality generally and non-maternal caregiving specifically (see Chapter 3). Behaviors were coded when the children were 54 months old. Eight qualitative ratings were made. Four assessed the caregivers' relationship with the children (sensitivity to nondistress, detachment, stimulation of cognitive development, and intrusiveness), and four assessed the classroom setting (chaos, overcontrol, positive emotional climate, and negative emotional climate).

Structural Measures of Child Care

We chose to focus on the two most policy-relevant indicators: caregivers' training and child–staff ratio. Information on caregivers' training in child development or early-childhood education was obtained from interviews with the caregivers. Child–staff ratios were recorded by child care observers at the beginning and end of each of the two ORCE cycles. An average across the four recordings was then computed.

Family Background

Two well-established measures of family background were selected: mothers' education in years and an income-to-needs ratio (i.e., total family income, including government payments, divided by the appropriate poverty threshold for the household, as determined by the U.S. Department of Labor).

Maternal Caregiving

Three measures of the quality of maternal caregiving were included. First, a composite measure of maternal sensitivity was created from observers' ratings of structured play sessions (see Chapter 17). When the children were 6, 15, and 24 months old, the score reflected the sum of the average ratings of sensitivity to nondistress, positive regard, and intrusiveness (reversed). When the children were 36 and 54 months old, the score reflected the average sum of ratings of supportive presence, respect for autonomy, and hostility (reversed). Second, overall quality of the physical and social resources available to the child in the family context was assessed through the Home

Observation for Measurement of the Environment (HOME; Caldwell & Bradley, 1984). The Infant/Toddler version was used at ages 6 and 15 months, and the Early Childhood version was used at ages 36 and 54 months. Third, when the infants were 1 month old, mothers completed a questionnaire that assessed nonauthoritarian childrearing attitudes and values (Schaefer & Edgerton, 1985).

Cognitive Competence

Seven measures of competence were used to form a latent variable. Two were from the Woodcock–Johnson Tests of Cognitive Ability (Woodcock & Johnson, 1989, 1990): incomplete words and memory for sentences; two were from the Woodcock–Johnson Tests of Achievement (Woodcock & Johnson, 1989): letter–word identification and applied problems; and two were from the Preschool Language Scale (Zimmerman, Steiner, & Pond, 1992): auditory competence and expressive language. The seventh measure was the number of omission errors (i.e., missed target stimuli) derived from the Continuous Performance Task (Rosvold, Mirsky, Sarason, Bransome, & Beck, 1956), a measure of sustained attention.

Caregivers' and Mothers' Ratings of Social Competence

Caregivers and mothers each completed the Child Behavior Checklist (Achenbach, 1991a), a measure of internalizing and externalizing behavior problems. In addition, caregivers completed the California Preschool Social Competence Scale (Levine, Elzey, & Lewis, 1969), and mothers completed the Social Skills Rating System (Gresham & Elliott, 1990), each yielding a measure of social skills.

RESULTS

Data Analysis Plan

Specified models were fitted in two stages. First, measurement models were fitted, yielding latent variables, and then hypothesized models were fitted, including both latent and manifest variables. Indirect paths were tested using a t statistic developed by Sobel (1982).

Multiple indices of fit were examined because the chi-square overall goodness-of-fit test statistic is adversely affected by a large sample size, model misspecification, or violation of distribution assumptions (Bollen, 1990). Following Hu and Bentler (1999), we selected three widely used measures to supplement the chi-square statistic: the standardized root mean squared residual (SRMR), the root mean square error of approximation (RMSEA; see Browne & Cudek, 1993; Steiger & Lind, 1980), and Bollen's Goodness-of-Fit Index (Bollen GFI; see Bollen, 1990).

Structural Equation Models

Six models were fitted to the data. Each model included one of the two structural measures of child care quality (training and child–staff ratio) and one of the three child outcomes (cognitive competence and caregivers' and mothers' ratings of social competence). The models also included mothers' education and family income-to-needs ratio, which were treated as exogenous variables, as well as maternal caregiving, a factor, and nonmaternal caregiving, a latent variable. For each model, the significance of 11 direct paths, 4 indirect paths with three variables, and 3 indirect paths with four variables was tested (outlined in Table 25.1). Six of the seven indirect paths concerned family selection of child care structure and process. Family selection was also assessed by contrasting the fit of each of the six models with the fit of a corresponding model that excluded these six indirect paths. The seventh indirect path concerned the hypothesized mediated path from child care structure to child care process to child outcome. Hypotheses regarding each of these indirect paths were directional and therefore one-tailed t tests were used to evaluate their fit.

Cognitive Competence

The two cognitive-competence models were fitted with data from 738 children. Figures 25.2a and 25.2b show the results of the analyses involving caregiver training and child–staff ratio, respectively, by displaying the estimated standardized path coefficients and loadings. Table 25.1 shows the unstandardized coefficients, which were used in the tests for indirect effects. The chi-square tests for training, $\chi^2(77) = 143.2$, $p < .001$, and for ratio, $\chi^2(77) = 155.6$, $p < .001$, were both significant, perhaps as a result of the large sample size. Because the other three indices indicated good fit for caregiver training (SRMR = .03, RMSEA = .03, and Bollen GFI = .98), as well as for child–staff ratio (SRMR = .03, RMSEA = .04, and Bollen GFI = .98), we argue that interpretation of the estimated paths is reasonable.

As expected, indicators of structural child care quality were related to nonmaternal caregiving. In addition, family variables as well as nonmaternal caregiving were related to child outcomes. There were significant paths in the model from training to nonmaternal caregiving (beta = .17) and from child–staff ratio to nonmaternal caregiving (beta = −.10). There were also significant paths from nonmaternal caregiving to cognitive competence (beta = .10 in the training and ratio models). The betas were relatively small. In contrast, there were larger direct paths between maternal caregiving and cognitive competence (beta = .46).

Next, we tested the indirect effects (see Table 25.1). As hypothesized, significant indirect paths were observed from training, beta = .071, $t(75)$ = 2.29, $p < .05$, and from child–staff ratio, beta = −.017, $t(75) = −1.81$, $p < .05$, to cognitive competence as mediated by nonmaternal caregiving. Of the six

TABLE 25.1. Unstandardized Coefficients Representing Direct and Indirect Paths for the Models

	Model			
	Cognitive competence		Caregiver ratings of social competence	
Path	Training	Child–staff ratio	Training	Child–staff ratio
Direct effects				
Maternal caregiving → O	2.407 (0.28)***	2.409 (0.28)***	0.126 (0.034)***	0.127 (0.034)***
Mothers' education → O	0.405 (0.126)***	0.406 (0.126)***	0.034 (0.020)	0.034 (0.020)*
Income → O	0.219 (0.089)**	0.219 (0.089)**	−0.015 (0.015)	−0.015 (0.015)
Nonmaternal caregiving → O	0.837 (0.306)**	0.818 (0.303)**	0.170 (0.050)***	0.167 (0.049)***
S → Nonmaternal caregiving	0.085 (0.019)***	−0.021 (0.008)**	0.095 (0.020)***	−0.021 (0.009)**
Maternal caregiving → Nonmaternal caregiving	0.088 (0.029)**	0.096 (0.029)***	0.034 (0.029)	0.039 (0.029)
Mothers' education → Nonmaternal caregiving	0.001 (0.016)	0.005 (0.016)	0.013 (0.016)	0.015 (0.017)
Income → Nonmaternal caregiving	0.004 (0.012)	0.012 (0.012)	0.011 (0.012)	0.019 (0.012)
Maternal caregiving → S	0.017 (0.056)	0.327 (0.129)	−0.026 (0.055)	0.325 (0.128)
Mothers' education → S	0.069 (0.031)*	−0.091 (0.073)	0.060 (0.031)*	−0.177 (0.074)**
Income → S	0.062 (0.022)**	0.131 (0.052)	0.049 (0.023)*	0.110 (0.005)
Indirect effects[a] with three variables				
S → Nonmaternal caregiving → O	0.071 (0.031)*	−0.017 (0.009)*	0.017 (0.006)**	−0.004 (0.002)*
Maternal caregiving → Nonmaternal caregiving → O	0.074 (0.04)*	0.079 (0.03)*	0.006 (0.005)	0.007 (0.005)
Mothers' education→ Nonmaternal caregiving → O	0.001 (0.014)	0.004 (0.014)	0.002 (0.003)	0.003 (0.003)
Income→ Nonmaternal caregiving → O	0.003 (0.011)	0.01 (0.011)	0.002 (0.002)	0.003 (0.002)
Indirect effects[a] with four variables				
Maternal caregiving → S → Nonmaternal caregiving → O	0.001 (0.004)	−0.006 (0.04)	−0.004 (0.001)	−0.001 (0.001)
Mothers' education → S → Nonmaternal caregiving → O	0.005 (0.003)	0.002 (0.002)	0.001 (0.0006)	−0.000 (0.0003)
Income → S → Nonmaternal caregiving → O	0.004 (0.002)*	−0.002 (0.002)	0.001 (0.0005)*	−0.000 (0.0003)

Note. Standard errors are given in parentheses. S, structural child care quality, in this case caregiver training (columns 1 and 3) and child–staff ratio (columns 2 and 4); O, outcome.

[a]Indirect paths computed as the product of the included direct paths (e.g., for two paths labeled b, c). The estimated unstandardized coefficient for the indirect path is $b \times c$. The estimated standard error is computed as the square root of $(c^2)(SE_b^2) + (b^2)(SE_c^2) + (SE_b^2)(SE_c^2)$. The t ratio is computed as the estimated coefficient divided by the estimated standard error.

*p < .05; **p < .01; ***p < .001.

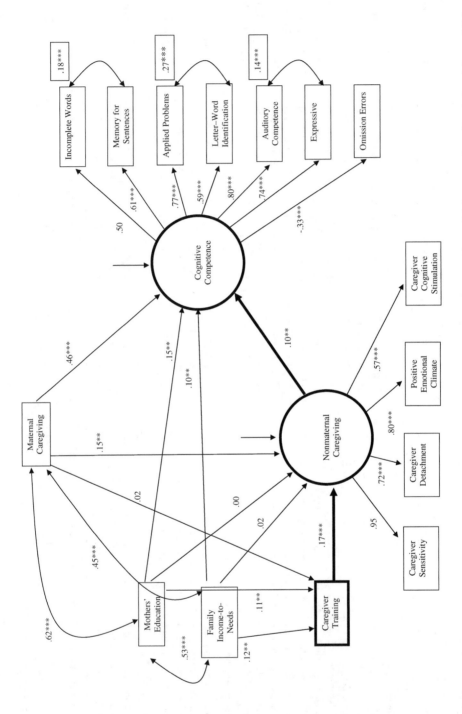

FIGURE 25.2. Structural equation models predicting cognitive competence from family variables, caregivers' training (a) or child–staff ratio (b), and nonmaternal caregiving. Significant paths are indicated by asterisks: $^{**}p < .01$; $^{***}p < .001$.

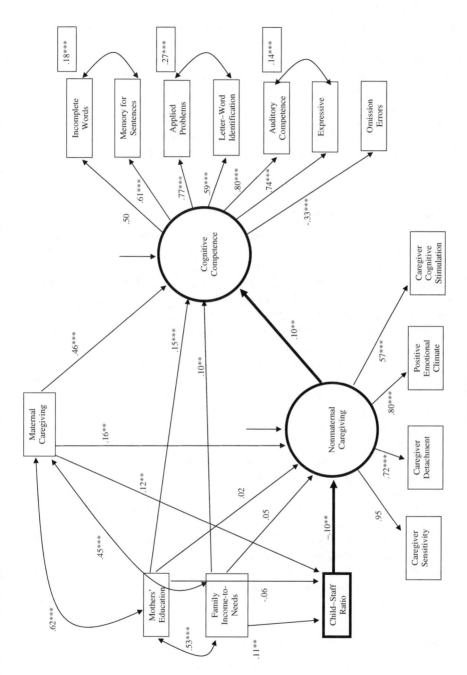

FIGURE 25.2. (*continued*)

371

indirect family paths tested for training and the six indirect family paths tested for child–staff ratio, three paths reached statistical significance: the path from maternal caregiving through nonmaternal caregiving to cognitive competence for training, beta = .074, $t(75)$ = 1.97, p < .05, and for ratio, beta = .079, $t(75)$ = 2.04, p < .05, and the path from income through training and nonmaternal caregiving to cognitive competence, beta = .004, $t(75)$=1.71, p < .05. Comparisons of models with and without these six indirect paths from family through nonmaternal caregiving to cognitive competence suggested that these paths taken together added significantly to the model including training, $\chi^2(6)$ = 50.2, p < .001, and the model including child–staff ratio, $\chi^2(6)$ = 45.6, p < .001.

Caregiver Report of Social Competence

A similar pattern of results emerged for the models predicting caregivers' ratings of social competence. These models were fitted with data from 656 children (see Figures 25.3a and 25.3b). Again, both chi-square tests were significant, $\chi^2(34)$ = 72.2, p < .001, for caregiver training and $\chi^2(34)$ = 101.0, p < .001, for child–staff ratio, and again the other three indices indicated good fit for training (SRMR = .027, RMSEA = .041, and Bollen GFI = .98), as well as for ratio (SRMR = .032, RMSEA = .055, and Bollen GFI = .97). Both caregiver training (beta = .19) and child–staff ratio (beta = –.10) were significantly associated with nonmaternal caregiving, which was associated with caregiver report of social competence (beta = .15). The direct path from maternal caregiving to social competence was larger and significant in both models (beta = .20).

Significant indirect paths from training, beta = .017, $t(34)$ = 2.73, p < .01, and child–staff ratio, beta = –.004, $t(34)$ = 1.86, p < .05, to social competence as mediated by nonmaternal caregiving were tested (see Table 25.1). For the training model, one indirect path from the family measures was statistically significant, namely, the path from income level through training and nonmaternal caregiving to social outcomes, beta = .001, $t(75)$ = 1.62, p < .05. None of the other indirect paths from the family measures through child care quality were significant in either the training or the ratio model. Comparisons of models with and without those six indirect paths from family to child outcomes showed that including family paths added to the overall fit of the model including training, $\chi^2(6)$ = 27.0, p < .001, and of the model including child–staff ratio, $\chi^2(6)$ = 28.9, p < .001.

Mother Report of Social Competence

The models predicting mothers' reports of social competence were fitted for 789 children. As before, both chi-square tests were significant, $\chi^2(34)$ = 120.2, p < .001, for caregiver training and $\chi^2(34)$ = 143.5, p < .001, for child–staff ratio. The other three indices indicated an adequate fit for the model

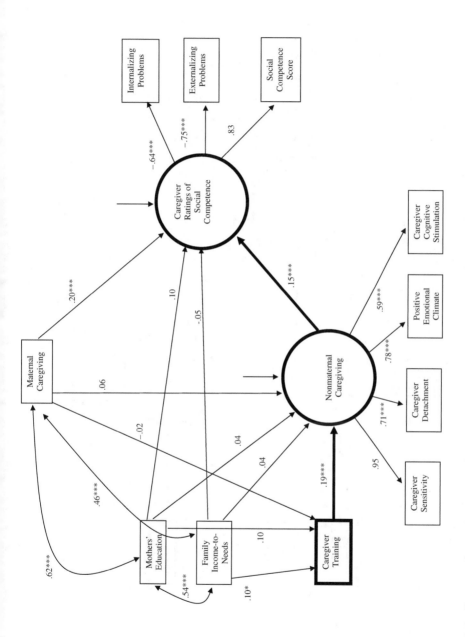

FIGURE 25.3. Structural equation models predicting caregivers' ratings of social competence from family variables, caregivers' training (a) or child–staff ratio (b), and nonmaternal caregiving. Significant paths are indicated by asterisks: * $p < .05$; ** $p < .01$; *** $p < .001$.

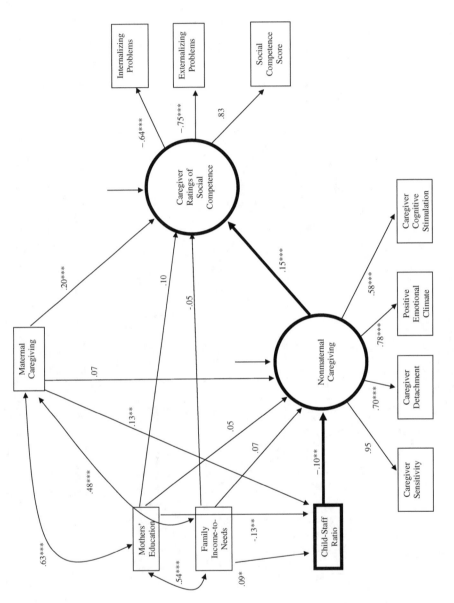

FIGURE 25.3. (continued)

that included caregiver training (SRMR = .048, RMSEA = .057, and Bollen GFI = .97) and for the model that included child–staff ratio (SRMR = .05, RMSEA = .064, and Bollen GFI = .96). These models did not provide evidence for a link from nonmaternal caregiving to this child outcome (beta = .01, $p > .05$). Thus, no tests of indirect effects were conducted.

DISCUSSION

The model that has guided child care researchers to date links structural indicators of quality through process indicators to child outcomes. Yet there have been no attempts to test this indirect or mediated path until now. SEM offers a method for testing mediation within a single analytic model. We computed six models, one for caregiver training and one for child–staff ratio for each of three outcomes. Note that these two structural variables are both potentially regulable by states.

There were three main findings. First, maternal caregiving was a strong predictor of cognitive competence and a moderate predictor of social competence as rated by caregivers. This finding is hardly surprising, given that contemporary studies on parenting, especially intervention studies, document the importance of sensitive parenting in young children's lives (see the review by Collins, Maccoby, Steinberg, Hetherington, & Bornstein, 2000).

The second finding from these models concerns the association between nonmaternal caregiving and both cognitive and social competence. These associations were revealed in our previous reports with 36-month outcomes (Chapters 19 and 20), as well as in other researchers' work (see reviews by Clarke-Stewart & Allhusen, 2002; Lamb, 1998).

The third finding concerns the heart of this investigation, specifically, the path from structure to process to outcome. This indirect or mediated path was tested for cognitive competence and caregivers' ratings of social competence in separate models for caregiver training and child–staff ratio. In all four models the indirect effect was significant. These models provide the first empirical evidence of a path from child care structure to process to outcomes. Although the arrows suggest a causal path, we recognize that causality cannot be inferred from structural equation models, which rely on correlational data as input.

The child care effects, both direct and indirect, do not appear to be due to family selection of child care quality per se. Indirect paths from the family variables to nonmaternal caregiving to each of the outcomes were tested, and only 4 of the 24 such paths were significant. We know that family selection exists, however, because the models were better fitted when indirect paths from family variables to child care variables were included than when they were not. It is probably safest to say that family selection into child care occurs but does not account entirely for the path from child care structure to process to outcome.

26

—

Early Child Care and Children's Development Prior to School Entry

NICHD Early Child Care Research Network

The placement of infants and young children in child care challenges deeply held beliefs and scientific theories that stress the importance of maternal care (Bowlby, 1973; Brazelton, 1986). Research on the effects of early child care on children's development has proven highly controversial (Fox & Fein, 1990), with researchers drawing vastly different conclusions about the direction of these effects. Some have contended that child care is a source of enrichment that promotes academic and social development (e.g., Clarke-Stewart, Gruber, & Fitzgerald, 1994; Lamb, 1998), whereas others have expressed concerns about the developmental risks associated with early child care (e.g., Belsky, 1999, 2001). A third group asserts that reports of both negative and positive consequences of child care are vastly exaggerated because discerned effects are negligible and do not endure over time (e.g., Blau, 1999; Scarr, 1998).

Increasingly, as nations move to raise educational standards for children's performance in school (National Education Goals Panel, 1997), experiences in child care settings are looked to as sources of variability in children's readiness for school (Pianta & Cox, 1999). Because the debate about the effects of child care on school readiness has implications for social and educational policy, clarification of the nature and extent of child care as a source of variability in children's developmental status is a pressing scientific concern.

From *American Educational Research Journal*, 2002, Vol. 39, pp. 133–164. Copyright 2002 by the American Educational Research Association. Reprinted by permission.

Consequently, in this report, we consider two basic questions: (1) are early-child care experiences positively or negatively related to child functioning prior to school entry? And, if so, (2) are statistical effects sufficiently large to be meaningful? In addressing these questions, we seek to move beyond a global characterization of early child care as good or bad for children to examine specific aspects of care that may foster or undermine children's development, by focusing on the cumulative amount or quantity of care from birth onward, the quality of the care received throughout these early years, and the types of care experienced (e.g. center-based vs. home-based care).

METHOD

Participants

Chapter 1 provides details about recruitment and participants, as well as an overview of data collection.

Overview of Data Collection

Children were followed from birth to age 54 months. Mothers were interviewed in person when infants were 1 month old. Detailed measures of home and family environments were obtained via interviews and observations when children were 6, 15, 24, 36, and 54 months old. Primary child care settings were observed at those same ages, for all children who were in nonmaternal care on a regular basis for 10 or more hours per week. Mothers were telephoned regularly to update reports on child care usage. Children's cognitive skills and social behavior were assessed at 4½ years.

child care Measures

During telephone interviews conducted at 3-month intervals through 36 months and at 4-month intervals thereafter, mothers reported types and hours of nonmaternal care that were being used.

Type of Care

For each 3–4-month interval (16 epochs in all), the child's primary care arrangement was classified as center, child care home (any home-based care outside the child's own home except care by grandparents), in-home care (any caregiver in the child's own home except father or grandparent), grandparent care, or father care. Epochs in which children were in non-maternal care for less than 10 hours/week were coded as exclusive maternal care. The proportion of epochs in which the child received care in a center and the proportion of epochs in a child care home were determined and included as type of care predictors in analyses.

Child Care Quantity

Parents were asked about the hours of routine nonmaternal care during the phone and personal interviews. The hours spent in all settings were summed for each of the 16 epochs.

Child Care Quality

Observational assessments of quality were obtained for primary nonmaternal arrangements that were used for 10 or more hours per week at 6, 15, 24, 36, and 54 months. Observations were conducted during two half-day visits scheduled within a 2-week interval at 6–36 months and one half-day visit at 54 months. At each half-day visit, observers completed two 44-minute cycles of the Observational Record of the Caregiving Environment (ORCE). (See Chapter 3 for detailed descriptions of the infant version of the ORCE assessments; see Chapter 6 for details about the toddler versions and preschool versions; complete observation manuals can be found at *http://public.rti.org/secc*.)

On average, four ORCE cycles at each eligible time period were completed for children from 6–36 months and two ORCE cycles were completed at 54 months. ORCE quality ratings were obtained at least one age period for 91% of the sample (985 of 1,083) and at least two ages for 779 children. Thirty-four children were never in nonmaternal care on a regular basis, and thus it was not possible to observe these children in a child care arrangement.

Positive caregiving composites were calculated for each age level. At 6, 15, and 24 months, positive caregiving composite scores were the mean of five 4-point qualitative ratings (sensitivity to child's nondistress signals, stimulation of cognitive development, positive regard for child, emotional detachment [reflected], flatness of affect [reflected]). Cronbach's alphas for the composite were .89 at 6 months, .88 at 15 months, and .87 at 24 months. At 36 months, these five scales plus two additional subscales, "fosters child's exploration" and "intrusive" (reflected), were included in the composite (Cronbach's alpha = .83). At 54 months, the positive caregiving composite was the mean of 4-point ratings of caregivers' sensitivity/responsivity, stimulation of cognitive development, intrusiveness (reflected), and detachment (reflected) (Cronbach's alpha = .72).

Maternal, Child, and Family Controls

Measures of maternal, child, and family characteristics were collected and used as controls for selection effects.

Demographic Variables

During home interviews at 1 month, mothers reported their own *education* (in years) and the study children's *race and ethnicity* (non-Hispanic African American, non-Hispanic European American, Hispanic, or other) and *sex*.

The *presence of a partner in the home* was reported in telephone interviews spaced every 3–4 months. *Partner status* was the proportion of 3–4-month intervals during which the mother reported a husband/partner was present. Mothers reported *family income* at 6, 15, 24, 36, and 54 months. *income-to-needs ratios* were calculated from U.S. Census Bureau tables as the ratio of family income to the appropriate poverty threshold for each household size and number of children under 18. In the current analyses, these ratios were averaged.

Maternal Depressive Symptoms

Maternal depressive symptoms were assessed at 6, 15, 24, 36, and 54 months, using the Center for Epidemiological Studies–Depression (CES-D) scale (Radloff, 1977), a self-report measure that assesses depressive symptomatology in the general population. Cronbach's alpha coefficients ranged from .88 to .91 in the present sample.

Mother–Child Interactions

Mother–child interactions were videotaped in semistructured 15-minute observations at 6, 15, 24, 36, and 54 months. The tasks provided a context for assessing age-appropriate qualities of maternal behavior. The observation task at the 6-month visit had two components. In the first 7 minutes, mothers were asked to play with their infants and were told that they could use any toy or object available in the home or none at all. For the remaining 8 minutes, mothers were given a standard set of toys they could use in play. At 15, 24, and 36 months, the observation procedures followed a three-boxes procedure in which mothers were asked to show their children age-appropriate toys in three containers in a set order (see Vandell, 1979). The mother was asked to have her child play with the toys in each of the three containers and to do so in the order specified.

At 6, 15, and 24 months, composite maternal sensitivity scores were created from the sums of three 4-point ratings (maternal sensitivity to child nondistress, intrusiveness [reversed], and positive regard). At 36 and 54 months, the maternal sensitivity composite was the sum of the three 7-point ratings of supportive presence, hostility (reversed), and respect for autonomy. Cronbach's alphas exceeded .70 at every age.

Home Observation for Measurement of the Environment

The Home Observation for Measurement of the Environment (HOME; Caldwell & Bradley, 1984) was administered during home visits at 6, 15, 36, and 54 months. The focus is on the child in the environment, child as a recipient of inputs from objects, events, and transactions occurring in connection with the family surroundings. The Infant/Toddler HOME (IT-HOME) is aimed for use during infancy (birth to age 3). It is composed of

45 items clustered into six subscales: (1) parental responsivity, (2) acceptance of child, (3) organization of the environment, (4) learning materials, (5) parental involvement, and (6) variety in experience. Each item is scored in binary fashion (yes/no). Information used to score the items is obtained during the course of the home visit by means of observation and semi-structured interview. The Early Childhood HOME (EC-HOME) is aimed for use during early childhood (age 3 to 6 years). It is composed of 55 items clustered into eight subscales. Both forms of the HOME are correlated with intellectual/academic performance and adaptive social behavior in the expected direction.

A centrally located system of training was used for data collectors at each age. Every 4 months, each observer coded videotaped visits and the coding was compared with gold standard codes. All observers were required to maintain a criterion of scoring like the master coder on 90% of the items. Cronbach's alphas for the total score at each age exceeded .77.

Parenting Quality

The HOME and maternal sensitivity ratings were standardized at each age and then averaged at each age to create a composite score. Together, these combined scores reflect parenting in two contexts: in the home and during semistructured play (also see Chapter 19).

Expanded List of Child and Family Covariates

Additional child and family measures were included as covariates in some analyses. These measures were maternal rating of *child temperament* obtained at 6 months measured by the 55-item Revised Infant Temperament Questionnaire (Carey & McDevitt, 1978), *maternal psychological adjustment* measured by three subscales (agreeableness, neuroticism, extraversion) of the Neuroticism Extraversion Openness (NEO) Personality Inventory (Costa & McCrae, 1985) collected at the 6-month home visit, maternal report of *social support* using 11 items that were rated with 6-point Likert scales collected at all visits (Marshall & Barnett, 1993), maternal report of *separation anxiety* using 21 items that were rated with 5-point Likert scales averaged from the 1–24-month visits (DeMeis, Hock, & McBridge, 1986), and maternal *beliefs about the benefits of employment* for children using 11 items collected at the 1-month visit (Greenberger, Goldberg, Crawford, & Granger, 1988). All measures were established measures with excellent psychometric properties.

Child Functioning at 4½ Years

Measures of child functioning were obtained during a laboratory visit, home visit, and child care visit at 4½ years.

Preacademic skills is a composite score from two subtests of the Woodcock–Johnson Achievement and Cognitive Batteries (1990). The letter–word identification test measures skills at identifying letters and words. The applied problems test measures skill in analyzing and solving practical problems in mathematics. Their correlation with each other was .57. Cronbach's alphas for the letter–word identification and applied problems were .86 and .85. The composite score was formed by averaging the standardized scores on the two subtests.

Short-term memory was assessed using the Woodcock–Johnson Cognitive Memory for Sentences subtest. Cronbach's alpha was .84 for this measure.

Language competence was assessed using the Preschool Language Scale (PLS-3; Zimmerman, Steiner, & Pond, 1979). It measures a range of language behaviors, including vocabulary, morphology, syntax, and integrative thinking, which are grouped into two subscales: auditory comprehension and expressive language (Cronbach's alpha = .89 and .92, respectively, in the current study). These scales were highly correlated (r = .70, p < .001).

Social competence was measured by having mothers complete the Social Skills Questionnaire (SSQ) from the Social Skills Rating System (Gresham & Elliott, 1990) for their children. This instrument is composed of 38 items describing child behavior. Mothers responded on a 3-point scale reflecting how often their child exhibited each behavior. Items are grouped into four areas: cooperation (e.g., keeps room neat and clean without being reminded), assertion (e.g., makes friends easily), responsibility (e.g., asks permission before using a family member's property), and self-control (controls temper when arguing with other children). The total score is the sum of all 38 items, with higher scores reflecting higher levels of perceived social competence. Cronbach's alpha in the current sample was .88.

For children who were in child care at least 10 hours per week at age 54 months (n = 833), caregivers completed the California Preschool Social Competency Scale (Levine, Elzey, & Lewis, 1969), a 30-item instrument assessing a range of social competencies especially relevant in child care settings (e.g., safe use of equipment, using names of others, greeting new child, and initiating group activities). Four items were added to index specific features of peer play (cooperation, following rules in games, empathy, and aggression). Items were rated on 4-point scales. Items scored as not applicable were set as missing. The total social competency score was the sum of the 34 items, with higher scores denoting greater social competence. Scores ranged from 46 to 135 (M = 104.88, SD = 13.6, alpha = .88).

Behavior problems were assessed by having mothers and caregivers complete the appropriate versions of the Child Behavior Checklist (Achenbach, 1991a). The parent version lists 113 problem behaviors. The parent rates each as not true (0), somewhat true (1), or very true (2) of her child. Caregivers (n = 768) in children's child care settings completed the 100-item caregiver–teacher version developed for children ages 2–5 years. Both the parent and teacher version contain two subscales: internalizing problems (e.g., too fearful and anxious) and externalizing problems (e.g., argues a lot). Cronbach's alphas for the mother version in the current sample were .81 for internalizing and .88 for externalizing. For the teacher version, Cronbach's alphas were .90 for internalizing and .95 for externalizing in the current sample. For both subscales as well as for the total problem score, raw scores were converted into standard T-scores, based on normative data for children of the same age.

Details about all data collection procedures are documented in manuals of operation of the study, which can be found at *http://public.rti.org/secc*.

RESULTS

Longitudinal Analyses of Child Care and Family Characteristics

Preliminary analyses summarized our longitudinal assessment of the children's child care experiences and family context. Using hierarchical linear model (HLM) analyses (Bryk & Raudenbush, 1987), two individual growth curve parameters were retained for subsequent analysis: the intercept (general tendency) of hours/week that nonmaternal care was used during the 16 intervals from 1 month through 4½ years and the linear slope of reported hours/week over time. Overall, at 24 months children experienced almost 25 hours of care per week ($M = 26.25$ hours/week; $SD = 17.4$) and showed modest increases in child care hours over time ($M = 1.90$ hours/week, $SD = 4.5$). In addition, two analysis variables representing the type of care were computed: the proportion of epochs that the child was in center care (% center care) and the proportion of epochs that the child was in a child care home (% child care home).

Observations of caregiver sensitivity also were summarized using HLM to describe longitudinal patterns of change. Analyses yielded significant individual differences in the positive caregiving quality intercept ($z = 10.21$, $p < .001$) and positive caregiving linear slope ($z = 5.68$, $p < .001$). On average, children experienced fair quality care ($M = 2.82$, $SD = .23$), with child care providers showing slightly more sensitivity to children when they were younger ($M = -.029$, $SD = .013$).

In addition, HLM analyses were used to summarize longitudinal assessments of maternal depression and parenting. An unconditional linear growth curve was fit to the repeated assessments of maternal depression. There were systematic individual differences in the intercept ($z = 20.9$, $p < .001$) and linear change over time ($z = 6.8$, $p < .001$). On average, mothers reported few symptoms overall (intercept $M = 9.35$, se = .18, $p < .0001$) and very modest gains over time ($M = .19$ symptoms per year, $se = .06$, $p < .003$). An unconditional linear model also was fit to the repeated assessments of parenting. Significant individual differences emerged in both the overall level ($z = 22.9$, $p < .001$) and linear change over time ($z = 8.2$, $p < .001$). The parenting variable was created as the mean of standardized variables, so it is not surprising that the group growth curve was characterized by intercepts and slopes that did not significantly vary from zero. Nevertheless, the substantial individual differences in the intercepts and slopes made these summary measures interesting as covariates in subsequent analyses. Finally, income was summarized as the mean income-to-needs ratio and partner status was summarized as the proportion of time the mother reported a partner in the household from the 6–54 assessments.

Is Child Functioning Associated with Child Care Quantity, Quality, and Type?

The primary analyses involved multivariate linear regression models that tested if child functioning at 4½ years varied as a function of child care quantity, quality, and type. Two quantity indicators (individual intercept and slope of reported hours per week in care from 3 months to 4½ years), two quality indicators (individual intercept and slope of positive caregiving ratings), and two type indicators (proportion of 3–4-month epochs in which children attended centers and proportion of epochs in which children were cared for in child care homes) were tested along with the following control variables: child sex (1 = male); child ethnicity (coded African American, European American, Hispanic American, and other); proportion of epochs in which a husband or partner was in the household; maternal education; average income-to-needs, maternal depression intercept and slope; and parenting quality intercept and slope.

Interactions between the child care parameters and each of the controls were tested to determine if child care effects were moderated by family characteristics. Interactions between the three child care parameters were tested to determine if these factors acted synergistically. These tests of interactions also served as tests of homogeneity of regression. None of these interactions was significant, so they are not presented or discussed further.

Tables 26.1 and 26.2 show results of the primary analyses. The second through fourth rows in Table 26.1 present the explained variance (R^2) for the models as a whole, the block of child care predictors, and the block of variables composed of the child and family controls. Also presented in this table are the multivariate test statistics for the child care and control blocks. The next six rows list the test statistics for the multivariate test and the standardized regression coefficients for each child care predictor, and the final rows list the standardized regression coefficients for each one-degree-of-freedom covariate and the p-value level for multiple-degree-of-freedom covariates.

Table 26.2 shows a complementary measure of association, the structural coefficients (Courville & Thompson, 2001). This measure reflects the relative predictive power of each predictor included in the analysis model without adjusting for shared variance among the predictors. The structural

TABLE 26.1. Prediction of Child Functioning at 4½ Years from Child Care Quantity, Quality, and Type: Tests and Standardized Coefficients (β)

| | Cognitive outcome (n = 737) | | | | Social Outcomes | | | | | |
| | | | | | Caregiver report (n = 533) | | | Mother report (n = 748) | | |
Predictor	MANOVA	Acad.	Lang.	Mem.	MANOVA	Skills	Prob.	MANOVA	Skills	Prob.
	F	R^2	R^2	R^2	F	R^2	R^2	F	R^2	R^2
Model fit										
Overall model	1.84*	.39***	.44***	.22***		.13***	.14***	.20	.18***	.17***
Child care block	11.39***	.02*	.01*	.01	2.95***	.02	.04***		.00	.00
Covariate block		.23***	.25***	.11***	3.02***	.07***	.07***	10.34***	.15***	.16***
	F	β	β	β	F	β	β	F	β	β
Child care										
Quantity intercept	1.48	.03	−.02	−.05	5.78**	−.07	.16**	.05	−.01	.01
Quantity slope	0.53	.03	−.01	−.00	2.40	−.08	.09*	.02	−.00	.01
Quality intercept	4.16**	.16***	.10*	.08	2.73	.11	−.00	.44	.01	.04
Quality slope	3.04*	.10*	.05	−.03	1.64	.09	−.01	.79	.03	.04
% Child care home	1.71	−.01	.06	.05	0.28	.04	−.02	.09	−.02	.01
% Centers	3.98**	.05	.11**	.11*	3.45*	.02	.11	.02	.00	−.01
	β	β	β	β	β	β	β	β	β	β
Covariates										
Site										
Male		−.06*	−.11***	.03		−.11**	.01		.17***	−.03
Ethnicity										
Maternal education		.16***	.09*	.06		.04	−.10		−.05	−.02
Partnered		−.08*	−.06	−.08*		.03	−.08		−.10*	.02
Income		.01	.07	.06		−.00	.07		.01	.04
Parenting intercept		.40***	.37***	.28***		.16*	−.16*		.28***	−.09
Parenting slope		.12***	.15***	.06		.08	−.14**		.06	−.15***
Depression intercept		.04	.00	−.06		−.06	−.03		−.20***	.33***
Depression slope		−.06	−.07*	−.08*		−.07	.04		−.02	.08*

Note. Acad., preacademic skills; Lang., language competence; Mem., memory; Skills, social skills; Prob., behavior problems.
*p < .05; **p < .01; ***p < .001.

384

TABLE 26.2. Prediction of Child Functioning at 4½ Years from Child Care Quantity, Quality, and Type: Structural Coefficients (r_s)

Predictor	Cognitive outcome (r_s)			Caregiver report on social outcome (r_s)		Mother report on social outcome (r_s)	
	Acad.	Lang.	Mem.	Skills	Prob.	Skills	Prob.
Child care							
Quantity intercept	.02	.01	−.05	−.19	.47	−.06	−.02
Quantity slope	−.13	−.18	−.14	−.30	.27	−.05	.02
Quality intercept	.43	.36	.45	.39	−.32	.18	−.08
Quality slope	−.13	−.11	−.27	−.05	.09	.00	.02
% Child care home	−.03	.02	−.04	.03	−.04	−.06	.00
% Centers	.18	.22	.23	−.09	.37	.08	−.03
Covariates[a]							
Male	−.14	−.20	.04	−.31	.00	.40	−.06
Maternal education	.69	.63	.60	.48	−.44	.35	−.35
Partnered	.25	.32	.24	.35	−.40	.19	−.21
Income	.51	.55	.54	.38	−.19	.33	−.23
Parenting intercept	.86	.84	.80	.66	−.56	.71	−.50
Parenting slope	.29	.31	.23	.36	−.43	.25	−.42
Depression intercept	−.27	−.30	−.38	−.39	.32	−.66	.86
Depression slope	−.16	−.17	−.25	−.24	.12	−.05	.24

Note. $r_s = r_{YX1}$, where r_{YX1} is the correlation coefficient for predictor X_1 and outcome Y and R_J is the square root of R^2 of the model.
Acad., preacademic skills; Lang., language competence; Mem., memory; Skills, social skills; Prob., behavior problems.
[a] Site and ethnicity were also included in the model, but are not listed because they are categorical predictors.

coefficient is computed as the zero-order correlation between a predictor and outcome measure divided by the multiple correlation. These coefficients are interpreted within the context of a given model (i.e., within each column in Table 26.2) by identifying the coefficients that are largest as the best unconditional predictors if the overall model provides significant prediction of the outcome. Examination of both the structural and standardized coefficients provides information about both the degree that a predictor is associated with the outcome and provides unique prediction.

Cognitive Outcomes

Three cognitive outcomes (preacademic skills, language, short-term memory) were considered. As shown in the first four columns of Table 26.1, the multivariate analysis indicated that cognitive functioning was significantly associated with child care, $F(18, 2008) = 1.80$, $p = .02$, and specifically with the quality intercept, $F(3, 710) = 4.13$, $p = .006$, the quality slope, $F(3, 710) = 2.92$, $p = .03$, and the proportion of center-care epochs,

$F(3, 710) = 3.97, p = .008$. Children who attended higher-quality child care scored higher on tests of preacademic skills and language than children who attended lower-quality child care. Children whose child care increased in quality over time had better preacademic skills, whereas preacademic skills were lower when child care decreased in quality over time. Children who had more center experience displayed better language skills and better performance on the memory test than did children with less center-type experience.

The structural coefficients in Table 26.2 show a similar pattern of results. These unconditional measures of association indicate that family characteristics such as parenting, maternal education, and income show the strongest association with the cognitive outcomes but that overall quality of child care (quality intercept) was a moderately strong predictor of these outcomes. In contrast, amount of center care was a stronger predictor in the regression model than when considered alone.

Social Outcomes

Four aspects of social functioning (social skills and behavior problems reported by mothers; social skills and behavior problems reported by caregivers) were considered in relation to child care quantity, quality, and type using multivariate hierarchical regression models that paralleled those used to predict cognitive functioning. Separate analyses were conducted for reports by mothers and caregivers because these reports were only minimally related. The correlation between maternal and caregiver reports of behavior problems was $r = .23, p < .001$, and the correlation between maternal and caregiver reports of social skills was $r = .21, p < .001$.

As shown in Table 26.1, caregiver reports of social behavior were significantly related to child care, $F(12, 1014) = 2.90, p < .001$, and specifically to overall quantity of care (individual intercept) from 3 months to 4½ years, $F(2, 507) = 5.64, p = .004$, and proportion of epochs of center care, $F(2, 507) = 3.38, p = .035$. The structural coefficients shown in Table 26.2 reveal a similar pattern of associations, although the various family measures not surprisingly show stronger associations with the structural coefficients than the standardized coefficients due to their shared variance. Both sets of coefficients indicated that children with more child care hours per week (quantity intercept) had more problem behaviors according to their caregivers than did children with fewer child care hours. Although the multivariate test indicated that proportion of center-care epochs was significantly related to caregivers reports of social outcomes and the structural coefficients identify amount of center care as a moderately strong predictor of behavior problems, the individuals betas associated with center care were not significant for either social skills or behavior problems. Similarly, quality of care shows a moderate association with the unadjusted structural coefficients but not with the adjusted standardized coefficients. Thus, among the child care variables, only quantity of care provides significant prediction when all covariates are considered but both type and quality of care are associated before adjusting for the extensive set of family characteristics.

To address the concern that the difference in caregiver reports was an artifact of differential familiarity with the study child, the length of time that the caregiver provided care to the child was added in a final analysis of the caregiver's ratings of social behaviors. Caregiver ratings of problem behaviors continued to be significantly related to overall amount of time the child spent in nonmaternal care (beta = .13, p < .05) and became significantly related to amount of center care that the child experienced (beta = .14, p < .05).

Analyses with Additional Covariates

To address the concern that selection factors were not adequately controlled for, analyses were reconducted with an expanded list of covariates consisting of the maternal rating of child temperament, maternal psychological adjustment, maternal report of social support, maternal separation anxiety, and maternal beliefs about the benefits of employment. These covariates were added to the nine child and family predictors in the previous model. The same significant child care findings were obtained with the expanded list of covariates, suggesting that the obtained findings were not an artifact of inadequate controls for family characteristics.

Analyses of the "Whole" Sample

Additional multivariate regressions were then conducted for all the children in the sample, including children without any nonmaternal care. In these additional analyses, two quantity indicators (hours intercept and slope) and two type indicators (proportion of epochs of center care and proportion of epochs of child care homes) were used as predictors. Child care quality was not included as a predictor in these analyses, because quality could not be assessed for children who were not in child care. Very similar findings regarding quantity and type of child care to those previously described were obtained in these follow-up analyses. Consequently, the quantity and type findings excluding quality controls are not presented or discussed further. They are available upon request from the authors.

How Large Are the Effects of Child Care Quantity, Quality, and Type?

Follow-up analyses were then conducted in order to evaluate the magnitude of the statistically significant child care effects reported earlier. Following the recommendation of McCartney and Rosenthal (2000), the obtained effects were evaluated in relation to two other well-established predictors of child outcomes—parenting quality and poverty. Effect sizes were computed as the difference between the adjusted means for high and low groups divided by the pooled standard deviation.

For these analyses, continuous variables were transformed to categorical ones so that differences between the mean scores for high- and low-risk groups could be compared. Child care quantity was categorized as < 10 hours/week, 10–29 hours/week, or 30+ hours/week using the estimated individual intercepts from the HLM analysis of quantity up to 54 months. Child care quality was categorized as the bottom, middle, and top third of the distribution of the estimated intercept from the HLM analysis of quality ratings from 6 to 54 months. Type of care variables (center and child care home) were categorized as 0 epochs, 1–32% of epochs, and 33%+ of epochs. Quality of parenting was categorized as the bottom, middle, and top third of the distribution of the estimated intercept from the HLM analysis of parenting quality from 6 to 54 months. Family income was categorized as poverty if the average income-to-needs ratio was 2.0 or lower (n = 301, 27.8% of sample). For analytic purposes, the same proportion of families was categorized as high income (n = 301, 27.8%). These families had income-to-needs ratios in excess of 4.43. "Middle-income" was categorized as income-to-needs ratios that were greater than 2.0 but less than 4.43.

Two sets of child care effect sizes were estimated, based on the number of family selection factors included in the analyses. The first analysis estimated effect sizes for parenting and child care variables and included all other variables as covariates as the regression analyses reported previously. The second analysis estimated effect sizes for poverty and child care variables and included fewer covariates. This approach was adopted because poverty is a widely recognized risk factor for child development and, therefore, an intuitively appealing comparison. However, the full array of family selection factors could not be used as controls in this analysis because inclusion of these factors eliminated poverty as a risk factor. This occurred because poverty is linked to child development through its negative association with parental beliefs and practices (McLoyd, 1998).

Quantity Effects

The analysis of covariance (ANCOVA) that included the full set of child care, child, and family covariates indicated that children who averaged 30 or more hours of child care per week during the first 4½ years had more problem behaviors according to their caregivers than did children who averaged less than 10 hours of care per week (effect size, d = .38). The high-quantity group scored, on average, 3.7 points higher on the behavior problem scale than the low-quantity group. In comparison, children who experienced parenting quality in the bottom tercile scored 2.2 points higher than did children in the top tercile (d = .23). The quantity effect size was 165% (i.e., .38/.23) as large as the parenting effect size.

The ANCOVA that included the more limited set of covariates indicated that caregivers reported more problem behaviors among children who had been in care for more than 30 hours per week than children with little or no early child care. The high-quantity group scored, on average, 4.2 points higher on the behavior problem scale than the low-quantity group (d = .43). In comparison, children in the poverty group scored 4.5 points higher than did children in the high-income group (d = .47). The quantity effect size was 91% as large as the poverty effect size.

Quality Effects

Children whose child care was in the highest tercile of quality obtained higher scores on tests of preacademic skills and language than children whose child care was in the bottom tercile. The ANCOVA that included the full set of family and child covariates indicated that the adjusted mean scores for children in higher quality care were 2.2 points (d = .24) higher on preacademic skills and 2.3 points (d = .15) higher on language skills than the scores for children in the low-quality tercile. In comparison, the adjusted means for children receiving high-quality parenting were 8.3 points (d = .88) higher on preacademic skills and 13.7 points (d = .87) higher on language skills than for children receiving low-quality parenting group. The effect sizes for child care quality were 27% and 17%, respectively, as large as the effect associated with parenting quality and poverty.

The ANCOVA that included the more limited set of covariates yielded differences of 3.8 points (d = .39) for preacademic skills and 4.8 points (d = .29) for language for children in high- and low-quality child care. In comparison, the adjusted means for children from the poverty group were 8.3 points (d = .83) lower on preacademic skills and 15.6 points (d = .95) lower on language skills than for children from high-income families. The effect sizes for child care quality were 47% and 31%, respectively, as large as the effect size for parenting quality and poverty.

Type Effects

The analysis with the full set of family and child covariates yielded differences between children who were in center care for at least one-third of the epochs versus children with no center experience: a difference of 4.4 points (d = .28) on language performance and 5.5 (d = .33) on memory. In comparison, the difference in adjusted means between children who received high- and low-quality parenting was 13.7 (d = .87) on language and 10.6 (d = .64) on memory. Center effect sizes comprised 32% and 52% of the parenting quality in these analyses.

Differences in adjusted means with the more limited set of covariates were 6.6 points for language performance (d = .41) and 7.1 points for memory performance (d = .41) for children with extensive versus no center-type experience. The comparable effects for poverty were 15.6 points (d = .95) for language and 9.6 points (d = .56) for memory. The center effect sizes were from 43% and 73% as large as poverty effect sizes in these analyses.

CONCLUSION

Results from the current analyses indicate that early child care is associated with both developmental risks and developmental benefits for children's functioning prior to school entry, even after controlling for a host of factors including gender, ethnicity, family socioeconomic status, maternal psychological adjustment, and parenting quality. The risk is that more hours in child care across the first 4½ years of life is related to elevated levels of problem behavior at 4½ years. The benefit is that higher-quality child care, quality that improves over time, and more experience in centers predicts better performance on measures of cognitive and linguistic functioning.

Importantly, each of these aspects of child care (quantity, quality, and type) was associated with child functioning when other aspects of child care were controlled. Higher-quality child care predicted better preacademic skills and language, regardless of hours and type of care. Larger amounts of child care were associated with behavior problems, even after quality of care was controlled. Center experience was a unique predictor of both language and memory performance. These child care findings at 4½ years are consistent with earlier findings involving this same sample, even though different measures of cognitive, language, and social functioning were used with younger children. The consistency of the earlier findings and the 4½-year results suggest robust associations, at least across the preschool period. Also, consistent with our prior findings when children were ages 2 and 3 years, effects associated with hours of care and with type of care were maintained when analyses were conducted for all of the children in the sample, including those with zero hours.

In the current analyses, amount of child care was related to caregiver but not mother report of behavior problems. This difference may well reflect the fact that mothers and caregivers observed the children in different contexts, one at home where the number of other people is rather limited (and have been known for a long time) and the other where there can be many children and adults (who may not be highly familiar). The modest correlations between maternal and caregiver report of the children's social behaviors obtained in the current study and in other research (Ablow et al., 1999) are consistent with the argument that mothers and caregivers offer different perspectives of child functioning.

To evaluate the practical importance of the 4½-year findings, we compared the effect sizes that were associated with child care with effects associated with two other well-recognized influences on young children's development: parenting quality and poverty. The obtained quantity effects on caregivers' reports of child behavior problems were larger than the effects on behavior problems that were associated with parenting ($d = .38$ vs. .23) and almost as large as the effects associated with poverty ($d = .43$ vs. .47). Effects of child care quality on children's preacademic skills and language ($d = .39$ and .29, respectively) and effects of center type experience on language and memory (d = .28 and .33) were comparable in size to quantity effects on behavior problems but smaller than effects of parenting on these cognitive and linguistic outcomes. Using these factors as benchmarks, we conclude that the detected child care effects were meaningful.

The results of the current study also underscored the importance of parenting and the home environment for young children. Children who received higher-quality parenting as indicated by more sensitive, stimulating, and supportive maternal behavior at home and in semistructured play displayed higher preacademic skills, better language skills, more social skills, and fewer behavior problems than did children who received lower-quality parenting. The effects associated with parenting and preacademic skills (d = .88) and language (d = .87), which include both shared genes and environmental influences, were among the largest effects obtained in the current study.

Although significant child care and parenting effects were obtained in this study, it is important to acknowledge that both may be underestimated. Our sampling plan excluded some high-risk families (adolescent mothers, non-English speakers, and those who lived in very dangerous neighborhoods) and children at biological risk such as children of low birthweight. It seems likely that these exclusions truncated the range in scores, resulting in lower effect sizes for parenting and poverty. It seems less likely that we have overestimated the effects associated with child care because of a failure to control adequately for family selection factors. Results were essentially the same when the additional covariates were included. We had anticipated that high-quality child care and center-based care would be most advantageous for children growing up in less advantageous circumstances, such as lower family income, maternal depression, and lower-quality parenting. We failed, however, to detect statistically significant child care and family interactions of this sort. We had anticipated that effects of child care quality would be magnified by child care hours. We failed, however, to detect dosage effects or other interactions between child care parameters. In future research, we plan to extend consideration of effects of early child care and family experiences to child developmental outcomes during elementary school. It remains to be determined whether the apparent consequences of child care remain, dissipate, or grow in time, and whether early schooling maintains or deflects developmental trajectories set in motion during the infant, toddler, and preschool years.

VII

Effects of Families on the Development of Children Who Are in Child Care

Our interest in families in a study of child care grows out of recent evidence that supports an ecological/systems model of growth and development. According to this model, the child's genetic endowment is expressed through interaction with an environment composed of intersecting influences, including the physical setting; individuals with whom the child interacts; and social relationships, institutions, and culture. The family system serves as a developmental nexus by sharing with its children genetic, environmental, cultural, and institutional influences and by transmitting these to them for most of the first two decades of their lives.

Extensive evidence shows that mothers, fathers, and other family members influence both cognitive and social development during early childhood. The sensitivity and responsiveness of the mother and the sense of trust these qualities build in the child are at the heart of emotional security and the acquisition of social and cognitive skills. Most modern theories about early child development stress that, through interaction with their mothers and fathers, infants come to know these individuals and to trust them as sources of emotional security and knowledge about the world.

Results reported in this book consistently support these notions regardless of any impact that nonmaternal child care may have on children's development. Most of this evidence, however, concerns the developmental significance of mother–child interaction and relationships; fathers have rarely been mentioned.

Consequently, in Chapter 27, we compensate for this shortcoming and present data concerning fathers' caregiving roles and the quality of their interactions with their children. Results reveal that fathering is constrained both by family circumstances and by the relationship between the father and the mother. For example, fathers are more involved in caregiving when they work fewer hours and mothers work more hours as compared to when things are the other way around. Fathers are more involved in caregiving when fathers and mothers are younger rather than older, when the personalities of the fathers are positive rather than negative, and when mothers report more rather than less intimacy between themselves and their husbands. Paternal sensitivity during interaction with the children is more characteristic of men with more modern childrearing beliefs than among men with more conservative beliefs, among men who report more rather than lesser marital intimacy, and men who are younger rather than older. And, finally, fathers are more involved with their sons than with their daughters.

Cultural beliefs in the United States and elsewhere specify that families have primary responsibilities for rearing the young. Some argue that when an infant or toddler is enrolled in child care, the family relinquishes some of this responsibility even though the family selects the child care provider and requires that certain standards of quality care be met. Because child care is regulated and sometimes subsidized by the state or the community, this argument goes, the family inevitably surrenders some of its unique responsibility to an outside institution whose childrearing values and goals may not be consistent with the family's own. The second chapter in this section asks whether family effects on child development are, in fact, different for children in child care than for children in exclusive maternal care. Family factors, including demographic characteristics, the mothers' sense of well-being, maternal attitudes, mothering behaviors, and the nature of the mother–child relationship, were used to predict the cognitive, language, school readiness, social competence, and problem behaviors of the children at 24 and 36 months of age. Results provide no evidence that these family variables predicted outcomes differently for the two groups of children. However, follow-up exploratory analyses described in Chapter 28 revealed a few instances of differential prediction but these need confirmation by other investigators.

In the final chapter of this section, we summarize our findings about the effects of family characteristics on the development of children who are in child care. Generally, child care effects on children's development were smaller than family effects. In some analyses, family effects were evident when child care effects were not. Maternal characteristics and behaviors were among the strongest family predictors of children's cognitive and social developmental outcomes.

27

Factors Associated with Fathers' Caregiving Activities and Sensitivity with Young Children

NICHD Early Child Care Research Network

In the last two decades, one of the major themes in child developmental research has been the "discovery" of the father. After abundant research on the importance of maternal sensitivity for the development of children, there is a realization that paternal sensitivity to the child's needs also is important (Lamb, 1997; Parke, 1996). Moreover, there is an appreciation that fathers often provide significant caregiving for their children, and that many fathers provide substantial hours of care for children while mothers work (Hofferth, Brayfield, Deich, & Holcomb, 1991). Scholarship on fathering has coalesced around the idea that fathering is multifaceted and multidetermined, that fathering tends to be more sensitive to contextual factors than mothering, and that future inquiry on fathers is likely to be more productive if viewed from the frame of responsible or generative fathering rather than from notions that accentuate paternal absence or inadequate parenting behaviors. There has been a spate of efforts to synthesize research on fathering, to explicate the nature of paternal involvement, and to offer conceptual models aimed at identifying the key determinants of fathering (cf. Doherty, Kouneski, & Erickson, 1998; Lamb, 1997; Parke, 1996).

From *Journal of Family Psychology*, 2000, Vol. 14, pp. 200–219. Copyright 2000 by the American Psychological Association. Reprinted by permission.

The conceptual model offered by Doherty and colleagues (1998) is, in most respects, representative and inclusive. It includes five major components: child characteristics, including gender, temperament, and age; father characteristics, including his employment, beliefs, and well-being; mother characteristics including her employment, beliefs, and well-being; coparental relationships, including marital support and intimacy; and contextual or sociodemographic characteristics, including income and ethnicity. In this chapter we examine elements of each of these components as they relate to two distinct aspects of fathers' parenting: engagement in caregiving activities and the quality (specifically, sensitivity) of fathers' interactions with their children.

First, we asked if child characteristics, sociodemographic factors, and father characteristics predict fathers' caregiving activities and sensitivity during interactions, and if the addition of mother characteristics improves the prediction of paternal behavior over and above the other factors. Second, we asked if associations between the predictor variables (child characteristics, sociodemographic factors, and father characteristics) and paternal behavior are moderated by maternal employment—that is, if associations differ for families in which mothers are not employed, employed part time, or employed full time.

We expected greater father involvement with sons as opposed to daughters and with firstborn children. We expected that the father's own adjustment and attitudes would relate to caregiving involvement and sensitivity in that fathers who are better adjusted and have less traditional beliefs would be more highly involved in the care of their young children and more sensitive in that care. We expected fathers who are employed for more hours to be less engaged in caregiving activities. More positive perceptions of the marriage were expected to predict more caregiving by fathers and greater sensitivity in play because (we suspect that) couples who perceive their marriage as more supportive are more likely to work as a team with greater similarity in their roles and responsibilities within the family. Finally, we hypothesized that fathers would be more involved in caregiving activities when mothers are employed for more hours and they have more positive views about maternal employment.

METHOD

Participants

Chapter 1 provides a detailed description of the participants. Six of the research sites (Arkansas, California, Kansas, Pittsburgh, North Carolina, & Wisconsin) obtained funding to collect additional information directly from fathers. After infants and mothers were enrolled in the study, households at these sites were invited to participate in the father protocol if a husband or partner was in residence (n = 816). In most cases, the men were married to the infants' mothers (87.7%). Of the eligible households, 585 agreed to participate in at least one data collection period. When children were 6 and 36 months old, a subsample of fathers at three sites (Kansas, North Carolina, & Wisconsin) participated in the observational component of the father protocol (n = 278 at 6 months and n = 184 at 36 months).

Table 27.1 shows the demographic characteristics of families who participated in the interview portion of the father protocol, those who participated in the observational component of the father protocol, and eligible households who did not participate in the father protocol. White, non-Hispanic fathers were more likely than black, non-Hispanic fathers to participate in the interview protocol, $\chi^2(3, n = 812) = 74.20, p < .001$, and the observational protocol at 6 and 36 months, $\chi^2(3, n = 509) = 12.03, p < .007$, and $\chi^2(3, n = 415) = 11.83, p < .008$, respectively. Fathers who had received at least a college degree were more likely to participate in interviews, $\chi^2(4, n = 812) = 25.04, p < .001$, and observations at 6 months, $\chi^2(4, n = 509) = 31.88, p < .001$, and at 36 months, $\chi^2(4, n = 415) = 25.13, p < .001$, than were fathers with a high school diploma or less. There were no significant differences between fathers who participated in the observational component of the study and fathers who participated only in the interview component of the study in terms of child gender, father ethnicity, or father education.

TABLE 27.1. Demographic Characteristics of the Father Sample and the Sample of Eligible Families

	Participants				Eligible nonparticipants[c]	
	Interview sample[a]		Observed sample[b]			
Variable	n	%	n	%	n	%
Child sex						
Male	299	51	143	51	81	58
Female	286	49	135	49	60	43
Paternal ethnicity						
White, non-Hispanic	506	87	247	89	108	77
Black, non-Hispanic	44	8	16	6	19	14
Hispanic	24	4	10	4	7	5
Other	10	2	5	2	7	5
Paternal education						
Less than 12 years	45	8	18	7	16	11
High school or GED	110	19	43	16	38	27
Some college	197	34	95	34	46	33
Bachelor's degree	125	22	60	22	21	15
Postgraduate work	97	17	60	22	20	14

[a]n = 585; [b]n = 278; [c] n = 231.

Overview of Data Collection Procedures

During home visits, fathers completed questionnaires concerning their personality, attitudes, beliefs, relationship with their partner, and involvement in caregiving activities. Thirty-seven percent of the fathers were interviewed at four visits, 34% at three visits, 15% at two visits, and 14% at one visit. At 6 and 36 months, a subset of fathers was videotaped playing with their child during 15-minute semistructured play procedures. During separate home visits, mothers were interviewed and completed questionnaires pertaining to their personality, attitudes, beliefs, family demographics, financial resources, child temperament, and their relationship with their partner. Mothers also were interviewed by phone every 3 months about their employment hours and their husband or partner's employment hours.

Measures of Fathers' Parenting

Caregiving Activities

When children were 6, 15, 24, and 36 months of age, fathers completed questionnaires describing their responsibilities for caregiving activities (Glysch & Vandell, 1992). The 15 items included bathing the child, feeding the child, diapering the child, dressing the child, putting the child to bed, attending to the child at night, playing with the child, reading to the child, buying clothes or toys for the child, taking the child to day care, taking the child to the doctor, and taking the child on outings. Some of these items changed for the infant, toddler, and preschool assessments, reflecting different developmental needs. A total score was calculated by averaging the 5-point ratings (1 = partner's job, 3 = we share equally, 5 = my job). A higher score indicated greater paternal responsibility for caregiving activities. Cronbach's alphas ranged from .72 to .80. Paternal reports of caregiving responsibilities over time were moderately correlated ($r = .54$ to .73, mean $r = .65$).

Observed Father Sensitivity

Fathers' sensitivity was assessed during 15-minute videotaped observations of father–child play. When children were 6 months old, fathers were asked to play with them for 7 minutes with any toy or object available in the home (or none at all). Then, they were asked to play for 8 minutes with a standard set of toys provided by an examiner (rattles, activity center, ball, rolling toy, book, and stuffed animal). At 36 months, fathers and children were provided with three numbered containers. A set of washable markers, stencils, and paper was in the first container, a set of dress-up clothes and a cash register was in the second, and a set of Duplo blocks with a picture of a model was in the third container. Fathers were instructed that the child play with the toys in all three containers and do so in the order specified (Vandell,

1979). Videotapes were coded at a single location by observers who knew nothing about the families' child care, parents' employment, or other family circumstances.

At 6 months, three aspects of father sensitivity were rated using 4-point scales: (1) father's responsivity to infant signals and needs, with high scores indicating consistent and appropriate responsiveness to the infant's social gestures, needs, moods, and interests; (2) positive regard, indicating the quality and quantity of positive feelings shown to the infant through facial, vocal, and physical expressions of affection; and (3) intrusiveness, the degree to which the father attempted to control the interaction, allowing the child little self-direction.

The global ratings were made after viewing the entire videotaped inter-action while taking notes on relevant behavior throughout the interaction. Coders were trained extensively and established good reliability on the coding of the larger National Institute of Child Health and Human Develop-ment (NICHD) study's videotaped mother–infant interactions prior to cod-ing the father–child interaction videotapes. Intercoder agreement on the 6-month father–child interactions on the basis of 27 of the cases (10% of the sample observed) was calculated as the intraclass correlation. Interrater agreement was .83, .82, and .86 for responsivity, positive regard, and intru-siveness, respectively. A paternal sensitivity composite score was created by averaging the individual scales after intrusiveness was reflected. Cronbach's alpha for the composite was .71.

At 36 months, coders rated three aspects of the father's sensitivity—supportive presence, respect for the child's autonomy, and hostility toward the child—using 7-point rating scales. Supportive presence was analogous to the 6-month responsivity rating scale; high scores indicated emotional sup-port, encouragement, and positive emotional regard. Hostility reflected the father's expression of anger, discounting, or rejection of the child. Respect for the child's autonomy (analogous to a reversed score of intrusiveness) was shown in acknowledging the child's intentions and displaying respect for the child's individuality. Low scores on this scale were given when the father was highly intrusive and controlling.

Interrater agreement on the father–child tapes on the basis of 38 (30%) of the 36-month cases was calculated using Winer's (1971) technique. Agree-ment was .90, .83, and .89 for the ratings of supportiveness, respect for autonomy, and hostility, respectively. The three ratings were averaged, after reversing hostility, to create a paternal sensitivity composite score. Cronbach's alpha for the composite score was .75.

The 6-month and 36-month sensitivity composites were not signifi-cantly correlated ($r = .15$). In contrast, the sensitivity composite ratings for mother–child interaction, using the same observation procedures and rat-ing scales, were moderately stable from 6 to 36 months ($r = .42$; see NICHD Early Child Care Research Network, 1999a).

Predictor Variables

Child Characteristics

At the 6-month home visit, mothers completed a modified Infant Temperament Questionnaire (Carey & McDevitt, 1978). Mothers rated their infants
on 55 items, using a 6-point response scale. The composite measure, difficult temperament, was created by calculating the mean of the nonmissing
items with a higher score reflecting a more "difficult" temperament.
Cronbach's alpha for the composite score was .81. Child gender and birth
order (scored here as firstborn yes–no) were reported by the mothers at the
1-month interview.

Sociodemographic Factors

Total family income, income from the father, and income from the mother
were reported by mothers at 6, 15, 24, and 36 months. Mothers reported
the race and ethnicity of the infants' fathers at the 1-month interview.

Father and Mother Characteristics

During telephone interviews conducted every 3 months, mothers reported
their own employment hours and their husband–partner's employment
hours. Average number of hours per week in all jobs was considered beginning at 3 months postpartum. Fathers and mothers who were not employed
during a given 3-month epoch were assigned scores of 0 hours for that
epoch.

At the 1-month visit, fathers and mothers completed a 30-item questionnaire about childrearing beliefs (Schaefer & Edgerton, 1985). Responses
were scored on a 5-point scale. Higher overall scores indicate more traditional, less progressive beliefs about childrearing. Cronbach's alphas were
.87 and .84 for men and women, respectively.

At the 6-month home visit, fathers and mothers completed three subscales of the Neuroticism Extraversion Openness (NEO) Five Factor Inventory, a short form of the NEO Personality Inventory (Costa & McCrae,
1989). Five-point ratings were used to assess neuroticism (12 items), extro-
version (12 items), and agreeableness (12 items). Summing scores for extro-
version, agreeableness, and neuroticism (reversed) created a positive personality composite. The alphas for the composites for men and women were
.82 and .63, respectively.

At 6, 15, 24, and 36 months, men's and women's beliefs about the
effects of maternal employment on children were assessed using 11 items
that were rated on 6-point scales (Greenberger, Goldberg, Crawford, &
Granger, 1988). The questionnaire yielded scores reflecting beliefs about
the benefits (5 items) and costs (6 items) of maternal employment for children. Summing the benefits subscale and cost subscale (reversed) created a

composite positive beliefs score that was internally consistent. The mean alpha was .89.

At 6, 15, 24, and 36 months, mothers and fathers also completed a 6-item scale assessing marital intimacy (Schaefer & Olson, 1981). Ratings were made on 5-point Likert scales (1 = strongly disagree, 5 = strongly agree). Higher scores indicated greater marital intimacy. Cronbach's alphas ranged from .80 to .87 (M = .85).

RESULTS

Tables presenting the means and standard deviations for predictor variables and outcome variables used in the data analyses and the correlations between cumulative scores of predictor variables at 36 months can be found in the unabridged version of the article. Tables summarizing correlations are available on request.

Fathers' Caregiving Activities

Are fathers' caregiving activities predicted by individual characteristics and sociodemographic factors? Table 27.2 presents the Pearson product–moment correlations between predictor variables (child characteristics, sociodemographic factors, father characteristics, and mother characteristics) and fathers' caregiving activities at 6 months, 15 months, 24 months, and 36 months. Also summarized in Table 27.2 are the results of simultaneous hierarchical linear models (HLMs) in which individual intercepts and slopes were estimated with respect to time and time squared. For Model 1, three blocks of predictors (child characteristics, sociodemographic factors, and father attributes) were entered simultaneously as predictors of paternal caregiving responsibilities. Interactions with time and time squared were tested for each block.

The HLM analyses showed that fathers' caregiving activities were related to child characteristics, $F(3, 485) = 3.53$, $p < .02$; sociodemographic factors, $F(3, 485) = 4.77$, $p < .01$; and father characteristics, $F(6, 485) = 4.78$, $p < .001$. In terms of significant individual predictors, fathers assumed more caregiving responsibilities for sons than for daughters. Fathers also assumed more caregiving responsibilities when they contributed lower proportions of family income, were employed for fewer hours, were younger, and had more positive personalities.

Next, we asked if the addition of mother characteristics to the model further improved the prediction. As shown in Table 27.2, the block of mother predictors also was associated with fathers' caregiving activities, $F(6, 483) = 7.95$, $p < .001$. Fathers reported being more involved in caregiving activities when mothers were younger, were employed for more hours, and reported more intimate marriages.

TABLE 27.2. Factors Associated with Father Involvement in Caregiving Activities

Variable	r				Hierarchical linear model analyses			
					Model 1[e]		Model 2[e]	
	6-month[a]	15-month[b]	24-month[c]	36-month[d]	β	SE	β	SE
Intercept					2.63	.06	2.57	.06
Time (years)					.042***	$.072 \times 10^{-2}$	.044***	.001
Time squared					-.024**	$.006 \times 10^{-2}$	-.023**	.000
Child characteristics								
Gender	NS	M > F*	M > F*	M > F*	.068*	.30	.060*	.029
Difficult temperament	-.07	-.08	-.04	-.14	-.062	.038	-.063	.039
Firstborn (firstborn = 1)	NS	NS	NS	NS	.048	.031	.032	.030
Test of block					F(3, 485) = 3.53, p = .015		F(3, 483) = 2.89, p = .035	
Sociodemographic factors								
Family income	-.15*	-.19**	-.07	-.12	-.0126	.012	-.020	.12
Father's income (%)	-.18**	-.27***	-.22**	-.32***	-.030**	.009	-.010	.010
Father's ethnicity	White < not*				-.103	.055	-.009	.054
Test of block					F(3, 485) = 4.77, p = .003		F(3, 483) = 2.18, p = .089	
Father characteristics								
Age	-.15**	-.16**	-.06	-.11	-.006*	.003	.003	.004
Work hours	-.18**	-.22***	-.23***	-.28***	-.003***	.001	-.003***	.001
Personality	.07	.08	.15*	.12*	.004**	.001	.005***	.001
Childrearing beliefs	.08	.08	-.09	.03	$.010 \times 10^{-2}$	$.100 \times 10^{-2}$	.001	.001
Beliefs about maternal employment	.09	.10	.07	.16*	.005	.003	.002	.003
Report of marital intimacy	.01	.02	.11	.02	-.010	.012	-.021	.012
Test of block					F(6, 485) = 4.78, p < .0001		F(6, 483) = 5.44, p < .0001	
Mother characteristics								
Age	-.24***	-.19**	-.12	-.15			-.013**	.004
Work hours	.18**	.25***	.19**	.27***			.002***	.001
Personality	-.00	-.20***	-.07	-.03			-.003	.001
Childrearing beliefs	.04	.09	-.03	.06			-.002	.001
Beliefs about maternal employment	.10	.12*	.13**	.22**			.008	.005
Report of marital intimacy	.11	.01	.18**	.15*			.042***	.012
Test of block							F(6, 483) = 7.95, p < .0001	

Note. M, male; F, female.
[a]n = 293; [b]n = 323; [c]n = 276; [d]n = 197; [e]n = 378.
*p < .05; **p < .01; ***p < .001.

To determine whether the associations between predictor variables and caregiving activities are moderated by maternal employment we crossed each predictor in the final HLM model with maternal work hours scored as a three-level categorical variable: full time, part time, or minimal (< 10 hours per week). Overall and block tests were conducted to see if patterns of associations varied across work groups. A significant interaction between maternal work group and the father characteristics block was found, $F(12, 448) = 2.02$, $p < .02$. When we examined interactions within the father characteristics block, we found that the association between fathers' childrearing beliefs and their caregiving activities was moderated by maternal employment, $F(2, 448) = 5.74$, $p < .003$. In households in which mothers were not employed or were employed part time, fathers who endorsed traditional childrearing beliefs were significantly less likely to participate in caregiving activities. In households in which mothers were employed full time, whether the father endorsed traditional childrearing beliefs was not significantly related to whether he participated in caregiving activities.

Fathers' Sensitivity during Play Interactions

In Table 27.3 we present results of Pearson product–moment correlations of the sociodemographic and individual factors with paternal sensitivity at 6 and 36 months. Also presented in Table 27.3 are the results of multiple regression analyses. In Model 1, paternal sensitivity was regressed on three blocks of predictors: child characteristics, sociodemographic factors, and father characteristics. In Model 2, the block of maternal characteristics was added as predictors. Separate regressions were conducted at 6 and 36 months instead of HLM analyses because different families were typically observed at the two ages.

As shown in Table 27.3, neither Model 1 nor Model 2 was significant at 6 months. At 36 months, paternal sensitivity was significantly predicted by Model 1, $F(12, 117) = 3.30$, $p < .001$. Within this model, both sociodemographic factors, $F(3, 117) = 2.68$, $p < .05$, and father characteristics, $F(6, 117) = 4.53$, $p < .001$, were associated with fathers' sensitivity during play interactions. Fathers who were older, who endorsed less traditional childrearing beliefs, and who reported more marital intimacy were more sensitive during the play interactions. In addition, paternal sensitivity was higher in households in which family income was lower. The addition of maternal characteristics in Model 2 did not improve the prediction of paternal sensitivity.

To determine whether paternal sensitivity is moderated by maternal employment, the maternal block was omitted because maternal characteristics did not add significantly to the overall model and its deletion reduced the number of parameters being estimated. Each predictor was crossed with the three-level maternal work hours variable—full time, part time, or minimal (< 10 hours per week) or no employment—to estimate a separate regres-

TABLE 27.3. Factors Associated with Paternal Sensitivity during Interaction

| | r | | Multiple regression analyses (βs) | | | |
| | | | Model 1 | | Model 2 | |
Variable	6-month[a]	36-month[b]	6-month[a]	36-month[b]	6-month[a]	36-month[b]
Child characteristics						
Gender (male = 1)	NS	NS	.009	-.011	.012	-.003
Difficult temperament	-.16*	-.07	-.129	-.037	-.143	-.009
Firstborn (firstborn = 1)	NS	First > not**	-.050	.184*	-.059	.166*
Test of block			$F(3, 178) = 1.19,$ $p = .314$	$F(3, 117) = 1.79,$ $p = .154$	$F(3, 172) = 1.31,$ $p = .272$	$F(3, 111) = 1.38,$ $p = .254$
Sociodemographic factors						
Family income	-.04	-.08	-.071	-.278**	-.082	-.282**
Father's income (%)	.08	.09	.044	-.025	.068	-.006
Father's ethnicity (white = 1)	White > not**	NS	.186*	.067	.191*	.037
Test of block			$F(3, 178) = 2.25,$ $p = .084$	$F(3, 117) = 2.68,$ $p = .049*$	$F(3, 172) = 2.36,$ $p = .073$	$IF(3, 111) = 2.39,$ $p = .073$
Father characteristics						
Age	-.01	.15	-.073	.214*	-.074	.281*
Work hours	-.004	.03	-.045	.101	-.062	.056
Personality	.15*	.03	.088	-.142	.100	-.152
Childrearing beliefs	-.12	-.31***	-.069	-.331***	-.025	-.257*
Beliefs about maternal employment	-.06	-.04	-.018	-.169	-.023	-.147
Report of marital intimacy	.09	.13	.065	.217	.079	.212
Test of block			$F(6, 178) = .87,$ $p = .52$	$F(6, 117) = 4.53,$ $p < .0004***$	$F(6, 172) = .75,$ $p = .613$	$F(6, 111) = 2.61,$ $p = .02*$
Mother characteristics						
Age	.01	.08			-.025	-.146
Work hours	.0002	-.07			.042	.019
Personality	.06	.21*			-.013	.152
Childrearing beliefs	-.10	-.31***			-.110	-.190
Beliefs about maternal employment	-.05	-.10			.0002	-.053
Report of marital intimacy	.04	.10			-.058	.002
Test of block					$F(6, 172) = .364,$ $p = .90$	$F(6, 111) = 1.47,$ $p = .20$
Full model			$F(12, 178) = 1.58,$ $p < .10, R^2 = .10$	$F(12, 117) = 3.30,$ $p < .001, R^2 = .25$	$F(18, 172) = 1.51,$ $p < .31, R^2 = .11$	$F(18, 111) = 2.74,$ $p < .001, R^2 = .31$

[a]$n = 191;$ [b]$n = 130.$
*$p < .05;$ **$p < .01;$ ***$p < .001.$

404

sion model for each of these three groups. Overall and block tests were conducted to see if observed patterns of associations varied across work groups.

At 6 months, there was an interaction between the overall model and maternal employment, $F(24, 152) = 1.74$, $p = .024$. When specific block interactions were examined, a significant interaction was found between maternal employment and sociodemographic factors, $F(6, 152) = 3.17$, $p = .006$. When mothers were not employed or were employed full time, families with higher incomes had more sensitive fathers; in contrast, in households in which mothers were employed part time, families with higher incomes had less sensitive fathers.

At 36 months, the overall model was not significantly different for the three maternal employment groups (none, part time, and full time), nor were there any block × maternal employment interactions.

How Large Are the Effects on Paternal Involvement?

In order to evaluate the size of the associations with paternal involvement, partial correlations (controlling for all other factors) were conducted. Because there is not a standard effect size from HLM analysis, we computed the partial correlations from the data from each age separately. The partial correlations between caregiving activities and individual significant predictors were of similar magnitude and small by Cohen's criterion ($pr = .10$). The median partial correlation between paternal caregiving activities and father work hours was −.16 (range = −.15 to −.21). Other partial correlations with caregiving activities were .16 (range = .15 to .21) for father personality, −.14 (range = −.11 to −.15) for mother age, .16 (range = .12 to .17) for mother work hours, −.06 (range = −.02 to −.23) for mother personality, and .09 (range = .10 to .18) for mother-reported marital intimacy. The partial correlations between paternal sensitivity at 36 months and individual predictors were moderate in size according to Cohen's criterion ($pr = .30$). The partial correlations were −.25 with family income, .21 with father's age, −.31 with traditional childrearing beliefs, and .21 with father-reported marital intimacy.

DISCUSSION

Fathers' involvement in caregiving activities and their sensitivity during play interactions were predicted by different factors. In particular, fathers were more involved in caregiving when fathers worked fewer hours and mothers worked more hours, when fathers and mothers were younger, when the fathers had more positive personalities, when mothers reported greater marital intimacy, and when the child being cared for was a boy. Fathers were more sensitive during play interactions when fathers had less traditional childrearing beliefs, were older, and reported more marital intimacy.

It was notable that no single predictor accounted for more than a small fraction of the variance in either the level of paternal caregiving or paternal sensitivity. As such, our results vouchsafe Pleck's (1997) conclusion that "no single predictor exerts a predominant influence [on paternal involvement]" (p. 95). Of importance, they also extended findings pertaining to two important components of fathers' parenting: fathers' engagement in caregiving activities and their sensitivity. The complexity of these findings, together with the differences observed between the sets of findings pertaining to engagement and sensitivity, suggests that neither set may be applicable to other components of paternal involvement.

Although we had suspected that maternal employment might be a pervasive moderator of fathers' caregiving activities and sensitivity, we did not find this to be the case. In most cases, the factors associated with fathers' involvement were not fundamentally altered by mothers' employment. At the same time, it should be noted that maternal employment modified the relation between fathers' childrearing beliefs and their caregiving activities. In households in which mothers did not work or worked only part time, fathers were more likely to participate in caregiving activities if they espoused less traditional childrearing philosophies, whereas in households in which mothers were employed full time, fathers were involved in caregiving activities regardless of their childrearing beliefs. This finding suggests that mothers' full-time employment creates demands on family life that necessitate fathers assuming more caregiving responsibilities regardless of their underlying beliefs The second significant interaction involved maternal employment and family income in the prediction of paternal sensitivity at 6 months. In households in which mothers were not employed or were employed full time, fathers were observed to be more sensitive when family incomes were higher. In households in which mothers were employed part time, fathers were less sensitive when family incomes were higher. We are cautious about placing too much emphasis on this interaction, however, because the overall prediction model was not significant at 6 months and because the interaction was not replicated at 36 months.

28

Relations between Family Predictors and Child Outcomes
Are They Weaker for Children in Child Care?

NICHD Early Child Care Research Network

When considered collectively, results from quite a diverse array of inquiries (i.e., Dunham & Dunham, 1992; Egeland & Hiester, 1995; Howes, 1990; Howes, Galluzo, Hamilton, Matheson, & Rodning, 1989; Howes, Matheson, & Hamilton, 1994; Oppenheim, Sagi, & Lamb, 1988; Pierrehumbert, 1994; van IJzendoorn, Kranenburg, Zwart-Woudstra, Van Busschbach, & Lambermom, 1991) raise the prospect that one consequence of extensive early child care experience is to shift at least some of the locus of influence on children's development from the family to the child care setting and, thereby, attenuate the expected impact of traditional family factors and processes on children's development (Belsky, 1990b). There is reason to be cautious about embracing such a sweeping and provocative interpretation, however. Most of the evidence regarding differential prediction from family measures for children with and without early-care experience is based on relatively small studies, especially once samples are divided on the basis of child care experience; as a result, a few extreme cases could exert disproportionate influence on the reported results. Second, at least one investigation with a relatively large sample ($n = 150$) failed to support the hypothesis that family factors (including demographic, behavioral, and attitudinal characteristics of the parents and physical characteristics of the home) would exert

From *Developmental Psychology*, 1998, Vol. 34, pp. 1119–1128. Copyright 1998 by the American Psychological Association. Reprinted by permission.

more influence on children in full-time parental care than on children in full-time child care (Clarke-Stewart, Gruber, & Fitzgerald, 1994). Third, in many of the pertinent investigations, no tests were carried out to determine whether relations between family predictors and child outcomes differed significantly across families using versus not using early child care. In several cases, it was only evidence documenting significant relations in one group and insignificant relations in another that raised the possibility of different developmental processes operating across child care niches. Clearly, then, there is a need for a more rigorous evaluation of the hypothesis that the power of family factors in predicting developmental outcomes differ across groups of families defined in terms of early-child care experience.

Data from the ongoing National Institute of Child Health and Human Development (NICHD) Study of Early Child Care were used to determine whether a representative set of family factors differentially predicted child socioemotional and cognitive functioning at 2 and 3 years of age based on child care experience. Toward this end, we identified two homogeneous early-care groups to implement a quasi-experimental research design. One consisted of children who had received 30 hours or more per week of care by someone other than their own parents during each month of their life from the age of 4 months onward. The second, contrasting group comprised children who, during the same developmental period, never averaged more than 10 hours per week of routine care by someone other than the mother. We hypothesized that family factors would predict child functioning more strongly in the mother-care group than in the full-time, nonparental-care group.

It should be noted that in this work designed to extend prior research, we draw upon a broader set of family factors than was included in any individual inquiry that has documented differential prediction across child care niches. In fact, we incorporate in the study design three discrete sets of family predictors—one comprising demographic indicators, a second comprising measures of maternal personality and childrearing attitudes, and a third comprising observational assessments of mothering and the infant–mother relationship. The question addressed was whether, in general, family factors would predict child outcomes more strongly in the case of children reared principally by their parents than in the case of children who experienced extensive nonparental care, and, if so, what specific associations are responsible for such a finding.

METHOD

Chapter 1 provides descriptions of the participants and of the general data collection procedure. Children were assigned to contrasting child care groups on the basis of information provided by mothers across the child's first 3 years of life. Children assigned to the full-time child care group experienced 30 hours or more of routine nonparental care per week each and every month, beginning by 4 months of age and continuing until the time at which the dependent variables were assessed. These children were similar, then, to those in other studies who had experienced nonparental care in prior research. At 24 and 36 months, 187 and 157 children, respectively, met the criterion for full-time nonparental care. Children assigned to the maternal-care group never averaged, during any month, more than 10 hours per week of routine care by someone other than the mother; 169 and 137 children met the criterion for full-time maternal care at 24 and 36 months. These children's care experiences were thus similar to those in prior work without extensive nonparental-care experience.

MEASURES

Predictor Variables

Demographic Variables

Two demographic variables were included. First, income-to-needs ratio was computed from maternal interview items collected at the 1-month visit. Family income (excluding government payments) was divided by the appropriate poverty threshold (U.S. Department of Labor, Bureau of Labor Statistics; as cited in U.S. Department of Labor, Women's Bureau, 1993) for each family size. The second demographic variable was 1-month marital status, coded as not currently married or living with a partner (0) or as married or living with a partner (1).

Maternal Personality and Attitudinal Variables

Four measures of maternal personality and psychological adjustment and attitudes were included. A composite measure of the mother's personality was created using three subscales from the Neuroticism Extraversion Openness (NEO) Personality Inventory (Costa & McCrae, 1985): (1) neuroticism, reflecting the extent to which the mother was anxious, hostile, and depressed (reversed); (2) extraversion, reflecting the extent to which the mother was sociable, fun loving, and optimistic; and (3) agreeableness, reflecting the extent to which the mother was trusting, helpful, and forgiving. Thus, higher scores indicated better adjustment. Maternal depression was assessed using the Center for Epidemiological Studies–Depression scale (Radloff, 1977), which was completed by mothers at 1, 6, 15, 24, and 36 months. Scores generated on all assessments up to the time that a child outcome was assessed (i.e., 24 or 36 months) were averaged to generate the measure of maternal depression used in the analyses of child outcomes at different ages. Thus, when it came to predicting 24-month outcomes, the depression score reflected the average of 1-, 6-, 15-, and 24-month depression scores. Cronbach's alphas for these measures ranged from .85 to .90.

A measure of maternal beliefs about the benefits of maternal employment was created by summing five 6-point items from the Attitude toward Employment Questionnaire (Greenberger, Goldberg, Crawford, & Granger, 1988) administered at the 1-month visit. Cronbach's alpha was .80. Higher scores reflected the belief that maternal employment was beneficial for children. Finally, nonauthoritarian childrearing attitudes and values were assessed with a questionnaire that discriminates between "modern" and "traditional" childrearing beliefs (Schaefer & Edgarton, 1985). Higher scores reflected more progressive and less authoritarian beliefs (alpha = .6).

Mothering and Relationship Variables

Two composite measures of mothering were created, one based on maternal behavior during free-play interactions videotaped in the home (at 6 and 15 months) or the lab (at 24 and 36 months) for subsequent coding and the second based on mothering observed and rated during home visits at 6, 15, and 36 months as part of the Home Observation for Measurement of the Environment (HOME; Caldwell & Bradley, 1984).

A composite score of maternal sensitivity in play was created at each age of measurement. At 6, 15, and 24 months, it reflected the sum of three 4-point ratings: sensitivity to nondistress, positive regard, and intrusiveness (reversed). At 36 months, three different 7-point ratings were composited: supportive presence, respect for autonomy, and hostility (reversed). Intercoder reliability on the composite was .87 at 6 months, .83 at 15 months, .85 at 24 months, and .84 at 36 months. Alphas were .75, .70, .79, and .78, respectively. (See Chapter 17 for details of the interaction assessment procedures and coding.)

Factor analyses of the items on the HOME were conducted separately for each age of assessment, and the first factor from each was retained for analysis. Variables with loadings of greater than .4 on this factor were summed at each age of measurement. The resulting HOME/positive involvement factor assessed the extent to which mother was positively responsive and affectionate to the child during the visit (e.g., mother spontaneously vocalizes, hugs/kisses child, praises child, and encourages child to talk and listen). At 6 months, the positive involvement factor consisted of six items with loadings of .40 or greater that were summed (i.e., mother spontaneously vocalizes, responds verbally to child, initiates verbal interaction with home visitor, voices positive feelings for child, hugs/kisses child, watches child; alpha = .52). At 15 months, the positive involvement factor consisted of the same six high-loading items (alpha = .55), except that "praises child" replaced "watches child." At 36 months, the positive involvement factor consisted of six somewhat different items (encourages child to talk and listen, maternal voice positive in tone, talks to child two or more times, answers child's question verbally, responds to child's speech, caresses/kisses/cuddles child; alpha = .65).

A third measure of the mother–child relationship was used in predicting child outcomes in this study when those outcomes were assessed at 24 and 36 months: infant–mother attachment security. Infant–mother attachment security was assessed at 15 months using the Ainsworth & Wittig (1969) Strange Situation procedure. Videotapes of all Strange Situations were scored independently by two coders using the standard classifications of insecure–avoidant (A), secure (B), insecure–resistant (C), disorganized (D), and unclassifiable (U). Disagreements were viewed by the group of coders, and a code was assigned by consensus. Across all coder pairs, before conferencing, agreement with the five-category classification system was 83% ([kappa] = .69) and agreement for the two-category system (secure–insecure) was 86% ([κ = .70). It is the binary secure–insecure scoring that is used in this report (1 = insecure, 2 = secure). (For further information on attachment scoring, see Chapter 14.)

Child Outcomes

When children were 2 years of age, the revised Bayley Scales of Infant Development (Bayley, 1993) were administered, yielding the Mental Development Index. At 36 months, subscales of the Bracken Basic Concept Scale were administered, yielding a measure of school readiness. Children were also tested at 36 months on the Reynell Developmental Language Scales (Reynell, 1991), from which measures of expressive vocabulary and receptive vocabulary were drawn.

The Bracken Basic Concept Scale (Bracken, 1984) consists of the Diagnostic Scale and two screening tests and is designed to assess a child's knowledge of basic concepts. Children were tested on the subscales that comprise the school readiness composite of the Diagnostic Scale during the home visit at 36 months. This composite consists of five categories and 51 items assessing children's knowledge of color, letter identification, number/counting, comparisons, and shape recognition.

Designed to test verbal comprehension and expressive language skills in young children (Reynell, 1991), the Reynell Developmental Language Scales comprise two 67-item scales and yield two scores: verbal comprehension and expressive language. For the Verbal Comprehension scale, children are presented with sets of objects, and the examiner gives the child instructions such as "Where's the spoon?" or "Put all the white buttons in the cup." For the Expressive Language scale, the examiner observes the structure of the child's speech (e.g., child has one or more appropriate uses of past tense and child uses complex sentences) and asks the child to label objects, describe objects or activities observed in a picture, and define words. The internal consistency for this test is very high, with alphas in excess of .85 for each of the two subscales.

At both 24 and 36 months, maternal-report questionnaires were used to generate composite measures of behavior problems and social competence. The 99-item Child Behavior Checklist–2/3 (CBCL; Achenbach, Edelbrock, & Howell, 1987) was used to assess problem behavior. Mothers rated how characteristic each behavior was of their child over the last 2 months (0 = not true; 1 = sometimes true; 2 = very true). In this chapter, we used the two broad-band factors derived from the original standardization sample (Achenbach & Edelbrock, 1991)—externalizing (aggressive and destructive) and internalizing (social withdrawal and depression)—as well as two narrow-band factors—sleep problems and somatic problems. Research indicates that the CBCL–2/3 shows good test–retest reliability and concurrent and predictive validity; it discriminates between clinically referred and nonreferred toddlers and predicts problem scores over a 3-year period (Achenbach et al., 1987).

Social competence and disruptive behavior were assessed with the Adaptive Social Behavior Inventory (ASBI; Hogan, Scott, & Bauer, 1992). The 30 items were rated in terms of frequency of occurrence (1 = rarely, 2 = sometimes, 3 = almost always). The express scale (13 items) taps sociability and empathy, and the comply scale (10 items) measures prosocial engagement and cooperation. The disrupt scale (7 items) assesses resistant and agonistic behavior. In the NICHD sample, the 24/36-month coefficient alphas for these scales were .77/.76 for express, .82/.82 for comply, and .60/.62 for disrupt.

When the aforementioned subscales from the CBCL and ASBI were factored (separately at 24 and 36 months) in an analysis that included many measures of social and emotional functioning, two clear factors emerged at each age reflecting mother-reported problem behavior and social competence (Chapter 19). The problem behavior factor included high loadings (> .65) on all four of the CBCL scales and on the ASBI disrupt scale. The social competence factor had high loadings (> .65) on the express and comply subscales from the ASBI. These high-loading scales were composited to generate measures of problem behavior and social competence at 24 and 36 months.

RESULTS

As a first step in determining whether associations between family predictors and child outcomes varied as a function of early-child care experience, we correlated each of the nine family predictors with each of the eight child outcomes separately for the two child care groups. This resulted in the generation of 144 coefficients of association, which are displayed in Tables 28.1 and 28.2. Two things should be noted. First, the coefficients of association between the family variables and attachment security are point-biserial correlations rather than Pearson correlations (because attachment security was a binary variable). Second, the predictors associated with dependent vari-

TABLE 28.1. Correlations of Family Variables with Child Outcomes at 24 Months by Child Care Group

Family variable	MDI		Social competence		Problem behavior	
	FT	MC	FT	MC	FT	MC
Demographic						
Marital status	.15*	.19*	*-.04*	*.26******	-.21**	-.21**
Income/needs	.36***	.24**	.12	.19*	-.18*	-.17*
Psychological well-being/attitudes						
Personality	.07	.16*	.26***	.23**	-.33***	-.39***
Depression	-.12	-.25**	-.25***	-.38***	.35***	.40***
Benefits of work	.07	-.11	*.19**	*-.14*	*-.08*	*.33******
Nonauthoritarian childrearing	.26***	.18*	.19*	.29***	-.04	-.10
Mothering/relationship						
Sensitivity play	.38***	.40***	.23**	.26***	-.16*	-.23**
HOME–positive involvement	.09	.08	.14	.10	-.02	-.00
Attachment security	.14	-.07	.06	.16*	-.04	.03

Note. Pairs of correlations in ***italicized boldface*** are significantly different. *n* = 184 for FT group; *n* = 164 for MC group. MDI, Mental Development Index; FT, full-time nonparental care; MC, maternal care; HOME, Home Observation for Measurement of the Environment.
* $p < .05$; ** $p < .01$; *** $p < .001$.

ables from different times of measurement are not always the same because they reflect the averaged repeated measurements of the predictor up to the point at which the outcome in question was measured (i.e., maternal sensitivity and HOME positive involvement).

To test whether the predictor–outcome associations displayed in Tables 28.1 and 28.2 varied across child care groups, we created predictor–outcome correlation matrices. The matrix in Table 28.1, generated for both child care groups, involved the nine family predictors and the three 24-month outcomes; the matrix in Table 28.2, also generated for both child care groups, included the nine family predictors and the five 36-month outcomes. It was then determined whether, at the matrix level, patterns of covariation differed across child care groups. Differences between the correlation matrices generated for the maternal-care and the nonparental-care groups were tested using a multiple group LISREL approach (Jöreskog & Sörbom, 1993). This approach tested whether the two sets of correlations were sufficiently different for us to conclude the observed differences were not due to chance. At neither age did the predictor–outcome matrices prove to be significantly different across the two child care groups: 24-month, $\chi^2(51, n = 348) = 49.30$, $p = .54$; 36-month, $\chi^2(73, n = 274) = 87.39$, $p = .12$.

Although the multivariate approach clearly provides no evidence of differential relations between family factors and child functioning across child care groups on the basis of the correlations in Tables 28.1 and 28.2, we

TABLE 28.2. Correlations of Family Variables with Child Outcomes at 36 Months by Child Care Group

Family variable	School readiness		Expressive vocabulary		Receptive vocabulary		Social competence		Problem behavior	
	FT	MC	FT	MC	FT	MC	FT	MC	FT	MC
Demographic										
Marital status	*.07*	.31***	.06	.16	.12	.26***	*.02*	.38***	*.02*	*-.26**
Income/needs	.42***	.34***	.25**	.16	.38***	.25**	.13	.22*	-.10	-.23**
Psychological well-being/attitudes										
Personality	.12	.16	.11	.17	.10	.23*	.39***	.16	-.24**	*-.44***
Depression	-.14	-.28*	-.12	-.25**	-.12	-.33***	-.33***	-.27**	.43***	.42***
Benefits of work	*.13*	*-.16*	-.07	-.03	.03	-.17	.21*	-.23***	*-.19**	*.33***
Nonauthoritarian childrearing	.20*	.15	.21**	.06	.25**	.08	.20*	.25**	-.02	-.26**
Mothering/relationship										
Sensitivity play	.34***	.37***	.29***	.35***	.43***	.52***	.18*	.27**	-.10	-.27**
HOME—positive involvement	.25**	.31***	.21**	.21*	.26**	.26**	.07	.26**	-.10	-.08
Attachment security	.08	-.03	-.03	.01	.16	.03	-.04	.13	.08	-.08

Note. Pairs of correlations in ***italicized boldface*** are significantly different. $n = 147$ for FT group; $n = 127$ for MC group. FT, full-time nonparental care; MC, maternal care; HOME, Home Observation for Measurement of the Environment.
*$p < .05$; **$p < .01$; ***$p < .001$.

adopted an exploratory approach to determine whether there were signifi-cant differences between pairs of correlations and whether there were patterns associated with identified differences. To this end, each of the cor-relations presented in Tables 28.1 and 28.2 was transformed, using the Fisher r-to-z transformation, to a z-score form, and all pairs of transformed correlations (i.e., correlations between the same two constructs at a given time period for the two different groups) were tested for statistical signifi-cance. Of the pairs of correlations presented in Tables 28.1 and 28.2, 11 were found to differ by a degree of magnitude greater than one would expect by chance. (It should be noted that the 75 tests so performed across Tables 28.1 and 28.2 [27 at 24 months and 45 at 36 months] are not inde-pendent and do not take into account the internal structure of correlation matrices [positive definiteness] and are offered only as a means of exploring the internal structure of the correlations.) The pairs of correlations that are significantly different are indicated in Tables 28.1 and 28.2 in italicized boldface.

Two main patterns of significant differences in correlations across the two child care groups emerged from these exploratory analyses. First, rela-tions between marital status and child functioning were larger in the maternal-care group than in the full-time-care group in the case of social competence at 24 and 36 months and school readiness and problem behav-ior at 36 months. These associations were in the expected direction and sta-tistically significant in the maternal-care group but not significant in the full-time-care group. Thus, living in a single-parent household predicted poorer child functioning, and living in a two-parent household predicted higher cognitive and socioemotional functioning only when children were reared principally by their mother, not when they received full-time nonparental care beginning early in the first year of life.

The second pattern visible in the data involved the mother's belief in the benefits of work. Five associations—between the mother's belief in the benefits of work and children's social competence and problem behavior at 24 and 36 months and 3-year school readiness—were in opposite directions in the two groups. Whereas a favorable view of the benefits of maternal employment for child functioning positively predicted child development for children in full-time care (i.e., greater social competence, fewer behavior problems, and greater school readiness), it negatively predicted child func-tioning for the full-time maternal-care group (i.e., less social competence, more behavior problems, and lower school readiness).

Two additional differences between pairs of correlations proved consis-tent with the hypothesis that relations between family predictors and child outcomes would be stronger in the maternal-care group. First, maternal per-sonality predicted child behavior problems at 36 months more strongly in the maternal-care group, although for both groups the correlation was sig-nificant and indicated that poorer maternal adjustment forecast more behavior problems. Second, the more the mother endorsed nonauthoritarian (i.e., progressive) childrearing attitudes and values, the fewer problems she reported the child having at 36 months, but only in the case of children in the maternal-care group. The correlation in the full-time-care group was not significantly different from zero.

Beyond these findings pertaining to group differences in predictor–outcome relations, it seems notable that the correlations displayed in Tables 28.1 and 28.2 are, in the main, consistent with findings widely reported in the developmental literature. That is, irrespective of child care group, higher levels of maternal sensitivity in play were associated with higher levels of positive child outcomes (e.g., Bayley Mental Development Index, social competence) and lower levels of negative outcomes (e.g., behavior problems). The same was true of nonauthoritarian childrearing attitudes, family income, maternal personality, and positive involvement as measured by the HOME. Higher levels of depression were associated with poorer functioning on the part of the child. Somewhat surprisingly, attachment security proved to be the weakest predictor variable, significantly predicting child functioning in only one instance (i.e., 24-month social competence for the maternal-care group).

DISCUSSION

On the basis of provocative findings from a number of studies, some with quite limited sample sizes, comparing children with and without experience in nonparental child care, we took advantage of a unique longitudinal investigation to examine the prospect that the predictive power of an array of family factors on child functioning would vary as a function of child care experience.

Results of the multivariate analyses that compared patterns of co-variation between family predictors and child outcomes at the level of correlation matrices provided no support for the hypothesis that associations between family factors and child functioning would vary across groups. Furthermore, when regression analyses not presented here were run to determine whether prediction equations varied across child care groups for each dependent variable, substantively similar results obtained. As a result, the general hypothesis that the effects of family predictors would be attenuated in the case of children experiencing full-time nonparental care beginning early in their first year compared with those cared for virtually exclusively by their mothers was not supported. These findings clearly suggest that developmental processes—defined for purposes of this inquiry in terms of predictor–outcome relations—operate similarly in the case of children with and without extensive early-care experience. In fact, in both child care and maternal-care groups, predictor–outcome relations were generally in accord with expectations derived from the general developmental literature.

Despite this general conclusion, it should be recalled that analyses testing the difference between each and every pair of correlations—after failing to discern significant group differences in multivariate analyses—did reveal several significant group differences. In light of the absence of significant group differences at the level of entire matrices, these findings from the exploratory analyses need to be interpreted cautiously. One set of group differences pertaining to the benefits-of-employment variable was consistent with other evidence in the field suggesting that when maternal attitudes toward employment coincide with mother's actual employment, then children benefit, whereas when attitudes and employment are at odds, the opposite is the case (e.g., Crockenberg & Litman, 1991; Gold & Andres, 1980). The second set of group differences that emerged from the exploratory analyses was consistent with the hypothesis that relations between family predictors and child outcomes would be stronger for children reared primarily by their parents. This was especially so with respect to family structure (i.e., one vs. two parents). Despite these comments, it is important to remember that the most consistent finding to emerge from this inquiry is that similarities in correlations between family predictors and child outcomes far exceeded differences.

29

Families Matter—
Even for Kids in Child Care

NICHD EARLY CHILD CARE RESEARCH NETWORK

In the United States and other developed countries, the economic and technological developments since World War II have carried with them a host of social and political changes affecting family life. For young children, few changes have been more significant than the dramatic increase in the number of women in the workforce and the concomitant increase in the number of children cared for by someone other than their parents while their parents are at work. This shift has given rise to feelings of uncertainty and discomfort on the part of parents, schools, policymakers, and leaders from a variety of social organizations. Do parents continue to have a meaningful effect on children's development when their children are out of their care for extended periods of time each week? This concern arises from deeply held cultural beliefs that families have the primary, if not sole, responsibility for childrearing (Steiner, 1981) and is fostered by psychological theory that gives parents the principal role in shaping children's futures (Bowlby, 1973; McCartney & Phillips, 1988). It remains at the forefront of public debate and private consciousness as the trends of the late 20th century become consolidated in the early decades of the 21st.

Among those who have followed the history of the National Institute of Child Health and Human Development (NICHD) Study of Early Child Care

From *Journal of Developmental and Behavioral Pediatrics*, 2003, Vol. 24, pp. 58–62. Copyright 2003 by Lippincott Williams & Wilkins. Reprinted by permission.

and Youth Development, most know that our efforts have mostly concentrated on addressing questions about children's experiences in child care (NICHD Early Child Care Research Network, 2001e). However, as a large-scale, comprehensive, and detailed natural history study of children's development, initiated shortly after their birth, the study's results also provide the opportunity to examine the associations between the family and children's developmental outcomes when the children receive considerable care outside the immediate family. Overall, the findings suggest that the role of families is not substantially weakened or changed with considerable child care experience in the earliest years. Specifically, when we controlled for both the quality and the quantity of child care, we still found statistically significant associations between family factors and children's cognitive, language, and socioemotional development similar to those reported for the past 50 years for children whose child care history was not taken into account (Bornstein & Tamis-LeMonda, 1989; Bradley, 1994; Friedman & Cocking, 1986; Hart & Risley, 1995; Kagan, 1984; Wachs & Chan, 1986).

To some, this general finding may come as something of a surprise in that there is evidence from several sources (Egeland & Hiester, 1995; Jaeger & Weinraub, 1990; Oppenheim, Sagi, & Lamb, 1988) to suggest that nonparental care experience might attenuate the link between parent–child relationships and children's development. Howes (1990) found that parents' management of children's behaviors was a consistently stronger predictor of cognitive and social development for preschool and kindergarten-age children in maternal care than for children who started care in infancy. Similarly, Dunham & Dunham (1992) found that maternal verbal behavior was predictive of children's vocabulary for children in exclusive maternal care but not for children in extensive child care. Our findings, however, do comport with findings from other studies. For example, Clarke-Stewart, Gruber, & Fitzgerald (1994) noted that, even for children who were in child care, family circumstances and specific maternal attributes, attitudes, and behaviors were associated with children's developmental outcomes. Their results linked family economic resources, maternal education, higher-quality home environments, and sensitive and cognitively stimulating parenting to better psychological outcomes for children with child care experience initiated in infancy.

In the NICHD Study of Early Child Care and Youth Development, (NICHD Early Child Care Research Network, 2001e) family, mothering, child care, and child-development measures were assessed by face-to-face interviews, observations, and questionnaires at predetermined intervals. Results reported here are based on data collected during face-to-face contacts at 1, 6, 15, 24, 36, and 54 months as well as on data collected during phone contacts made every 3 months over the first 3 years and, later, every 4 months through kindergarten. Family assessments pertained to family structure, parental employment, income, psychosocial characteristics of the mother, attitudes and beliefs about parenting and child care, maternal depression, maternal sensitivity in observed interaction with her child, and quality of the home environment. The assessment of the quality of the home environment was based on both observations by study staff and maternal reports. Assessments captured the physical characteristics of the home and the opportunities it provides for social and cognitive enrichment, as well as observed parental involvement/support. The child care measures pertained to both the child care provider and the child care environment. The child care provider's education, training, philosophy, and the quality of her interaction with the target child were recorded. Children's behavior and development were assessed in the social, emotional, cognitive, language, academic readiness, and health domains using well-known assessment methods (NICHD Early Child Care Research Network, 2001e).

A question of considerable importance to parents is whether children are likely to be less securely attached to parents if they begin child care early and spend many hours in child care each week. Some studies have found an increased likelihood of an insecure–avoidant attachment when children experienced extensive nonmaternal care in the first year (see the multistudy analysis of Belsky & Rovine, 1988, and the recent study by Sagi, Koren-Karie, Gini, Ziv, & Joels, 2002). In the NICHD study, however, the child care effects with respect to attachment at both 15 and 36 months were conditioned by the mother's involvement and her sensitive parenting of her child (NICHD Early Child Care Research Network 1997b, 2001b). Greater maternal sensitivity in observed mother–child interactions and maternal responsiveness in home observations were associated with an increased probability of children being classified as securely attached to their mothers when children were 15 and 36 months of age. Moreover, maternal sensitivity moderated effects of the amount of child care (at 15 and 36 months of age), quality of child care (at 15 months), and number of child care arrangements (at 15 months). Children whose mothers were relatively low in sensitivity (relative to the sample studied) when the children were 15 months and 36 months of age and were in more than 10 hours of child care per week had an increased probability of being insecurely attached to mother. In addition, children whose mothers were low in sensitivity had an increased probability of being insecurely attached at 15 months of age when child care quality was lower and when more than one child care arrangement had been used in the first year, which was the norm for children in child care. For example, the proportion of secure children at 15 months of age among those with mothers receiving low scores on maternal sensitivity and with lower scores on our measures of quality of care was between .44 and .51. The mean proportion of secure attachment for the rest of the children was .62. These findings indicate that maternal behavior predicts attachment security when children experience nonmaternal care and that responsive and sensitive mothering moderates the effects of child care on attachment security.

The NICHD Study of Early Child Care and Youth Development also looked at the development of self-control, cooperation, and problem behavior. Specifically, we examined the link between family predictors and children's psychosocial functioning, both independent of child care experience and in combination with child care experience (NICHD Early Child Care Research Network, 1998a, 2002a, 2003). The findings showed that better psychological adjustment of mothers was related to greater compliance and self-control and fewer behavior problems in their children. When mothers were more involved with their children and behaved in a more sensitive manner when interacting with them, their children were more compliant and self-controlled and displayed fewer behavior problems when they were 2 and 3 years of age and were more cooperative at age 2. These findings thus highlight the mother's role in fostering cooperation, compliance, and self-control in early childhood. More sensitive parenting throughout the preschool years was linked to better social skills and less problem behavior of 4½-year-old and kindergarten-age children who had experienced varying degrees of child care throughout the preschool years. For example, when the children were 4½ years of age, those whose mothers were in the lowest tercile in terms of parenting quality scored 2.2 points higher on a 100-item scale of behavior problems than did children with parents in the highest quartile of parental quality. These findings, though small in magnitude, are important given that problem behavior at this early age is significantly predictive of future behavior problems (Richman, Stevenson, & Graham, 1986; Rose, Rose, & Feldman, 1986).

Parenting was also linked to peer competence when the children were 2 and 3 years old (NICHD Early Child Care Research Network, 2001c). Assessments of peer competence were based on mothers' and child care providers' ratings of children's positive and negative peer-related behaviors, data collectors' observations of the positive and negative peer-related behaviors in child care, and ratings of videotaped positive, negative, and self-assertive dyadic peer interaction in semistructured settings. Maternal sensitivity predicted more competent interactions with peers across all measures, highlighting the family's role in the development of early emerging individual differences in peer relations among children with early child care experience.

Because children who attend child care spend a significant proportion of their waking hours out of contact with their parents, there are also questions pertaining to the impact of parents on children's language and cognitive development. The broader literature indicates that direct efforts by parents to stimulate language and learning are associated with better scores on measures of language, intelligence, and achievement (Friedman & Cocking, 1986; Hart & Risley, 1995; Hoff-Ginsberg, 1991; Tomasello & Farrar, 1986). Likewise, there is evidence that providing children with a rich array of materials and broadening experiences is associated with higher scores on such measures (Bradley, Caldwell, Rock, Ramey, & Johnson, 1989; Wachs & Chan, 1986). However, few of these studies have examined the impact of these family and home environment factors while controlling for time spent in child care, the quality of child care, and the type of care used (e.g., center and child care home).

In a publication about the links between childrearing experience and cognitive outcomes of children over the first 3 years of life (NICHD Early Child Care Research Network, 2000b), we reported that the richness of maternal vocabulary, cumulative assessments of maternal level of cognitive stimulation when interacting with her child, and, as anticipated, other sources of cumulative experiential enrichment provided by parents in the home environment were significant predictors of cognitive and language development of the children, especially when they were 36 months of age. These associations with parenting were found even after controlling for the cumulative effects of the quality, quantity, and type of child care. Similar findings were reported in a publication about preacademic and language skills when the children were 4½ years of age (NICHD Early Child Care Research Network, 2002a). Children receiving high-quality parenting scored 8.3 points higher on preacademic skills (mean for all children in the study = 98.9; SD = 11.6) and 13.7 points higher on language skills (mean for all children in the study = 99.8; SD = 10.3) than children receiving low-quality parenting.

The findings from the NICHD Study of Early Child Care and Youth Development demonstrate that family characteristics and the quality of parenting are related to the cognitive, language, and socioemotional development of young children throughout the preschool years regardless of the number of hours they spend in child care over the early years, the quality of their child care, or the type of child care (center, child care home, relative care) they experienced (NICHD Early Child Care Research Network, 2001g). We found that parenting, like child care, plays a role in the development of children who spend time in child care early in life. These findings corroborate and bolster conclusions about early childhood experience found in *From Neurons to Neighborhoods* (Shonkoff & Phillips, 2000), the recent publication of the National Research Council/Institute of Medicine.

To address more decisively the question about parental impact on children's development for children who attend child care, we compared the two most extreme groups of children in terms of their early child care experience: those exclusively reared at home and those in extensive (more than 30 hours per week) nonparental care across their first 3 years (NICHD Early Child Care Research Network, 1998b). When the children were 2 and 3 years of age, we examined child outcomes in both the cognitive and social domains, including mental development, expressive and receptive language, social competence, and problem behavior. Family predictors included an index of family income, maternal depression, maternal beliefs in the benefits of work, maternal nonauthoritarian childrearing beliefs, infant attachment security, and maternal sensitivity in mother–child interactions and maternal positive involvement as evaluated in the family home. Comparisons of the matrices of correlations between family predictors and child outcomes of the group with extensive nonparental care and the group without nonparental care experience provided no evidence for differences. Overall, the correlations of child developmental outcomes with family demographics, maternal personality and beliefs, and parenting were quite consistent with the findings widely reported in the developmental literature. Moreover, none of the correlations between the measures of mother's observed parenting and children's social and cognitive development were significantly different for the children in the full-time maternal care and full-time child care groups across the first 3 years. Examinations of this question at later ages have not yet been undertaken.

In our publications, statistically significant prediction from parenting to developmental outcomes was more frequent than prediction from child care. When both parenting and child care were predictive of outcomes to a statistically significant extent, the link between parenting and outcomes tended to be stronger than the link between child care and outcomes. For example, we observed that family characteristics (i.e., parenting, maternal education, and income) were more strongly linked with preacademic skills, language, and short-term memory assessed at 4½ years than were the same child outcomes (e.g., preacademic skills) and child care quality, hours in child care, or type of care. The effect sizes of child care quality were reported to be 27% as large as the effect associated with parenting quality (NICHD Early Child Care Research Network, 2002a). The findings in the socioemotional domain were more mixed, with comparable effects of family and child care experiences on some outcomes and stronger family effects on others. For example, we found that maternal sensitivity was the strongest and most consistent predictor of maternal, caregiver, and teacher reports of both social competence and problem behavior when children were 4½ years of age and when they were in kindergarten; higher levels of observed maternal sensitivity across early childhood predicted higher levels of adult-reported social competence and caregiver reports of less conflict and fewer behavior problems (NICHD Early Child Care Research Network, 2003). In our study, the assessments of the family environment and the child care environment, though comparable in terms of their focus on adult sensitivity, responsivity, and the provision of cognitive stimulation while interacting with young children, were not identical. This means that we are not in a position to test the extent to which the above-mentioned differences are statistically significant. Others, in their own research, may wish to examine the lead proposed by our observations.

Overall, our findings indicate that the important role of families was apparent for children with extensive child care experience as well as for those without child care experience. Yet, one needs to be aware of the fact that the associations between parenting and children's developmental outcomes discerned throughout the preschool years in this large and diverse sample of children, most of whom have experienced early nonmaternal care, may be partly due to factors that we could not account for in our analyses. Ninety-four percent of the children participating in our study were not in extremely poor quality of care (see Chapter 6), and we cannot be sure that the parenting of children in extremely poor quality care is not compromised. Likewise, our analyses could not address the role of a genotype–environment confound in contributing to our findings (Collins, Maccoby, Steinberg, Hetherington, & Bornstein, 2000; Scarr & McCartney, 1983). Nevertheless, the findings reinforce a body of knowledge about the merits of positive qualities of parenting—sensitivity, involvement, and cognitive stimulation—for children's development. These qualities appear to benefit all children, those exclusively reared by their parents and those with extensive child care experience.

Parents, policymakers, and those who work with parents to help them in the task of caring for their children will undoubtedly continue to be concerned about families and children in the 21st century. Findings from our study suggest that families clearly do matter in the lives of children. Considered as a whole, findings from our study indicate that experience at home and in child care affects children's well-being. Such findings are in agreement with propositions about environmental influences on behavior stipulated in most current ecological–developmental theories (Bronfenbrenner, 1995). Although the findings do not offer direct support for any particular type of parenting intervention, they reinforce proposals for investing in educating current and future parents about the importance of their role in the psychological well-being of their children (U.S. Department of Health and Human Services, 2001).

VIII

—

Commentary

Given the diverse contents of this volume, the editors arranged for a commentary to be written by a qualified scientist who has had no role in conducting the study. We were fortunate to obtain the commentary that follows from Sharon L. Ramey, Susan H. Mayer Professor of Child and Family Studies at Georgetown University, and Director of the Georgetown University Center on Health and Education. Professor Ramey, whose credentials include extensive research and teaching in the fields of early child development and child care, has written a commentary that focuses on the strategies and findings of the study itself as well as her views concerning their social implications.

30

—

Human Developmental Science Serving Children and Families

Contributions of the NICHD Study of Early Child Care

SHARON LANDESMAN RAMEY

This volume is a wonderful gift to the field of human developmental science. Contained in this book are chapters derived from scientific journal articles, each focused on a distinct topic and set of findings; each subjected to rigorous internal and external peer review; and each reflecting years of investment in the design, conduct, analysis, and interpretation of this landmark 10-site study launched by the National Institute of Child Health and Human Development (NICHD) with the endorsement of the U.S. Congress. This a gift that has the potential to realize a multiplier effect, by informing readers in a timely way about the major findings concerning the impact of children's early care experiences on their development. This book is a "must read" for anyone seeking to be informed about the latest scientific knowledge in the field of child care and early human experience. The findings present a compelling portrait of the realities of child care and its contribution to the course of young children's lives.

My commentary on this study concentrates on three topics. The first concerns "big science" and the ushering in of a new era of scientific inquiry about the processes of human development. Conducting projects on the scale of the NICHD Study of Early Child Care represents a fundamentally new style of research, guided by a newly emerging set of assumptions about how to advance our knowledge of human development. The controversies and uncertainties about this divergent approach abound; their resolution will be of great consequence for all of the branches of science and practice classified under life sciences, social and behavioral sciences, and education.

The second topic for commentary concerns those findings that I have identified as "call to action" findings—findings so impressive that parents and politicians, scientists and social analysts, governmental agencies and child care providers must respond to them and use these findings to inform the future course of child care in our nation. I do not seek to provide a survey-like review of the contents of this book here. Neither do I mean that only a few findings matter. I simply have chosen to write about those findings that I judge to be most worthy of vigorous, concerted, and timely action to improve the lives of millions of young children and their families.

The third topic is a more subjective and diffuse topic, which I have difficulty naming. The topic concerns the need to place children first and the dangers of institutionalized uncertainty. Too many examples of inaction, contradictory actions, and divisive politics crowd the field of early child development and family policy. Blatant instances abound of placing politics and programs first, rather than children's well-being. There is no established pathway from reliable information to well-informed practices and policies, despite what the public is often told by leading agencies, politicians, and advocacy organizations. When scientific findings challenge what is popular, profitable, or politically advantageous, the pathway to effective action requires strategic planning and coalitions, along with dedication and cooperation. The NICHD Study of Early Child Care has engaged the attention of the media and the public; this study may also provide an inroad into studying patterns of information dissemination and utilization.

THE ERA OF BIG SCIENCE AND LANDMARK STUDIES

The era of "big science" is upon us, and the results are impressive. In the life sciences, the Human Genome Project supported by the National Institutes of Health (NIH) is a truly unprecedented effort, bringing together leading investigators from diverse areas of specialization, familiar with cutting-edge technology, to achieve a single and gigantic task—the mapping of the human genome. The Human Genome Project was so unlikely in its birth, its nurturance, and its timely completion (ahead of schedule) that its story and efforts to evaluate its impact are likely to reverberate for a long time. The Human Genome Project also has helped other fields to "think big." For the field of child and family development, large-scale scientific inquiry is uniquely able to advance our understanding for topics that meet these criteria: (1) there is a compelling single question or issue to be resolved; (2) the methods to gather critical data are diverse and specialized; (3) a huge quantity of information must be gathered within a short time period to inform the answer; (4) the best thinkers and the best empiricists must work closely together in the design, conduct, and analysis of the study; and (5) a new working style of research collaboration is vital to success of the endeavor.

The 10-site NICHD Early Child Care Study met the aforementioned criteria. The research findings in this book represent some of the products of the newly emerging "big science" in the field of child development. They are worthy of close scrutiny, widespread dissemination, thoughtful discussion, and timely action. Like the Human Genome Project, this landmark study necessitated obtaining funding at levels far greater than the typical single-site, single-investigator-led style of research (although the absolute amounts for the NICHD Early Child Care Study pale in comparison to the Human Genome Project). Similarly, its launching engendered controversy, skepticism, and frank jealously from some in the field. Significant delays in launching this study, due to the need to resolve crucial design and multisite training issues, fueled further concern among the critics. And, undoubtedly, there must have been doubts among the participating scientists themselves about the direction, the feasibility, and the ultimate value of this large-scale, multisite study. The most remarkable similarity of the NICHD Early Child Care Study to the Human Genome Project is that the actual productivity of each landmark study has advanced their respective fields to new levels of understanding and to a new way of preparing the next generation of scientists, practitioners, and policymakers. The junior colleagues and the students associated with these studies, as well as the senior leaders, now have unprecedented knowledge about these topics, as well as new research strategies and support for the importance of collaboration; their experiences will shape the vision for future investigation in each field.

My reflections on the NICHD Early Child Care Study are grounded in this historical perspective about the life sciences, especially human development. "Big science" is not inherently good or even better than other styles of investigation; the same can be said of research that is interdisciplinary, collaborative, longitudinal, and complex. Yet there is no substitute for big science when it is the best match approach for the questions being asked. After several decades of well-conducted but small, scattered, and usually short-term studies about the impact of early child care on the development of young children, there was no doubt that the conclusions—when critically reviewed—were weak, flawed, and inadequate to answer the urgent question, "How important and consequential is child care in the lives of young children and families in the United States?" Infants and young children are vulnerable; protecting them from harm and neglect, and actively promoting their physical, mental, and psychosocial well-being is at the heart of our nation and its future. Parents have the right to make informed decisions about how to maximize the well-being of their children. Communities must know what can be done to sustain a citizenry that is healthy, productive, and perhaps even happy. Our country must understand how the allocation of resources and the establishment of standards for child care affect our ability

430 COMMENTARY

to realize the goals of our democracy and sustain an economically viable nation.

A summit of concerned scientists and professionals, held in Bethesda, Maryland, on the campus of the NIH, set the stage for this landmark study. The unresolved issues were explicated in clear and competent ways. Further, the option of conducting new scientific studies that could provide answers that would be more trustworthy in their rigor and objectivity, more complete in their scope, and more relevant to the many changes in the landscape of American families and the workforce was immediately available. Both NIH—through the NICHD and its director, Dr. Duane Alexander—and Congress strongly endorsed the idea of this large national research program to bring in scientifically robust answers to this compelling question. No matter what one's own personal best guess was about this highly charged topic of babies and toddlers in the care of nonparents, everyone appeared to agree that the time was right to act.

The story of the launching of this study and the early decision making about its course is told, in part, in the early chapters of this book. What is particularly instructive is how thoroughly the investigators considered the multiple competing theories and the real-world observations in assembling the plan to obtain the study's sample of newborns and families and to apply multiple and refined measures, some old and others newly developed, of key factors hypothesized to shape the course of children's development. The reader who studies the conceptual framework and the history of the NICHD Early Child Care Study will receive the equivalent of an advanced scholarly course in the current views about the nature of human development and how to identify what matters in the lives of young children. The dominant 20th-century way of thinking endorsed thinking about constructs in terms of cause and effect and creating equations whose elements have differing weights to designate their relative importance. Indeed, the statistics scientists use rely on explicit assumptions about how the world works, which in turn determine how the mathematics are applied to the gathered observations (data). Over time, both the conceptualization of human development and the statistics used to analyze the information collected by a study have evolved, so that things are far less linear, simplistic, and mechanistic. The fresh framing of the compelling question that guided this study recognized explicitly that there is a highly dynamic and large set of influences, including contextual and counterbalancing factors, that contribute to the course of children's development. Appropriately, most of the questions are framed in terms of increased or decreased probabilities of outcomes that occur within the context of multiple and changing sets of life circumstances; and the answers are fine-tuned to the emergence and differentiation of children's individuality and their competencies from the early period of infancy through the transition into school.

This study's findings are not simply an affirmation of what wise grandparents could have told us; nor are they so fine-grained and complex that no one will be able to remember exactly what does matter, and why, in the final analysis. The findings from this 10-site study are deeply substantive and well-supported; and the contents of this book should be viewed as a mandatory, fundamental basis for future policy, practice, and research.

I want to affirm the value of this study. I repeat: The findings from this 10-site study are deeply substantive and well supported; and the contents of this book should be viewed as a mandatory, fundamental basis for future policy, practice, and research. At the same time, I recognize that the study's limitations are considerable, and these are remarkably well detailed in most of the articles. The two most serious limitations I discern are these: First, the study includes a relatively small number of children and families from historically marginalized groups of families living in poverty; second, there is a lack of linguistic diversity in the study sample (because of the requirement that parents were sufficiently proficient in English to complete extensive questionnaires and interviews). Perhaps a third limitation that will become increasingly noticed in future years is the relative inattention to children's individual biology and the complex influence of physical environmental and intergenerational influences on outcomes. A predictable criticism that can be issued with commanding authority is, "This study does not delineate the precise mechanisms by which differential courses of human development are obtained." All these limitations and criticisms are legitimate. Yet none diminishes the integrity of the science conducted, nor lessens the contributions to advancing knowledge about children from working poor through middle- and upper-middle-class families. The limitations can be corrected by the timely conduct of studies that focus on children from very poor families, from linguistically diverse families, and from places in our country that represent especially high and low risk in terms of hypothesized environmental and biological risks. Currently, a multiyear planning effort is under way—again with strong leadership from the NICHD and support from many other institutes within the NIH—to design a far larger, far broader, and far more biologically sophisticated study of a birth cohort of 100,000 children. Known as the National Children's Study, this study is being informed by scientists from many fields. Many of the interdisciplinary work committees include scientists from this NICHD study. The pathway of thinking afresh in the life sciences is being vigorously forged in these ambitious planning efforts; yet at times, the serious challenges associated with the need for compromise and inadequacy of measures for important topics seem overwhelming. The recent experiences from the current 10-site longitudinal study are among those informing the National Children's Study in valuable ways. Thus, when reflecting on the magnitude of the contributions from the current study, we should temper our expectations by realizing that even "big science" contains a range of bigness. What is so exciting to contemplate is that the life sciences are on the cusp of a revolution in understanding how biological, behavioral, social, and environmental variables become intertwined and contribute to the health and well-being of future generations.

THE CALL-TO-ACTION FINDINGS

There are four sets of findings that I classify as major call-to-action findings. The first call-to-action finding is generated by basic descriptive data about current American family life. *Simply stated, babies born in the United States face an uncertain and highly fluctuating future regarding who will care for them and when.* Many parents in the study stated plans for caregiving that did not come true; that is, they could not accurately predict what they themselves would choose in terms of child care arrangements over the first year or two of their child's life. In the first 5 years of life, many children experienced multiple changes in their caregiving arrangements, for a large number of reasons. As young as 6 months of age, more than 60% of the babies were in nonparental care for at least 30 hours per week. Although we may think and hope that children are highly adaptable and resilient, and we strongly believe that young children benefit from the love and care of many people beyond the immediate family home, the fact is that child care in the United States is highly fragmented and erratic. This uncertain system of care is stressful for families and careproviders alike, and inadequate to provide the desired and likely beneficial levels of support and continuity that children and families need.

The second major finding is that the vast majority of child care is of unacceptably low quality and in the first 3 years of life does not meet even minimal recommended guidelines. This finding is supported by a variety of different measures and different criteria; interestingly, I judge that the basic descriptive findings about the generally low quality of care that children experience are minimized in the scientific articles about this project. That is, many of the studies emphasize the relationship between quality and child outcome and tend to gloss over the basic finding that so many children spend so much time in low to medium quality care, and such a small percentage are in consistently high quality care. It is true that there is no single measure of child care quality, but there are multiple and solid methods for measuring aspects of the child care environment that have undeniable face validity. Indeed, the measures generated and evaluated by this network of investigators represent a major contribution to the field of early child development and child care. The direct observations obtained in child care settings are remarkably consistent with parental values. These include an overall rating of positive caretaking quality, including subscales for the caregiver's sensitivity to the child's nondistress signals, stimulation of the child's development, positive regard toward the child, and lack of detachment and flatness of affect, as well as quantitative measurement of the amounts of language stimulation, positive talk, positive physical contact, positive interaction with other children, and interaction with stimulating physical materials. These measures closely match what parents and child care regulators can readily observe. Positive caregiving by nonparents in child care settings is rare. In the first 3 years of life, only 12% of the children studied in these 10 sites received child care that fit the definition of "highly characteristic" of positive care! When extrapolated to the United States as a whole, only 9% of children are estimated to receive such levels. In contrast, at every age, well over 50% of the children receive care that is either "very uncharacteristic" or "somewhat uncharacteristic" of positive care. *This is shocking and intolerable; it also is well concealed from most parents and the general public.* This finding warrants action, regardless of the magnitude and type of long-term consequences that care has on the children. Infants and young children should not be subjected to care that is nonresponsive, nonstimulating, indifferent, and/or neglectful. This is a very precious time in the lives of children, when they are inclined to be highly trusting, highly curious and exploratory, ready to receive language and learning stimulation, and increasingly independent and mobile. This is the age when a sense of self emerges and when children try to make sense of their world. Please remember, the responsive care measured by the NICHD Early Child Care Research Network was not unrealistically high or unattainable; *nothing less should be acceptable to families or our nation.*

The third major set of findings provides the answer to the major question that drove the study—namely, does child care really matter in a young child's development? The answer is a resounding, "It does matter." The findings about precisely which indicators about child care predict particular outcomes at particular ages are somewhat detailed and complex. But collectively, this study unequivocally demonstrates that both the quality and the quantity of nonparental care influence children's development. Stated directly and summatively, poor quality care is harmful. Conversely, high-quality care can be somewhat beneficial, particularly for somewhat older children and particularly for children whose own family home environments do not consistently provide high levels of stimulation. Further, children in extended care—for more than 30 hours per week and starting very early in life—do show outcomes that are in a nonoptimal direction. This is not uplifting news; it means that no one can credibly claim that we do not know whether child care really matters. Child care makes a difference—and given the overall low levels of high-quality child care and the long hours many children spend in nonparental care, the risks are real.

As the findings from this study emerged over the years, I have shared them with writers and editors of leading family and child magazines, with the general media, and with policymakers, as have many other scientists. No one seems to like hearing about these findings. Everyone wants to find the flaws in the study and its measures, because this would be much easier than confronting the call-to-action findings. Not only will parents become worried and anxious, but careproviders will feel criticized. Yet this study indicates that if young children were to receive high-quality, responsive care from others, and probably not for more than 30 hours per week, our nation would have many more children who are, in everyday terms, highly capable, cooperative, and caring young citizens. I too wish the "news" had been better; it is not easy for anyone to fully contemplate the implications of this research.

Finally, the fourth set of findings that represents a call to action comprises an affirmation of the family unit in our society. Parents continue to matter. The quality of care parents provide, just like the quality of care provided by nonparents, influences the course of their children's development in important domains such as language and literacy development and social responsiveness. In fact, parental and home variables influence a child's development even more than child care does. Alas, the home influence is neither strongly enhanced nor negated by most child care (except perhaps for the children from the lowest-quality home environments who may be fortunate enough to receive high-quality child care).

PLACING CHILDREN FIRST AND THE DANGERS OF INSTITUTIONALIZED UNCERTAINTY

To what extent the scientific community will focus on discovering effective ways to communicate and collaborate with those who shape and implement public policy, as well as those who are engaged in the everyday transactions that affect parents' decisions and children's care, is far from certain. What is certain is that there are major barriers that have forcefully kept our scientific and professional fields from acting in ways that truly place children at the center of the agenda. I have spent more than 35 years encountering the zone that is betwixt and between science and policy, observing firsthand the different ways in which reliable information generated can be used versus ignored or denigrated by special interest groups.

The NICHD Early Child Care Network has produced the data that our country needs to move forward, with strong evidence, to overhaul the standards of care for young children, as well as to provide for supports to assist families in providing high-quality care at home and in making well-informed choices about nonparental child care. The lobbying efforts to ignore child care issues or to continue to settle for poor-quality care, based on pleas that high-quality child care is unattainable and unaffordable, must be strongly countered.

The scientific and academic community is surprisingly conservative when confronted with findings that are politically unpopular and somewhat fearful about taking scientific data to the next level of action. Yet some of the essential next steps to achieve much better child care options and much greater flexibility in the workforce for parents are not obscure. Poor-quality child care, along with the associated stressors for families and communities, represents a national crisis. Only an elite group of families readily attains consistent high-quality care, and high family income is not a guarantee that high-quality care will be available. Innovative and thoughtful solutions must be brought to bear. Old territorial issues, profit motives, and perceptions of cultural bias must be overcome so that young children do not suffer.

In the professional and political circles I know best, there is a culture of silence and defeatism that has crept in. People and groups are frankly fearful that criticism of existing standards and the quality of publicly funded programs, such as subsidized child care for welfare-to-work families and Head Start and pre-K public school programs, will lead to a total withdrawal of any public support for very low-income families or those with two working parents. A number of recent books and articles identify literally scores of independently funded public and private initiatives—at many billions of dollars—to help young children get ready for school and to improve the quality of child care. Yet there is little indication that things really have improved. To the contrary, many of us suspect that poor-quality care may be increasing, and that many parents remain ignorant about how really bad the child care is that their children are receiving.

The culture of silence among scientists and professionals is this: We dare not inflict even more guilt upon parents, or ask that they consider forgoing much needed outside income or spending more of their limited economic resources to obtain better quality care. As a result, many people become paralyzed by the magnitude of reforming our nation's standards for care and the critical supports needed to educate, sustain, and monitor the child care system. We earnestly and naively hope things will get better; that parents will somehow figure out solutions on their own. We choose to ignore that the United States remains an outlier in its lack of attention to this urgent national crisis; and we fail to place our children truly at the center of our agenda.

I often think about conducting a survey of the leading experts in the field of child development, to find out how they personally resolved the child care dilemma that faces every family today. When I probe more privately, I learn that most of my colleagues did not place their very young infants in nonparental care for more than 30 hours per week in the first 3 years of life; and that many had the freedom and the money to rearrange both their work hours and their support systems to create what is unattainable for the majority of citizens in our country. I also have dear friends who still start to cry when they describe some of the child care situations they encountered, either for their own children or when conducting research in their local communities.

Please read this book from cover to cover. Think carefully about the results that have come in and know that they have already been peer-reviewed and presented with the utmost caution and professional care. Talk with others about the study and its findings. Use the publicly available database and continue to analyze for important relationships. But never forget, this landmark study is a description about the lives of real children and their families, and the consequences are not merely minor statistical deviations that are irrelevant to everyday life. Hand-in-hand with parents, providers, politicians, and policymakers, we must create a uniform and universal set of standards that will protect every child from neglect and unresponsive care, whether in the care of nonparents or parents. Let us look, yet again, to the countries and the communities that have solved this problem well; and let us adopt the practices that are needed to increase our nation's strength and the competence and integrity of our country's families and young children.

When viewed in context, child care represents a set of experiences for children that impinge upon and afford them with learning opportunities, that provide their introduction to trustworthy relationships with adults and often other children, and that directly contribute to their health and safety on a frequent basis. Poor-quality child care must be eliminated; and parents must be able to earn livable incomes without subjecting their children to excessively long hours away from their responsible and loving parents.

References

Abbott-Shim, M., & Sibley, A. (1987). *Assessment Profile for Early Childhood Programs.* Atlanta, GA: Quality Assist.

Abbott-Shim, M., & Sibley, A. (1993). *Assessment Profile for Homes with Young Children–research version.* Atlanta, GA: Quality Assist.

Abbott-Shim, M., Sibley, A., & Neel, J. (1992). *Assessment Profile for Early Childhood Programs–research version.* Atlanta, GA: Quality Assist.

Abidin, R. R. (1983). *Parenting Stress Index manual.* Charlottesville, VA: Pediatric Psychology Press.

Ablow, J. C., Measelle, J. R., Kraemer, H. C., Harrington, R., Luby, J., Smider, N., Dierker, L., Clark, V., Dubick, B., Heffelfinger, A., Essex, M. J., & Kupfer, D. J. (1999). The MacArthur Three-City Outcome Study: Evaluating multi-informant measures of young children's symptomatology. *Journal of the American Academy of Child and Adolescent Psychiatry, 38,* 1580–1590.

Achenbach, T. M. (1991a). *Manual for the Child Behavior Checklist 4-18 and 1991 Profile.* Burlington, VT: Author.

Achenbach, T. M. (1991b). *Manual for the Child Behavior Checklist Revised Child Behavior Profile.* Burlington: University Associates in Psychiatry.

Achenbach, T. M. (1991c). *Manual for the Teacher's Report Form and 1991 Profile.* Burlington: University of Vermont Department of Psychiatry.

Achenbach, T. M. (1992). *Manual for the Child Behavior Checklist 2/3 and 1992 Profile.* Burlington: University of Vermont Department of Psychiatry.

Achenbach, T. M., & Edelbrock, C. (1991). *Manual for the Child Behavior Checklist and Revised Child Behavior Profile.* Burlington: University Associates in Psychiatry.

Achenbach, T. M., Edelbrock, C., & Howell, C. T. (1987). Empirically based assessment of behavioral/emotional problems of 2- and 3-year-old children. *Journal of Abnormal Child Psychology, 15,* 629–650.

Ackerman-Ross, S., & Khanna, P. (1989). The relationship of higher quality day care to middle-class three-year-olds' language performance. *Early Childhood Research Quarterly, 4,* 97–116.

Adamson, L. (1995). *Communication development during infancy.* Madison, WI: WCB Brown & Benchmark.

Administration on Children, Youth, and Families. (1996). *An annotated bibliography of*

Head Start research: 1985-1995. Washington, DC: U.S. Department of Health and Human Services.

Ainsworth, M. D. (1973). The development of infant–mother attachment. In B. Caldwell & H. Ricciuti (Eds.), *Review of child development research* (Vol. 3, pp. 1–94). Chicago: University of Chicago Press.

Ainsworth, M. D., Blehar, M., Waters, E., & Wall, S. (1978). *Patterns of attachment: A psychological study of the Strange Situation*. Hillsdale, NJ: Erlbaum.

Ainsworth, M. D., & Wittig, B. (1969). Attachment and exploratory behavior of one-year-olds in a Strange Situation. In B. M. Foss (Ed.), *Determinants of infant behavior* (Vol. 4). London: Methuen.

Allhusen, V. D. (1992). *Differences in day care experiences of infants in three different teacher-child ratio groups: Variations in caregiving quality*. Unpublished doctoral dissertation, Cornell University, Ithaca, NY.

Amato, P., & Ochiltree, G. (1986). Family resources and the development of child competence. *Journal of Marriage and the Family, 48,* 47–56.

American Public Health Association and American Academy of Pediatrics. (1992). *Caring for our children: National health and performance standards: Guidelines for out-of-home child care programs*. Ann Arbor, MI: Author.

Anderson, L., Parker, R., Strikas, R., Farrar, J., Gangarosa, E., Keyserling, H., & Sikes R. (1988). Day care center attendance and hospitalization for lower respiratory tract illness. *Pediatrics, 82,* 300–308.

Arnett, J. (1989). Caregivers in day-care centers: Does training matter? *Journal of Applied Developmental Psychology, 10,* 541–552.

Asher, S., Hymel, S., & Renshaw, P. D. (1984). Loneliness in children. *Child Development, 55,* 1456–1464.

Atkinson, A. M. (1994). Rural and urban families' use of child care. *Family Relations, 43,* 16–22.

Axtell, S. A. M., Garwick, A. W., Patterson, J., Bennett, F. C., & Blum, R. W. (1995). Unmet service needs of families of young children with chronic illnesses and disabilities. *Journal of Family and Economic Issues, 16,* 395–411.

Azure, S. L. (1996). *Child:staff ratios and group size requirements in child care licensing: A comparison of 1989 and 1996*. Boston: Center for Career Development in Early Care and Education, Wheelock College.

Azure, S. L., & Eldred, D. (1997). *Training requirements in child care licensing regulations*. Boston: Center for Career Development in Early Care and Education, Wheelock College.

Bailey, D. B., Blasco, P. M., & Simeonsson, R. J. (1992). Needs expressed by mothers and fathers of young children with disabilities. *American Journal on Mental Retardation, 97,* 1–10.

Ball, T., Holberg, C., Aldous, M., Martinez, F., & Wright, A. (2002). Influence of attendance at day care on the common cold from birth through 13 years of age. *Archives of Pediatric and Adolescent Medicine, 156,* 121–126.

Barglow, P., Vaughn, B., & Molitor, N. (1987). Effects of maternal absence due to employment on the quality of infant–mother attachment in a low-risk sample. *Child Development, 58,* 945–954.

Barnett, R. C., & Marshall, N. L. (1991). The relationship between women's work and family roles and their subjective well-being and psychological distress. In M. Frankenhauser, M. Chesney, & U. Lundberg (Eds.), *Women, work, and health: Stress and opportunities* (pp. 111–136). New York: Plenum Press.

Barnett, R. C., Marshall, N. L., & Singer, J. D. (1992). Job experiences over time, multiple roles, and women's mental health: A longitudinal study. *Journal of Personality and Social Psychology, 62,* 634–644.

Barnett, W. S. (1995). Long-term effects of early childhood programs on cognitive and school outcomes. *Future of Children, 5,* 25–50.

Baron, R. M., & Kenny, D. A. (1986). The moderator–mediator variable distinction in social psychological research: Conceptual, strategic, and statistical considerations. *Journal of Personality and Social Psychology, 51,* 1173–1182.

Bates, J., Marvinney, D., Kelly, T., Dodge, K., Bennett, R., & Pettit, G. (1994) Child care history and kindergarten adjustment. *Developmental Psychology, 30,* 690–700.

Baydar, N., & Brooks-Gunn, J. (1991). Effects of maternal employment and child care arrangements on preschoolers' cognitive and behavioral outcomes: Evidence from the children of the national longitudinal survey of youth. *Developmental Psychology, 27,* 932–945.

Bayley, N. (1969). *Bayley Scales of Infant Development.* New York: Psychological Corporation.

Bayley, N. (1993). *Bayley Scales of Infant Development* (2nd ed.). San Antonio, TX: Psychological Corporation.

Beardslee, W. R., Bemporad, J., Keller, M. B., & Klerman, G. L. (1983). Children of parents with major depressive disorder: A review. *American Journal of Psychiatry, 54,* 1254–1268.

Becerra, R. M., & Chi, I. (1992). Child care preferences among low-income minority families. *International Social Work, 35,* 35–47.

Beckwith, L. (1990). Adaptive and maladaptive parenting—implications for intervention. In S. J. Meisels & J. P. Shonkoff (Eds.), *Handbook of early intervention* (pp. 53–77). New York: Cambridge University Press.

Belsky, J. (1984). Two waves of day care research: Developmental effects and conditions of quality. In R. Ainslie (Ed.), *The child and the day care setting* (pp. 1–34). New York: Praeger.

Belsky, J. (1986). Infant day care: A cause for concern? *Zero to Three, 6,* 1–6.

Belsky, J. (1988). The "effects" of infant day care reconsidered. *Early Childhood Research Quarterly, 3,* 235–272.

Belsky, J. (1990a). Developmental risks associated with infant day care: Attachment insecurity, noncompliance and aggression? In S. Chehrazi (Ed.), *Psychosocial issues in day care* (pp. 37–68). Washington, DC: American Psychiatric Press.

Belsky, J. (1990b). Parental and nonparental child care and children's socioemotional development. *Journal of Marriage and the Family, 52,* 885–903.

Belsky, J. (1994, September). *The effects of infant day care: 1986–1994.* Invited plenary address to the British Psychological Association Division of Developmental Psychology, University of Portsmouth.

Belksy, J. (1999). Quantity of nonmaternal care and boys' problem behavior/adjustment at 3 and 5: Exploring the mediating role of parenting. *Psychiatry: Interpersonal and Biological Processes, 62,* 1–21.

Belsky, J. (2001). Developmental risks (still) associated with early child care. *Journal of Child Psychology and Psychiatry, 42,* 845–859.

Belsky, J., & Cassidy, J. (1994). Attachment: Theory and evidence. In M. Rutter, D. Hay, & S. Baron-Cohen (Eds.), *Developmental principles and clinical issues in psychology and psychiatry* (pp. 373–402). London: Blackwell.

Belsky, J., & Eggebeen, D. (1991). Early and extensive maternal employment and young children's socioemotional development: Children of the National Longitudinal Survey of Youth. *Journal of Marriage and Family, 53,* 1083–1110.

Belsky, J., & Most, R. (1981). From exploration to play: A cross-sectional study of infant free play behavior. *Developmental Psychology, 17,* 630–639.

Belsky, J., Rosenberger, K., & Crnic, K. (1995). The origins of attachment security: Classical and contextual determinants. In S. Goldberg, R. Muir, & J. Kerr (Eds.), *Attachment theory: Social, developmental and clinical perspectives* (pp. 153–184). Hillsdale, NJ: Analytic Press.

Belsky, J., & Rovine, M. J. (1988). Nonmaternal care in the first year of life and the security of infant–parent attachment. *Child Development, 59,* 157–167.

Belsky, J., & Steinberg, L. (1978). The effects of day-care: A critical review. *Child Development, 49,* 929–949.

Belsky, J., Woodworth, S., & Crnic, K. (1996). Trouble in the second year: Three questions about family interaction. *Child Development, 67,* 556–578.

Berk, L. E. (1985). Relationship of caregiver education to child-oriented attitudes, job satisfaction, and behaviors toward children. *Child Care Quarterly, 14,* 103–129.

Berndt, T., & Ladd, G. (Eds.). (1989). *Peer relationships in child development.* New York: Wiley.

Birch, S., & Ladd, G. (1997). The teacher–child relationship and children's early school adjustment. *Journal of School Psychology, 35,* 61–80.

Blau, D. (1999). The effects of child care characteristics on child development. *Journal of Human Resources, 34,* 786–822.

Bohlin, G., & Hagekull, B. (2000). Behavior problems in Swedish four-year-olds: The importance of maternal sensitivity and social context. In P. M. Crittenden & A. H. Claussen (Eds.), *The organization of attachment relationships: Maturation, culture, and context* (pp. 75–96). New York: Cambridge University Press.

Bolger, K. E., & Scarr, S. (1995). *Not so far from home: How family characteristics predict child care quality.* Unpublished manuscript. Charlottesville: University of Virginia.

Bollen, K. A. (1990). *Structural equations with latent variables.* New York: Wiley.

Booth, A. (Ed.). (1992). *Child care in the 1990s: Trends and consequences.* Hillsdale, NJ: Erlbaum.

Booth, A., Carver, K., & Granger, D. (2000). Biosocial perspectives on the family. *Journal of Marriage and the Family, 62,* 1018–1034.

Bornstein, M. H., & Tamis-LeMonda, C. S. (1989). Maternal responsiveness and cognitive development in children. In M. H. Bornstein (Ed.), *Maternal responsiveness: Characteristics and consequences. New directions for child development* (No. 43, pp. 49–61). San Francisco: Jossey-Bass.

Bowlby, J. (1973). *Separation: Anxiety and anger. Vol. 2: Attachment and loss.* New York: Basic Books.

Bracken, B. A. (1984). *Bracken Basic Concept Scale.* San Antonio, TX: Psychological Corporation.

Bradley, R. H. (1994). The HOME Inventory: Review and reflections. In H. Reese (Ed.), *Advances in child development and behavior* (pp. 241–288). San Diego, CA: Academic Press.

Bradley, R. H., & Caldwell, B. M. (1984). The relation of infants home environment to achievement test performance in first grade: A follow-up study. *Child Development, 55,* 803–809.

Bradley, R. H., Caldwell, B. M., Rock, S. L., Ramey, C., & Johnson, D. L. (1989). Home environment and cognitive development in the first 3 years of life: A collaborative study involving six sites and three ethnic groups in North America. *Developmental Psychology, 25,* 217–235.

Braiker, H., & Kelly, H. (1979). Conflict in the development of close relationships. *Developmental Psychology, 28,* 1048–1055.

Brayfield, A. A., Deich, S. G., & Hofferth, S. L. (1993). *Caring for children in low-income families: A substudy of the National Child Care Survey, 1990.* Washington, DC: The Urban Institute.

Brazelton, T. B. (1985). *Working and caring.* New York: Basic Books.

Brazelton, T. B. (1986). Issues for working parents. *American Journal of Orthopsychiatry, 56,* 14–25.

Bredekamp, S., & Glowacki, S. (1996). NAEYC accreditation. The first decade of NAEYC accreditation: Growth and impact on the field. *Young Children, 51,* 38–44.

Broberg, A., Wessels, H., Lamb, M., & Hwang, P. (1997). Effects of day care on the cognitive abilities in 8-year-olds. *Developmental Psychology, 33,* 62–69.

Bronfenbrenner, U. (1979). *The ecology of human development.* Cambridge, MA: Harvard University Press.

Bronfenbrenner, U. (1995). Developmental ecology through space and time: A future perspective. In P. Moen, G. H. Elder Jr., & K. Lscher (Eds.), *Examining lives in context: perspectives on the ecology of human development* (pp. 619–647). Washington, DC: American Psychological Association.

Bronfenbrenner, U. (1999). Environments in developmental perspective: theoretical and operational models. In S. L. Friedman & T. D. Wachs (Eds.), *Measuring environment across the life span: emerging methods and concepts* (pp. 3–28). Washington, DC: American Psychological Association.

Bronfenbrenner, U., & Crouter, A. C. (1982). Work and family through time and space. In S. B. Kamerman & C. D. Hayes (Eds.), *Families that work: Children in a changing world* (pp. 39–83). Washington, DC: National Academy Press.

Bronfenbrenner, U., & Morris, P. A. (1998). The ecology of developmental processes. In W. Damon (Series Ed.) & R. M. Lerner (Vol. Ed.), *Handbook of child psychology: Vol. 1. Theoretical models of human development* (5th ed., pp. 993–1028). New York: Wiley.

Brooks-Gunn, J., Duncan, G. J., & Maritato, N. (1997). Poor families, poor outcomes: The well-being of children and youth. In G. J. Duncan & J. Brooks-Gunn (Eds.), *Consequences of growing up poor* (pp. 1–17). New York: Russell Sage.

Browne, M. W., & Cudek, R. (1993). Alternative ways of assessing model fit. In K. A. Bollen & J. S. Long (Eds.), *Testing structural equation models* (pp. 136–162). Newbury Park, CA: Sage.

Brownell, C., & Brown, E. (1992). Peers and play in infants and toddlers. In V. Van Hasselt & M. Hersen (Eds.), *Handbook of social development* (pp. 183–200). New York: Plenum Press.

Bryk, A. S., & Raudenbush, S. W. (1987). Application of hierarchical linear models to assessing change. *Psychological Bulletin, 101*, 147–156.

Bryk, A. S., & Raudenbush, S. W. (1992). *Hierarchical linear models for social and behavioral research: applications and data analysis methods.* Newbury Park, CA: Sage.

Burchinal, M. R., Campbell, F. A., Bryant, D. M., Wasik, B. H., & Ramey, C. T. (1997). Early intervention and mediating processes in cognitive performance of children of low-income African-American families. *Child Development, 68,* 935–954.

Burchinal, M. R., Peisner-Feinberg, E., Bryant, D. M., & Clifford, R. (2000). Children's social and cognitive development and child care quality: Testing for differential associations related to poverty, gender, or ethnicity. *Applied Developmental Science, 4,* 149–165.

Burchinal, M., Roberts, J. E., Nabors, L. A., & Bryant, D. (1996). Quality of center child care and infant cognitive and language development. *Child Development, 67,* 606–620.

Bureau of Labor Statistics. (2000). Washington, DC: U.S. Department of Labor.

Caldwell, B. M., & Bradley, R. H. (1984). *Home Observation for Measurement of the Environment.* Little Rock: University of Arkansas at Little Rock.

Campbell, F. A., Pungello, E. P., Miller-Johnson, S., Burchinal, M. R., & Ramey, C. (2001). The development of cognitive and academic abilities: Growth curves from an early intervention educational experiment. *Developmental Psychology, 37,* 231–242.

Campbell, F. A., & Ramey, C. T. (1994). Effects of early intervention on intellectual and academic achievement: A follow-up study of children from low-income families. *Child Development, 65,* 684–698.

Campbell, S. B., Cohn, J. F., & Meyers, T. (1995). Depression in first-time mothers: Mother–infant interaction and depression chronicity. *Developmental Psychology, 31,* 349–357.

Carey, W., & McDevitt, S. (1978). Revision of the Infant Temperament Questionnaire. *Pediatrics, 61,* 735–739.

Carnegie Corporation. (1994). *Starting points: Meeting the needs of our youngest children.* New York: Author.

Casper, L. M. (1995). *What does it cost to mind our preschoolers?* Washington, DC: U.S. Bureau of the Census.

Casper, L. M. (1996). Who's minding our preschoolers? *Current Population Reports* (Series 70, No. 53). Washington, DC: U.S. Bureau of the Census.

Casper, L. M., Hawkins, M., & O'Connell, M. (1994). *Who's minding the kids? Child care arrangements, Fall 1991.* Washington, DC: U.S. Bureau of the Census.

Cassidy, J., Marvin, R. S., & MacArthur Attachment Working Group. (1992). *Attachment organization in preschool children: Procedures and coding manual.* Unpublished coding manual, Pennsylvania State University.

Caughy, M., DiPietro, J. A., & Strobino, D. M. (1994). Day care participation as a protective factor in the cognitive development of low-income children. *Child Development, 65,* 457–471.

Chilman, C. S. (1993). Parental employment and childcare trends: Some critical issues and suggested policies. *Social Work, 38,* 451–460.

Chin-Quee, D. S., & Scarr, S. (1994). Lack of early child care effects on school-age children's social competence and academic achievement. *Early Development and Parenting, 3,* 103–112.

Churchill, R., & Pickering, L. (1997, October). *Health issues in the context of out-of-home child care: diarrheal disease in infants and toddlers.* Paper presented at the first synthesis conference of the National Center for Early Development and Learning, Chapel Hill, NC.

Cillessen, A. H. N., Terry, R. A., Coie, J. D., & Lochman, J. E. (1998). *Accuracy of teacher-identification of children's sociometric status positions.* Unpublished manuscript, University of Connecticut.

Clark, R., Hyde, J., Essex, M., & Klein, M. (1997). Length of maternity leave and quality of mother–infant interactions. *Child Development, 68,* 364–383.

Clarke-Stewart, K. A. (1986). Family day care: A home away from home? *Children's Environment Quarterly, 3,* 34–46.

Clarke-Stewart, K. A. (1987). Predicting child development from child care forms and features: The Chicago study. In D. Phillips (Ed.), *Quality in child care: what does research tell us?* (pp. 21–42). Washington, DC: National Association for the Education of Young Children.

Clarke-Stewart, K. A. (1988). The effects of infant day care reconsidered: Risks for parents, children, and researchers. *Early Childhood Research Quarterly, 3,* 293–318.

Clarke-Stewart, K. A. (1989). Infant day-care: Maligned or malignant? *American Psychologist, 44,* 266–273.

Clarke-Stewart, K. A. (1993). *Daycare.* Cambridge, MA: Harvard University Press.

Clarke-Stewart, K. A., & Allhusen, V. (2002). Nonparental caregiving. In M. H. Bornstein (Ed.), *Handbook of parenting* (2nd ed., Vol. 3, pp. 215–252). Mahwah, NJ: Erlbaum.

Clarke-Stewart, K., & Fein, G. (1983). Early childhood programs. In P. H. Mussen (Gen. Ed.) and M. Haith & J. Campos (Vol. Eds.), *Handbook of child psychology: Vol. 2. Infancy and developmental psychobiology* (pp. 917–999). New York: Wiley.

Clarke-Stewart, K. A., Gruber, C. P., & Fitzgerald, L. M. (1994). *Children at home and in day care.* Hillsdale, NJ: Erlbaum.

Clarke-Stewart, K. A., Vandell, D. L., Burchinal, M., O'Brien, M., & McCartney, K. (2002). Do regulable features of child care homes affect children's development? *Early Childhood Research Quarterly, 17,* 52–86.

Cohen, J. (1988). *Statistical power analysis for the behavioral sciences* (2nd ed.). Hillsdale, NJ: Erlbaum.

Cohen, J., & Cohen, P. (1983). *Applied multiple regression/correlation analysis for the behavioral sciences* (2nd ed.). New York: Erlbaum.

Cohn, J. F., & Campbell, S. B. (1992). Influence of maternal depression on infant affect regulation. In D. Cicchetti & S. Toth (Eds.), *Rochester symposium on developmental psychopathology, Vol. 4: A developmental approach to affective disorders* (pp. 103–130). Rochester, NY: University of Rochester Press.

Cohn, J. F., Campbell, S. B., Matias, R., & Hopkins, J. (1990). Face-to-face interactions of postpartum depressed and nondepressed mother–infant pairs at 2 months. *Developmental Psychology, 26,* 15–23.

Coie, J., Terry, R., Lenox, K., & Lochman, J. (1995). Childhood peer rejection and aggression as predictors of stable adolescent disorder. *Development and Psychopathology, 7,* 697–713.

Collier, A., & Henderson, F. (1997, October). *Respiratory disease in infants and toddlers.* Paper presented at the first synthesis conference of the National Center for Early Development and Learning, Chapel Hill, NC.

Collins, W. A., Maccoby, E. E., Steinberg, L., Hetherington, E. M., & Bornstein, M. H. (2000). Contemporary research on parenting. *American Psychologist, 55,* 218–232.

Conger, R. D., Conger, K. J., & Elder, G. (1997). Family economic hardship and adolescent academic performance: Mediating and moderating processes. In G. J. Duncan & J. Brooks-Gunn (Eds.), *Consequences of growing up poor* (pp. 288–310). New York: Russell Sage.

Corcoran, M. E., & Chaudry, A. (1997). The dynamics of childhood poverty. *Future of Children, 7,* 40–54.

Costa, P. T., & McCrae, R. R. (1985). *The NEO Personality Inventory manual.* Odessa, FL: Psychological Assessment Resources.

Costa, P. T., & McCrae, C. C. (1989). *The NEO Five Factor Inventory.* Odessa, FL: Psychological Assessment Resources.

Cotterell, J. I. (1986). Work and community influences on the quality of child rearing. *Child Development, 57,* 362–374.

Courville, T., & Thompson, B. (2001). Use of structure coefficients in published multiple regression articles: β is not enough. *Educational and Psychological Measurement, 61,* 229–248.

Crittenden, P. M. (2000). A dynamic-maturational approach to continuity and change in pattern of attachment. In P. M. Crittenden & A. H. Claussen (Eds.), *The organization of attachment relationships: Maturation, culture, and context* (pp. 343–357). New York: Cambridge University Press.

Crockenberg, S., & Litman, C. (1990). Autonomy as competence in 2-year-olds: Maternal correlates of child defiance, compliance, and self-assertion. *Developmental Psychology, 26,* 961–971.

Crockenberg, S., & Litman, C. (1991). Effects of maternal employment on maternal and two-year-old child behavior. *Child Development, 62,* 930–953.

Cummings, E. M., & Cicchetti, D. (1990). Towards a transactional model of relations between attachment and depression. In M. T. Greenberg, D. Cicchetti, & E. M. Cummings (Eds.), *Attachment in the preschool years: Theory, research, and intervention* (pp. 339–372). Chicago: University of Chicago Press.

Cummings, E. M., & Davies, P. T. (1994). Maternal depression and child development. *Journal of Child Psychology and Psychiatry, 35,* 73–112.

Currie, J. (2000). *Early childhood intervention programs: What do we know?* (Working paper from the Children's Roundtable). Washington, DC: Brookings Institution.

Currie, J., & Thomas, D. (1995). Does Head Start make a difference? *The American Economic Review, 85,* 341–364.

Demchak, M., Kontos, S., & Neisworth, J. T. (1992). Using a pyramid model to teach management procedures to childcare providers. *Topics in Early Childhood Special Education, 12*, 458–477.

DeMeis, D. K., Hock, E., & McBride, S. L. (1986). Balance of employment and mother-hood: Longitudinal study of mothers feelings about separation from their first born infants. *Developmental Psychology, 22*, 627–632.

DeMulder, E. K., & Radke-Yarrow, M. (1991). Attachment with affectively ill and well mothers: Concurrent behavioral correlates. *Development and Psychopathology, 3*, 227–242.

Desai, S. P., Chase-Lansdale, P. L., & Michael, R. T. (1989). Mother or market? Effects of maternal employment on the intellectual ability of 4-year-old children. *Demography, 26*, 545–561.

Dettling, A., Gunnar, M., & Donzella, B. (1999). Cortisol levels of young children in full-day child care centers. *Psychoneuroendocrinology, 24*, 519–536.

Deutsch, M. (1967). *An evaluation of the effectiveness of an enriched curriculum in overcoming the consequences of environmental deprivation.* New York: Institute for Developmental Studies, New York University.

Dinnebeil, L. A., McInerney, W., Fox, C., & Juchartz-Pendry, K. (1998). An analysis of the perceptions and characteristics of child care personnel regarding inclusion of young children with special needs in community-based programs. *Topics in Early Childhood Special Education, 18*, 118–128.

Doherty, W. J., Kouneski, E. F., & Erickson, M. F. (1998). Responsible fathering: An over-view and conceptual framework. *Journal of Marriage and the Family, 60*, 277–292.

Duncan, G. J., & Brooks-Gunn, J. (1997). Income effects across the life span: Integration and interpretation. In G. J. Duncan & J. Brooks-Gunn (Eds.), *Consequences of growing up poor* (pp. 596–610). New York: Russell Sage.

Duncan, G. J., & Brooks-Gunn, J. (2000). Family poverty, welfare reform, and child devel-opment. *Child Development, 71*, 188–196.

Duncan, G. J., Yeung, W. J., Brooks-Gunn, J., & Smith, J. R. (1998). How much does childhood poverty affect the life chances of children? *American Sociological Review, 63*, 406–423.

Dunham, P., & Dunham, F. (1992). Lexical development during middle infancy: A mutu-ally driven infant–caregiver process. *Developmental Psychology, 28*, 414–420.

Dunn, L. (1993). Proximal and distal features of day care quality and children's develop-ment. *Early Childhood Research Quarterly, 8*, 167–192.

Dunn, L. M., & Dunn, L. M. (1981). *Peabody Picture Vocabulary Test–Revised.* Circle Pines, MN: American Guidance Service.

Ebb, N. (1994). *Child care tradeoffs: States make painful choices.* Washington, DC: Children's Defense Fund.

Edwards, C. P., Logue, M. E., Loehr, S., & Roth, S. (1986). The influence of model infant–toddler group care on parent–child interaction at home. *Early Childhood Research Quarterly, 1*, 317–332.

Egeland, B., & Hiester, M. (1995). The long-term consequences of infant day-care and mother–infant attachment. *Child Development, 66*, 474–485.

Eichman, C., & Hofferth, S. (1993, April). *Family strategies for managing work and family life.* Paper presented at the meeting of the Population Association of America, Cincinnati, OH.

Elder, G., Van Nguyen, T., & Caspi, A. (1985). Linking family hardship to children's lives. *Child Development, 56*, 361–375.

Elder, G. H., Jr. (1998). The life course and human development. In W. Damon (Series Ed.) & R. M. Lerner (Vol. Ed.), *Handbook of child psychology: Vol. 1. Theoretical models of human development* (5th ed., pp. 939–991). New York: Wiley.

Elder, G. H., Jr. (1999). *Children of the great depression: social change in life experience* (25th anniversary ed.). Boulder, CO: Westview Press.

Elicker, J., & Fortner-Wood, C. (1995). Adult–child relationships in early childhood programs. *Young Children, 51,* 69–78.

Elicker, J., Noppe, I. C., Noppe, L. D., & Fortner-Wood, C. (1997). The parent–caregiver relationship scale: Rounding out the relationship system in infant child care. *Early Education and Development, 8,* 83–100.

Elman, J. L., Bates, E. A., Johnson, M. H., Karmiloff-Smith, A., Parisi, D., & Plunkett, K. (1996). *Rethinking innateness.* Boston: MIT Press.

Entwisle, D. R., Alexander, K. L., & Olson, L. S. (1997). *Children, schools, and inequality.* Boulder, CO: Westview Press.

Erdwins, C. J., & Buffardi, L. C. (1994). Different types of day care and their relationship to maternal satisfaction, perceived support, and role conflict. *Child and Youth Care Forum, 23,* 41–54.

Fabes, R. A., Martin, C. L., Hanish, L. D., & Updegraff, K. A. (2000). Criteria for evaluating the significance of developmental research in the twenty-first century: Force and counterforce. *Child Development, 71,* 212–221.

Fagot, B. I., & Pears, K. C. (1996). Changes in attachment during the third year: Consequences and predictions. *Development and Psychopathology, 8,* 325–344.

Feagans, L. V., & Farran, D. C. (1983). *The Adaptive Language Inventory.* Chapel Hill: University of North Carolina, Frank Porter Graham Child Development Center.

Feagans, L. V., Fendt, K., & Farran, D. C. (1995). The effects of day care intervention on teachers ratings of the elementary school discourse skills in disadvantaged children. *International Journal of Behavioral Development, 18,* 243–261.

Fein, G. G., & Fox, N. (1988). Infant day care: A special issue. *Early Childhood Research Quarterly, 3,* 227–234.

Fenson, L., Dale, P. S., Reznick, J. S., Bates, E., Thal, D. J., & Pethick, S. J. (1994). Variability in early communicative development. *Monographs of the Society for Research in Child Development, 59*(Serial No. 173).

Feshbach, L. E. (1989). *Aggression-conduct problems, attention-deficits, hyperactivity, play, and social cognition in four year old boys.* Unpublished doctoral dissertation, University of Washington, Seattle.

Field, T. (1991). Quality infant day care and grade school behavior and performance. *Child Development, 62,* 863–870.

Field, T. M. (1992). Infants of depressed mothers. *Development and Psychopathology, 4,* 49–66.

Field, T., Masi, W., Goldstein, S., Perry, S., & Park, S. (1988). Infant day care facilitates preschool social behavior. *Early Childhood Research Quarterly, 3,* 341–359.

Flanagan, C. A., & Eccles, J. S. (1993). Changes in parents work status and adolescents adjustment at school. *Child Development, 64,* 246–257.

Ford, D. H., & Lerner, R. M. (1992). *Developmental system theory: An integrative approach.* Newbury Park, CA: Sage.

Fosburg, S. (1981). *Family day care in the United Stoles. National Day Care Home Study: Vol. 1. Summary of findings* (DHHS Publication No. OHDS 80-30282). Washington, DC: U.S. Department of Health and Human Services.

Fosburg, S., Hawkins, P. D., Singer, J. D., Goodson, B. D., Smith, J. M., & Brush, L. R. (1980). *National Day Care Home Study.* Cambridge, MA: Abt.

Fox, N., & Fein, G. (1990). *Infant day-care: The current debate.* Norwood, NJ: Ablex.

Fraley, R. C. (1999). *Attachment continuity from infancy to adulthood: Meta-analysis and dynamic modeling of developmental mechanisms.* Unpublished doctoral dissertation, University of California, Davis.

Freedman, R., Litchfield, L., & Warfield, M. E. (1995). Balancing work and family responsibilities: Perspectives of parents of children with developmental disabilities. *Families in Society: Journal of Contemporary Human Services, 76,* 507–514.

Friedman, S., & Amadeo, J. (1999). The child care environment: Conceptualizations, assessments, and issues. In S. L. Friedman & T. D. Wachs (Eds.), *Measuring environment across the lifespan* (pp. 127–165). Washington, DC: American Psychological Association.

Friedman, S. L., & Cocking, R. R. (1986). Instructional influences on cognition and on the brain. In S. L. Friedman, K. A. Klivington, & R. W. Peterson (Eds.), *The brain, cognition, and education* (pp. 319–346). New York: Academic Press.

Frodi, A., Grolnick, W., & Bridges, L. (1985). Maternal correlates of stability and change in infant–mother attachment. *Infant Mental Health Journal, 6,* 60–67.

Fuller, B., Holloway, S. D., & Liang, X. (1995). *Which families use nonparental child care and centers? The influence of family structure, ethnicity, and parental practices.* Cambridge, MA: Department of Human Development and Psychology, Harvard University.

Galambos, N. L., & Silbereisen, R. K. (1987). Income change, parental life outlook, and adolescent expectations for job success. *Journal of Marriage and the Family, 49,* 141–149.

Galinsky, E. (1988). Parents and teacher-caregivers: Sources of tension, sources of support. *Young Children, 43,* 2–39.

Galinsky, E., Howes, C., Kontos, S., & Shinn, M. (1994). *The study of children in family child care and relative care: Highlights of findings.* New York: Families and Work Institute.

Galluzzo, D., Matheson, C., Moore, J., & Howes, C. (1990). Social orientation to adults and peers in infant day care. In N. Fox & G. Fein (Eds.), *Infant day care: The current debate* (pp. 183–192). Norwood, NJ: Ablex.

Garcia Coll, C., Lamberty, G., Jenkins, R., McAdoo, H. P., Crnick, K., Wasik B. H., & Garcia, H. V. (1996). An integrative model for the study of developmental competencies in minority children. *Child Development, 67,* 1891–1914.

Gelfand, D. M., & Teti, D. M. (1990). The effects of maternal depression on children. *Clinical Psychology Review, 10,* 329–353.

Gerstadt, C. L., Hong, Y. J., & Diamond, A. (1994). The relationship between cognition and action: performance of children 3½–7 years old on a Stroop-like day–night test. *Cognition, 53,* 129–153.

Goelman, H., & Pence, A. (1987). Effects of child care, family, and individual characteristics on children's language development. In D. Phillips (Ed.), *Quality in child care: What does research tell us?* (pp. 89–104). Washington, DC: National Association for the Education of Young Children.

Gold, D., & Andres, D. (1980). Maternal employment and development of 10-year-old Canadian Francophone children. *Canadian Journal of Behavioral Science, 12,* 233–240.

Gottfried, A. E., Gottfried, A. W., & Bathurst, K. (1995). Maternal and dual-earner employment status and parenting. In M. H. Bornstein (Ed.), *Handbook of parenting: Vol. 2. Biology and ecology of parenting* (pp. 139–160). Mahwah, NJ: Erlbaum.

Greenberger, E., & Goldberg, S. (1989). Work, parenting, and the socialization of children. *Developmental Psychology, 25,* 22–35.

Greenberger, E., Goldberg, W., Crawford, T. J., & Granger, J. (1988). Beliefs about the consequences of maternal employment for children. *Psychology of Women Quarterly, 12,* 35–59.

Greenspan, S. I. (1997, October 19). The reasons why we need to rely less on day care. *Washington Post,* pp. CI–C2.

Greenstein, T. (1993). Maternal employment and child behavioral outcomes: A household economics analysis. *Journal of Family Issues, 14,* 323–354.

Gresham, F., & Elliott, S. (1990). *The Social Skills Rating System.* Circle Pines, MN: American Guidance Service.

Gunnar, M., Mangelsdorf, S., Larsen, M., & Herstgaard, L. (1998). Attachment, temperament, and adrenocortical activity in infancy. *Developmental Psychology, 25,* 355–363.

Halperin, J. M., Sharma, V., Greenblatt, E., & Schwartz, S. T. (1991). Assessment of the continuous performance test: Reliability and validity in a nonreferred sample. *Journal of Consulting and Clinical Psychology, 3*, 603–608.

Hamre, B., & Pianta, R. C. (2001). Early teacher–child relationships and the trajectory of children's school outcomes through eighth grade. *Child Development, 72*, 625–638.

Hanson, S. M. H., Heims, M. L., Julian, D. J., & Sussman, M. B. (1995). Single parent families: Present and future perspectives. *Marriage and Family Review, 20*, 1–26.

Harms, T., & Clifford, R. (1980). *Early childhood environmental rating scale.* New York: Teachers College Press, Columbia University.

Harms, T., & Clifford, R. (1984). *The family day care raring scale.* New York: Teachers College Press, Columbia University.

Hart, B., & Risley, T. R. (1995). *Meaningful differences in the everyday experience of young American children.* Baltimore: Brookes.

Hartup, W. (1983). Peer relations. In P. Mussen & E. Hetherington (Eds.), *Handbook of child psychology: Vol. 4. Socialization, personality, and social development* (pp. 103–196). New York: Wiley.

Hartup, W. (1996). The company they keep: Friendships and their developmental significance. *Child Development, 67*, 1–13.

Haskins, R. (1985). Public school aggression among children with varying day-care experience. *Child Development, 56*, 689–703.

Hayes, C. D., Palmer, J. L., & Zaslow, M. J. (Eds.). (1990). *Who cares for America's children? Child care policy for the 1990's.* Washington, DC: National Academies Press.

Helburn, S. W., (Ed.). (1995). *Cost, quality, and child outcomes in child care centers.* (Tech. Rep.). Denver: University of Colorado at Denver, Department of Economics.

Herman, S. E., & Thompson, L. (1995). Families' perceptions of their resources for caring for children with developmental disabilities. *Mental Retardation, 33*, 73–83.

Hock, E., DeMeis, D., & McBride, S. (1988). Maternal separation anxiety: Its role in the balance of employment and motherhood in mothers of infants. In A. E. Gottfried & A. W. Gottfried (Eds.), *Maternal employment and children's development: Longitudinal research* (pp. 191–229). New York: Plenum Press.

Hock, E., Gnezda, M., & McBride, S. (1983, April). *The measurement of maternal separation anxiety.* Paper presented at the biennial meeting of the Society for Research in Child Development, Detroit, MI.

Hoff-Ginsberg, E. (1991). Mother–child conversation in different social classes and communication settings. *Child Development, 62*, 782–796.

Hofferth, S. L. (1995). Caring for children at the poverty line. *Children and Youth Services Review, 17*, 1–31.

Hofferth, S. L. (1996). Child care in the United States today. *Future of Children, 6*, 41–61.

Hofferth, S. L., Brayfield, A., Deich, S., & Holcomb, P. (1991). *National child care survey, 1990.* Washington, DC: Urban Institute Press.

Hofferth, S. L., Shauman, K. A., Henke, R. R., & West, J. (1998). *Characteristics of children's early care and education programs: Data from the 1995 National Household Education Survey, National Center for Education Statistics, 98–118.* Washington, DC: U.S. Department of Education.

Hofferth, S. L., & Wissoker, D. A. (1992). Price, quality, and income in child care choice. *Journal of Human Resources, 27*, 70–111.

Hoffman, H., Overpeck, M., & Hildesheim, J. (1996). Factors in the United States affecting risk of frequent ear infections, deafness, or trouble hearing and related conditions. *Proceedings of the Sixth International Symposium on Recent Advances in Otitis Media* (pp. 71–75). Hamilton, ON, Canada: BC Decker.

Hoffman, L. W. (1989). Effects of maternal employment in the two-parent family. *American Psychologist, 44*, 283–292.

Hogan, A. E., Scott, K. G., & Bauer, C. R. (1992). The Adaptive Social Behavior Inventory (ASBI): A new assessment of social competence in high-risk three-year-olds. *Journal of Psychoeducational Assessment, 10*, 230–239.

Hojat, M. (1990). Can affectional ties be purchased? Comments on working mothers and their families. *Journal of Social Behavior and Personality, 5*, 493–502.

Horner, M., Rawlins, P., & Giles, K. (1987). How parents of children with chronic conditions perceive their own needs. *American Journal of Maternal Child Nursing, 12*, 40–43.

Hosmer, D. W., & Lemeshow, S. (1989). *Applied logistic regression.* New York: Wiley.

Howes, C. (1983). Caregiver behavior in centers and family day care. *Journal of Applied Developmental Psychology, 4*, 99–107.

Howes, C. (1988a). Peer interaction of young children. *Monographs of the Society for Research in Child Development, 53* (1, Serial No. 217).

Howes, C. (1988b). Relations between early child care and schooling. *Developmental Psychology, 25*, 53–57.

Howes, C. (1990). Can the age of entry into child care and the quality of child care predict adjustment in kindergarten? *Developmental Psychology, 26*, 292–303.

Howes, C. (1997). Children's experiences in center-based child care as a function of caregiver background and adult:child ratio. *Merrill-Palmer Quarterly, 43*, 404–425.

Howes, C., Galluzzo, D., Hamilton, C., Matheson, C., & Rodning, C. (1989, April). *Social relationships with adults and peers within child care and families.* Paper presented at the biennial meetings of the Society for Research in Child Development, Kansas City, MO.

Howes, C., & Hamilton, C. E. (1993). The changing experience of child care: Changes in teachers and in teacher–child relationships and children's social competence with peers. *Early Childhood Research Quarterly, 8*, 1532.

Howes, C., Matheson, C., & Hamilton, C. (1994). Maternal, teacher, and child care history correlates of children's relationships with peers. *Child Development, 65*, 264–273.

Howes, C., & Olenick, M. (1986). Family and child care influences on toddler's compliance. *Child Development, 57*, 202–216.

Howes, C., Phillips, D., & Whitebook, M. (1992). Thresholds of quality: Implications for the social development of children in center-based child care. *Child Development, 63*, 449–460.

Howes, C., Smith, E., & Galinsky, E. (1995). *The Florida child care quality improvement study.* New York: Families and Work Institute.

Howes, C., & Stewart, P. (1987). Child's play with adults, peers, and toys. *Developmental Psychology, 23*, 423–430.

Hu, L., & Bentler, P. M. (1999). Cutoff criteria for fit indexes in covariance structure analysis: Conventional criteria versus new alternatives. *Equation Modeling, 6*, 1–55.

Hurwitz, E., Gunn, W., Pinsky, P., & Shonberger, L. (1991). Risk of respiratory illness associated with day care attendance: A nationwide study. *Pediatrics, 87*, 62–69.

Huston, A. C., McLoyd, V. C., & Garcia Coll, C. (1994). Children and poverty: Issues in contemporary research. *Child Development, 65*, 275–282.

Hyson, M. C., Hirsh-Pasek, K. and Rescorla, L. (1990). An observation instrument based on NAEYC's guidelines for developmentally appropriate practices for 4- and 5-year-old children. *Early Childhood Research Quarterly 5*, 475–494.

Jaeger, E., & Weinraub, M. (1990). Early maternal care and infant attachment: In search of process. In K. McCartney (Ed.), *Child care and maternal employment: A social ecology approach* (pp. 71–90). San Francisco: Jossey-Bass.

Jeffrey, R. (1989). Risk behaviors and health: Contrasting individual and population perspectives. *American Psychologist, 44*, 1194–1202.

Jenrich, R. I., & Schluchter, M. (1986). Unbalanced repeated-measures models with structured covariance matrices. *Biometrics, 42*, 805–820.

Johnson, D. J., Chung, K. J., & Levy, M. (1998). *Ethnic preferences and Euro-American children presented with three representations of ethnic minority groups.* Unpublished manuscript, University of Wisconsin–Madison.

Jöreskog, K., & Sörbom, D. (1993). *LISREL: Analysis of linear structural relationship by the method of maximum likelihood*. Chicago: National Educational Resources.

Kagan, J. (1984). *The nature of the child*. New York: Basic Books.

Kamerman, S. (2000). Parental leave policies: An essential ingredient in early childhood education and care policies. *Social Policy Report, 14*, 3–15.

Karen, R. (1994). *Becoming attached*. New York: Warner.

Kisker, E. E., Hofferth, S. L., Phillips, D. A., & Farquhar, E. (1991). *A profile of child care settings: Early education and care in 1990* (Final report for U.S. Department of Education, Rep. No. LC88090001). Princeton, NJ: Mathematics.

Klaus, R., & Gray, S. (1968). The Early Training Project for Disadvantaged Children: A report after five years. *Monographs of the Society for Research in Child Development, 33*(4, Serial No. 120).

Kochanska, G. (1991). Socialization and temperament in the development of guilt and conscience. *Child Development, 62*, 1379–1392.

Kontos, S. (1987). The attitudinal context of family-day care relationships. In D. L. Peters & S. Kontos (Eds.), *Continuity and discontinuity of experience in child care. Annual advances in applied developmental psychology* (pp. 91–113). Norwood, NJ: Ablex.

Kontos, S., & Dunn, L. (1989). Attitudes of caregivers, maternal experiences with day care, and children's development. *Journal of Applied Developmental Psychology, 10*, 37–51.

Kontos, S., & Wells, W. (1986). Attitudes of caregivers and the day care experiences of families. *Early Childhood Research Quarterly, 1*, 47–67.

Kopp, C. B. (1989). Regulation of distress and negative emotions: A developmental view. *Developmental Psychology, 25*, 343–354.

Kopp, C. B. (1997). Young children: Emotion management, instrumental control, and plans. In S. L. Friedman & E. K. Scholnick (Eds.), *Why, how, and when do we plan? The developmental psychology of planning* (pp. 103–124). Hillsdale, NJ: Erlbaum.

Kotch, J., & Bryant, D. (1990). Effects of day care on the health and development of children. *Current Opinion in Pediatrics, 2*, 883–894.

Kramer, U., Wjst, J., & Wichman, H. E. (1993). Age of entry to day nursery and allergy in later childhood. *Lancet, 353*, 450–454.

Ladd, G. W. (1983). Social networks of popular, average, and rejected children in school settings. *Merrill-Palmer Quarterly, 29*, 283–307.

Laird, N. M., & Ware, J. H. (1982). Random-effects models for longitudinal data. *Biometrics, 38*, 963–974.

Lamb, M. E. (Ed.). (1997). *The role of the father in child development* (3rd ed.). New York: Wiley.

Lamb, M. E. (1998). Nonparental child care: Context, quality, correlates, and consequences. In W. Damon (Series Ed.) & I. E. Sigel & K. A. Renninger (Vol. Eds.), *Handbook of child psychology: Vol. 4. Child psychology in practice* (5th ed., pp. 73–133). New York: Wiley.

Lamb, M. E., & Easterbrooks, M. A. (1981). Individual differences in parental sensitivity: Origins, components, and consequences. In M. E. Lamb & L. R. Sherrod (Eds.), *Infant social cognition: Empirical and theoretical considerations*. Hillsdale, NJ: Erlbaum.

Lamb, M., & Sternberg, K. (1990). Do we really know how day-care affects children? *Journal of Applied Developmental Psychology, 11*, 351–379.

Landis, L. J. (1992). Marital, employment, and childcare status of mothers with infants and toddlers with disabilities. *Topics in Early Childhood Special Education, 12*, 496–507.

Laughlin, T. (1995). The school readiness composite of the Bracken Basic Concept Scale as an intellectual screening instrument. *Journal of Psychoeducational Assessment, 13*, 294–302.

Lazar, I., & Darlington, R. (1982). Lasting effects of early education: A report from the

Consortium for Longitudinal Studies. *Monographs of the Society for Research in Child Development, 47*(2–3, Serial No. 195).

Lazar, I., Darlington, R., Murray, H., Royce, J., & Snipper, A. (1982). Lasting effects of early education. *Monographs of the Society for Research in Child Development, 47*(Serial No. 195).

Lazarus, R. S. (1991). *Emotion and adaptation.* New York: Oxford University Press.

Leach, P. (1994). *Children first: What our society must do–and is doing–for our children today.* New York: Knopf.

Lee, M., & Burchinal, M. (1987). *Children of poverty: A multi-level analysis of the determinants of intellectual development.* Chapel Hill: University of North Carolina, Frank Porter Graham Child Development Center.

Lehrer, E. (1983). Determinants of child-care mode choice: An economic perspective. *Social Science Research, 12,* 69–80.

Leibowitz, A., Klerman, L. A., & Waite, L. J. (1992). Employment of new mothers and child care choice: Differences by children's age. *Journal of Human Resources, 27,* 112–133.

Levine, S., Elzey, F. F., & Lewis, M. (1969). *California Preschool Social Competency Scale.* Palo Alto, CA: Consulting Psychologists Press.

Lewis, M., & Michalson, L. (1983). *Children's emotions and moods.* New York: Plenum Press.

Liang, K. Y., & Zeger, S. L. (1986). Longitudinal data analysis using generalized linear models. *Biometrika, 73,* 13–22.

Little, R. J. A., & Rubin, D. (1987). *Statistical analysis with missing data.* New York: Wiley.

Louhiala, P., & Jaakkola, N., Ruotsalainen, R., & Jaakkola, J. (1997). Day care centers and diarrhea: a public health perspective. *Journal of Pediatrics, 131,* 476–479.

Love, J. M., Schochet, P. Z., & Meckstroth, A. L. (1996). *Are they in any real danger? What research does–and doesn't–tell us about child care quality and children's well-being.* Princeton, NJ: Mathematica Policy Research.

Luster, T., & McAdoo, H. (1996). Family and child influences on educational attainment: A secondary analysis of the High/Scope Perry preschool data. *Developmental Psychology, 32,* 26–39.

Maccoby, E. E., & Martin, J. (1983). Socialization in the context of the family: Parent–child interaction. In E. M. Hetherington (Ed.) & P. H. Mussen (Series Ed.), *Handbook of child psychology: Vol. 4. Socialization, personality, and social development* (pp. 1–101). New York: Wiley.

Macrae, J., & Herbert-Jackson, E. (1976). Brief reports: Are behavioral effects of infant day care program specific? *Developmental Psychology, 12,* 269–270.

Main, M., & Solomon, J. (1990). Procedures for identifying disorganized/disoriented infants in the Ainsworth Strange Situation. In M. Greenberg, D. Cicchetti, & M. Cummings (Eds.), *Attachment in the preschool years: Theory, research, and intervention* (pp. 121–160). Chicago: University of Chicago Press.

Marshall, N. L., & Barnett, R. C. (1991). Race and class and multiple role strains and gains among women employed in the service sector. *Women and Health, 17,* 1–19.

Marshall, N. L., & Barnett, R. C. (1993). Work–family strains and gains among two-earner couples. *Journal of Community Psychology, 21,* 64–78.

Marvin, R. S. (1977). An ethological–cognitive model for the attenuation of mother–child attachment behavior. In T. M. Alloway, L. Krames, & P. Piner (Eds.), *Advances in the study of communication and affect: Vol. 3. The development of social attachments* (pp. 25–60). New York: Plenum Press.

McBride, S., & Belsky, J. (1988). Characteristics, determinants, and consequences of maternal separation anxiety. *Developmental Psychology, 24,* 407–414.

McCartney, K. (1984). The effect of quality of day care environment upon children's language development. *Developmental Psychology, 20,* 244–260.

McCartney, K., & Galanoupoulos, A. (1988). Child care and attachment: A new frontier the second time around. *American Journal of Orthopsychiatry, 58*, 16–24.

McCartney, K., & Phillips, D. (1988). Motherhood and child care. In B. Birns & D. Hay (Eds.), *The different faces of motherhood* (pp. 157–183). New York: Plenum Press.

McCartney, K., & Rosenthal, S. (1991). Maternal employment should be studied within social ecologies. *Journal of Marriage and the Family, 53*, 1103–1106.

McCartney, K., & Rosenthal, R. (2000). Effect size, practical importance, and social policy for children. *Child Development, 71*, 173–180.

McCartney, K., Scarr, S., Phillips, D., Grajek, S., & Schwartz, J. C. (1982). Environmental differences among day-care centers and their effects on children's development. In E. F. Zigler & E. W. Gordon (Eds.), *Daycare: Scientific and social policy issues.* Boston: Auburn House.

McGurk, H., Caplan, M., Hennessy, E., Martin, S., & Moss, P. (1993). Controversy, theory, and social context in contemporary day care research. *Journal of Child Psychology and Psychiatry 34*, 3–23.

McKey, R. H., Condelli, L., Ganson, H., Barrett, B., McConkey, C., & Plantz, M. (1985). *The impact of Head Start on children, families, and communities: Final report of the Head Start evaluation, synthesis, and utilization project.* Washington, DC: US Department of Health and Human Services.

McLoyd, V. C. (1990). The impact of economic hardship on black families and children: Psychological distress, parenting, and socioemotional development. *Child Development, 61*, 311–346.

McLoyd, V. C. (1997). Children in poverty: Development, public policy, and practice. In W. Damon, I. E. Sigel, & K. A. Renninger (Eds.), *Handbook of child psychology: Vol. 4. Child psychology in practice* (5th ed., pp. 135–210). New York: Wiley.

McLoyd, V. C. (1998). Socioeconomic disadvantage and child development. *American Psychologist, 53*, 185–204.

McLoyd, V. C., Jayaratne, T. E., Ceballo, R., & Borquez, J. (1994). Unemployment and work interruption among African American single mothers: Effects on parenting and adolescent socioemotional functioning. *Child Development, 65*, 562–589.

Medoff-Cooper, B., Carey, W. B., & McDevitt, S. C. (1993). Early Infancy Temperament Questionnaire. *Journal of Developmental and Behavioral Pediatrics, 14*, 230–235.

Melhuish, E. C., Mooney, A., Hennesy, E., & Martin, S. (1992, September). *Characteristics of child care in early childhood and child development in middle childhood.* Paper presented at the European Conference on Developmental Psychology in Seville, Spain.

Messer, D. (1994). *The development of communication: From social interaction to language.* New York: Wiley.

Meyers, M. K., and van Leuwen, K. (1992). Child care preferences and choices: Are AFDC recipients unique? *Social Work Research and Abstracts, 28*, 28–34.

Mischel, W., Ebbesen, E., & Zeiss, A. (1972). Cognitive and attentional mechanisms in delay of gratification. *Journal of Personality and Social Psychology, 21*, 204–218.

Morison, P., & Masten, A. (1991). Peer reputation in middle childhood as a predictor of adaptation in adolescence: A 7-year follow-up. *Child Development, 62*, 991–1007.

Moskowitz, D. S., Schwarz, J. C., & Corsini, D. A. (1977). Initiating day care at three years of age: Effects on attachment. *Child Development, 48*, 1271–1276.

Murray, L. (1992). The impact of postnatal depression on infant development. *Journal of Child Psychology and Psychiatry, 33*, 543–561.

Myers, J. K., & Weissman, M. M. (1980). Use of a self-report symptom scale to detect depression in a community sample. *American Journal of Psychiatry, 137*, 1081–1084.

Nafstad, P., Hagen, J., Magnus, P., & Jaakkola, J. (1999). Day care centers and respiratory health. *Pediatrics, 103*, 753–758.

National Center for Education Statistics. (1995, October). *Statistics in brief: Child care and early education program participation of infants, toddlers, and preschoolers* (NCES Report 95-824). Washington, DC: U.S. Department of Education.

National Center for Health Statistics. (1991). *Incidence and impact of selected infectious dis-eases in childhood* (Series 10, No. 180). Hyattsville, MD: Centers for Disease Control, Department of Health and Human Services.

National Education Goals Panel. (1997). *The national education goals report: Building a nation of learners.* Washington, DC: Author.

National Institute of Child Health and Human Development Early Child Care Research Network. (1993). *The NICHD Study of Early Child Care: A comprehensive longitudi-nal study of young children's lives.* (ERIC Document Reproduction Service No. ED353087).

National Institute of Child Health and Human Development Early Child Care Research Network. (1994). Child care and child development: The NICHD Study of Early Child Care. In S. Friedman & H. C. Haywood (Eds.), *Developmental follow-up: Con-cepts, domains, and methods.* New York: Academic Press.

National Institute of Child Health and Human Development Early Child Care Research Network. (1996). Characteristics of infant child care: Factors contributing to posi-tive caregiving. *Early Childhood Research Quarterly, 11,* 269–306.

National Institute of Child Health and Human Development Early Child Care Research Network. (1997a). Child care in the first year of life. *Merrill-Palmer Quarterly, 43,* 340–360.

National Institute of Child Health and Human Development Early Child Care Research Network. (1997b). The effects of infant child care on infant–mother attachment security: Results of the NICHD Study of Early Child Care. *Child Development, 68,* 860–879.

National Institute of Child Health and Human Development Early Child Care Research Network. (1997c). Familial factors associated with characteristics of nonmaternal care for infants. *Journal of Marriage and the Family, 59,* 389–408.

National Institute of Child Health and Human Development Early Child Care Research Network. (1997d, April). *Mother–child interaction and cognitive outcomes associated with early child care: Results from the NICHD Study.* Poster symposium presented at the biennial meeting of the Society for Research in Child Development, Washing-ton DC.

National Institute of Child Health and Human Development Early Child Care Research Network. (1997e). Poverty and patterns of child care. In J. Brooks-Gunn & G. Duncan (Eds.), *Consequences of growing up poor* (pp. 100–131). New York: Russell Sage.

National Institute of Child Health and Human Development Early Child Care Research Network. (1998a). Early child care and self-control, compliance, and problem behavior at 24 and 36 months. *Child Development, 69,* 1145–1170.

National Institute of Child Health and Human Development Early Child Care Re-search Network. (1998b). Relations between family predictors and child out-comes: Are they weaker for children in child care? *Developmental Psychology, 34,* 1119–1128.

National Institute of Child Health and Human Development Early Child Care Research Network. (1999a). Child care and mother–child interaction in the first three years of life. *Developmental Psychology, 35,* 1399–1413.

National Institute of Child Health and Human Development Early Child Care Research Network. (1999b). Child outcomes when child-care center classes meet recom-mended standards for quality. *American Journal of Public Health, 89,* 1072–1077.

National Institute of Child Health and Human Development Early Child Care Research Network (1999c). Chronicity of maternal depressive symptoms, maternal sensitivity, and child functioning at 36 months. *Developmental Psychology, 35,* 1297–1310.

National Institute of Child Health and Human Development Early Child Care Research Network. (2000a). Characteristics and quality of child care for toddlers and pre-schoolers. *Applied Developmental Science, 4,* 116–135.

National Institute of Child Health and Human Development Early Child Care Research Network. (2000b). The relation of child care to cognitive and language development. *Child Development, 71,* 960–980.

National Institute of Child Health and Human Development Early Child Care Research Network. (2001a). Child care and common communicable illnesses: Results from the National Institute of Child Health and Human Development Study of Early Child Care. *Archives of Pediatric and Adolescent Medicine, 155,* 481–488.

National Institute of Child Health and Human Development Early Child Care Research Network. (2001b). Child care and family predictors of preschool attachment and stability from infancy. *Developmental Psychology, 37,* 847–862.

National Institute of Child Health and Human Development Early Child Care Research Network. (2001c). Early child care and children's peer relationships at 24 and 36 months: The NICHD Study of Early Child Care. *Child Development, 72,* 1478–2000.

National Institute of Child Health and Human Development Early Child Care Research Network. (2001d). Further explorations of the detected effects of quantity of early child care on socioemotional adjustment. In *Early childcare and children's development prior to school entry.* Symposium conducted at biennial meeting of the Society for Research in Child Development.

National Institute of Child Health and Human Development Early Child Care Research Network. (2001e). Nonmaternal care and family factors in early development: An overview of the NICHD study of early child care. *Journal of Applied Developmental Psychology, 22,* 457–492.

National Institute of Child Health and Human Development Early Child Care Research Network. (2001f). Overview of early child care effects at 4.5 years. In *Early childcare and children's development prior to school entry.* Symposium conducted at biennial meeting of the Society for Research in Child Development.

National Institute of Child Health and Human Development Early Child Care Research Network. (2001g). Parenting and family influences when children are in child care: Results from the NICHD Study of Early Child Care. In J. Borkowski, S. Ramey, & M. Bristol-Power (Eds.), *Parenting and the child's world: Influences on intellectual, academic, and social-emotional development* (pp. 99–123). Mahwah, NJ: Erlbaum.

National Institute of Child Health and Human Development Early Child Care Research Network. (2001h). Type of care and children's development at 54 months. In *Early childcare and children's development prior to school entry.* Symposium conducted at biennial meeting of the Society for Research in Child Development.

National Institute of Child Health and Human Development Early Child Care Research Network. (2002a). Early child care and children's development prior to school entry: Results from the NICHD Study of Early Child Care. *American Educational Research Journal, 39,* 133–164.

National Institute of Child Health and Human Development Early Child Care Research Network. (2002b). Structure→ process→ outcome: Direct and indirect effects of caregiving quality on young children's development. *Psychological Science, 13,* 199–206.

National Institute of Child Health and Human Development Early Child Care Research Network. (2003). Does amount of time spent in child care predict socioemotional adjustment during the transition to kindergarten? *Child Development, 74,* 976–1005.

Nicholson, J., Atkins-Burnett, S., & Meisels, S. J. (1997). *Academic Rating Scale* (field trial ed.). Washington, DC: US Department of Education, National Center for Education Statistics.

O'Connor, S. (1991). *ASQ: Assessing school-age child care quality.* Wellesley, MA: Wellesley College, Center for Research on Women.

Oppenheim, D., Sagi, A., & Lamb, M. (1988). Infant–adult attachments on the kibbutz and their relation to socioemotional development 4 years later. *Developmental Psychology, 24,* 427–433.

Owen, M. T., & Cox, M. J. (1988). Maternal employment and the transition to parenthood: Family functioning and child development. In A. E. Gottfried & A. W. Gottfried (Eds.), *Maternal employment and children's development: Longitudinal research* (pp. 85–119). New York: Plenum Press.

Palfrey, J. S., Walker, D. K., Butler, J. A., & Singer, J. D. (1989). Patterns of response in families of chronically disabled children: An assessment in five metropolitan school districts. *American Journal of Orthopsychiatry, 59,* 94–104.

Paradise, J., Rockette, H., Colborn, D., Bernard, B., Smith, C., Kurs-Lasky, M., & Janosky, J. (1997). Otitis media in 2253 Pittsburgh-area infants: Prevalence and risk factors during the first two years of life. *Pediatrics, 99,* 318–333.

Park, K., & Honig, A. (1991). Infant child care patterns and later teacher ratings of preschool behaviors. *Early Child Development and Care, 68,* 89–96.

Parke, R. D. (1996). *Fatherhood.* Cambridge, MA: Harvard University Press.

Peisner-Feinberg, E., & Burchinal, M. (1997). Concurrent relations between child care quality and child outcomes: The Study of Cost, Quality, and Outcomes in Child Care Center. *Merrill-Palmer Quarterly, 43,* 451–477.

Phillips, D. (Ed.). (1987). *Quality in child care: What does research tell us?* Washington, DC: National Association for the Education of Young Children.

Phillips, D. A. (Ed.). (1995). *Child care for low-income families: Summary of two workshops.* Washington, DC: National Academy Press.

Phillips, D. A., & Bridgman, A. (Eds.). (1995). *New findings on children, families, and economic self-sufficiency.* Washington, DC: National Academy Press.

Phillips, D., & Howes, C. (1987). Child care quality and children's social development. *Developmental Psychology, 23,* 537–543.

Phillips, D. A., McCartney, K., & Scarr, S. (1987). Child care quality and children's social development. *Developmental Psychology, 23,* 537–543.

Phillips, D., McCartney, D., Scarr, S., & Howes, C. (1987). Selective review of infant day care research: A cause for concern. *Zero to Three, 7,* 18–21.

Phillips, D. A., Voran, M., Kisker, E., Howes, C., & Whitebook, M. (1994). Child care of children in poverty: Opportunity or inequity? *Child Development, 65,* 472–492.

Pianta, R. C. (1992). *Student–Teacher Relationship Scale.* Charlottesville: University of Virginia.

Pianta, R. C. (1994). *Child–Parent Relationship Scale.* Charlottesville: University of Virginia.

Pianta, R. C. (1995). *Getting ready for school.* Charlottesville: University of Virginia.

Pianta, R. C. (2001). *The Student–Teacher Relationship Scale.* Odessa, FL: Personality Assessment Research.

Pianta, R. C., & Cox, M. J. (1999). *The transition to kindergarten.* Baltimore: Brookes.

Pianta, R. C., & Egeland, B. (1994). Predictors of instability in children's mental test performance at 24, 48, and 96 months. *Intelligence, 18,* 145–165.

Pierce, K. M., Hamm, J. V., & Vandell, D. L. (1999). Experiences in after-school programs and children's adjustment in first-grade classrooms. *Child Development, 70,* 756–767.

Pierrehumbert, B. (1994, September). *Socioemotional continuity through the preschool years and child care experience.* Paper presented at the meeting of the British Psychological Society, Developmental Section Conference, Portsmouth, UK.

Ponka, A., Nurmi, R., Salminen, E., & Nykyri, E. (1991). Infections and other illnesses in day-care centers in Helsinki, I: Incidences and effects of home and day-care center variables. *Infection, 19,* 230–236.

Portnoy, F. C., & Simmons, C. H. (1978). Day care and attachment. *Child Development, 49,* 239–242.

Posner, J. K., & Vandell, D. L. (1994). Low-income children's after-school care: Are there beneficial effects of after-school programs? *Child Development, 65,* 440–456.

Powell, D. R. (1978). The interpersonal relationship between parents and caregivers in day care settings. *American Journal of Orthopsychiatry, 48,* 680–689.

Powell, D. R. (1989). *Families and early childhood programs.* Washington, DC: National Association for the Education of Young Children.

Power, T. G., & Chapieski, M. (1986). Child-rearing and impulse control in toddlers: A naturalistic investigation. *Developmental Psychology, 22,* 271–275.

Prodromidis, M., Lamb, M., Sternberg, K., Hwang, C., & Broberg, A. (1995). Aggression and noncompliance among Swedish children in center-based care, family day care, and home care. *International Journal of Behavioral Development, 18,* 43–62.

Radke-Yarrow, M., Cummings, E. M., Kuczynski, L., & Chapman, M. (1985). Patterns of attachment in two- and three-year-olds in normal families and in families with parental depression. *Child Development, 56,* 884–893.

Radloff, L. (1977). The CES-D scale: A self-report depression scale for research in the general population. *Applied Psychological Measurement, 1,* 385–410.

Ramey C. T., & Ramey S. L. (1998). Early intervention and early experience. *American Psychologist, 58,* 109–120.

Reves, R., Morrow, A., Bartlett, A., Caruso, C., Plumb, R., Lu, B., & Pickering, L. (1993). Child care increases the risk of clinic visits for acute diarrhea and diarrhea due to rotavirus. *American Journal of Epidemiology, 137,* 97–107.

Reynell, J. (1991). *Reynell Developmental Language Scales (U.S. edition).* Los Angeles: Western Psychological Service.

Reynell, J. K., & Gruber, C. P. (1977). *Reynell Developmental Language Scales.* Los Angeles: Western Psychological Services.

Richman, N., Stevenson, J., & Graham, P. (1986). *Preschool to school: A behavioural study.* London: Academic Press.

Richters, J., & Zahn-Waxler, C. (1990). The infant day care controversy: Current status and future directions. In. N. Fox & G. Fein (Eds.), *Infant day care: The current debate* (pp. 87–106). Norwood, NJ: Ablex.

Rimm-Kaufman, S. E., Pianta, R. C., & Cox, M. J. (2000). Teacher's judgments of success in the transition to kindergarten. *Early Childhood Research Quarterly, 15,* 147–166.

Roberts, J. E., Rabinowitch, S., Bryant, D. M., & Burchinal, M. R. (1989). Language skills of children with different preschool experiences. *Journal of Speech and Hearing Research, 32,* 773–786.

Rogoff, B., Mistry, J., Goncu, A., & Mosier, C. (1993). Guided participation in cultural activity by toddlers and caregivers. *Monographs of the Society for Research in Child Development, 58* (8, Serial No. 236).

Roggman, L., Langlois, J., Hubbs-Tait, L., & Rieser-Danner, L. (1994). Infant day-care, attachment, and the "file drawer problem." *Child Development, 65,* 1429–1443.

Rogosa, D. (1995). Myths and methods: "Myths about longitudinal research" plus supplemental questions. In J. M. Gottman (Ed.), *The analysis of change* (pp. 3–66). Mahwah, NJ: Erlbaum.

Roopnarine, J. L., & Lamb, M. E. (1978). The effects of day care on attachment and exploratory behavior in a strange situation. *Merrill-Palmer Quarterly, 24,* 85–95.

Rose, S. L., Rose, S. A., & Feldman, J. (1986). Stability of behavior problems in very young children. *Developmental Psychopathology, 1,* 5–19.

Rosenthal, R. (1994). Parametric measures of effect size. In H. Cooper & L. V. Hedges (Eds.), *The handbook of research synthesis.* New York: Russell Sage.

Rosenthal, R., & Vandell, D. L. (1996). Quality of care at school-aged care programs: Regulatable features, observed experiences, child perspectives, and parent perspectives. *Child Development, 67,* 2434–2445.

Rosnow, R. L., & Rosenthal, R. (1988). Focused tests of significance and effect size estimation in counseling psychology. *Journal of Counseling Psychology, 35,* 203–208.

Rosvold, H. E., Mirsky, A. F., Sarason, I., Bransome, E. D., & Beck, L. H. (1956). A continuous performance test of brain damage. *Journal of Consulting Psychology, 20,* 343–350.

Rothbart, M. K. (1986). Temperament and development. In G. Kohnstamm, J. E. Bates, & M. Rothbart (Eds.), *Temperament in childhood* (pp. 187–247). New York: Wiley.

Rothbart, M. K., Ahadi, S. A., & Hershey, K. L. (1994). Temperament and social behavior in childhood. *Merrill-Palmer Quarterly, 40,* 21–39.

Rovine, M. J., & Molenaar, P. C. M. (1998). A nonstandard method for estimating a linear growth model in LISREL. *International Journal of Behavioral Development, 22,* 453–473.

Rubin, K. H. (1983). *The social problem-solving test–revised.* Unpublished manual.

Ruopp, R., Travers, J., Glantz, F., & Coelen, C. (1979). *Children at the center.* Cambridge, MA: Abt.

Rutter, M. (1981). Socioemotional consequences of day-care for preschool children. *American Journal of Orthopsychiatry, 51,* 4–28.

Sagi, A., Koren-Karie, N., Gini, M., Ziv, Y., & Joels, T. (2002). Shedding further light on the effects of various types and quality of early child care on infant–mother attachment relationship: The Haifa Study of Early Child Care. *Child Development, 73,* 1166–1186.

Sameroff, A. J., & Seifer, R. (1983). Familial and child competence. *Child Development, 54,* 1254–1268.

Sameroff, A. J., Seifer, R., Baldwin, A., & Baldwin, C. (1993). Stability of intelligence from preschool to adolescence: The influence of social and family risk factors. *Child Development, 64,* 80–97.

Sarason, I. G., Johnson, J. A., & Siegel, J. M. (1978). Assessing the impact of life changes: Development of the life experiences survey. *Journal of Consulting and Clinical Psychology, 46,* 932–946.

Scarr, S. (1992). Developmental theories for the 1990s: Development and individual differences. *Child Development, 63,* 1–19.

Scarr, S. (1998). American child care today. *American Psychologist, 53,* 95–108.

Scarr, S., & Eisenberg, M. (1993). Child care research: Issues, perspectives, and results. *Annual Review of Psychology, 44,* 613–644.

Scarr, S., Eisenberg, M., & Deater-Deckard, K. (1994). Measurement of quality in child care centers. *Early Childhood Research Quarterly, 9,* 131–151.

Scarr, S., & McCartney, K. (1983). How people make their own environments: A theory of genotype–environment effects. *Child Development, 54,* 424–435.

Schaefer, E. S., & Edgerton, M. (1985). Parent and child correlates of parental modernity. In I. E. Siegel (Ed.), *Parental belief systems* (pp. 287–318). Hillsdale, NJ: Erlbaum.

Schaefer, M., & Olson, D. (1981). Assessing intimacy: The PAIR Inventory. *Journal of Marital and Family Therapy, 7,* 640–653.

Shonkoff, J. P., & Meisels, S. J. (Eds.). (2000). *Handbook of early childhood intervention* (2nd ed.). New York: Cambridge University Press.

Shonkoff, J., & Phillips, D. (Eds.). (2000). *From neurons to neighborhoods: The science of early childhood development.* Washington, DC: National Academy Press.

Siegel, G., & Loman, L. A. (1991). *Child care and AFDC recipients in Illinois (Report).* St. Louis, MO: Institute of Applied Research.

Singer, J. D. (1998). Using SAS PROC MIXED to fit multilevel models, hierarchical models, and individual growth models. *Journal of Educational and Behavioral Statistics, 23,* 323–355.

Smith, S. (1998, April). *The past decade's research on child care quality and children's development: What we are learning, directions for the future.* Paper prepared for a meeting on Child Care in the New Policy Context, sponsored by the Office of the Assistant Secretary for Planning and Evaluation. Bethesda, MD: U.S. Department of Health and Human Services.

Sobel, M. E. (1982). Asymptotic confidence intervals for indirect effects in structural equation models. In S. Leinhart (Ed.), *Sociological methodology* (pp. 290–312). San Francisco: Jossey-Bass.

Sonenstein, F. L., & Wolf, D. A. (1991). Satisfaction with child care: Perspectives of welfare mothers. *Journal of Social Issues, 47,* 15–31.

Spieker, S. J., & Booth, C. L. (1988). Maternal antecedents of attachment quality. In J. Belsky & T. Nezworski (Eds.), *Clinical implications of attachment* (pp. 95–135). Hillsdale, NJ: Erlbaum.

Sroufe, L. A. (1988). A developmental perspective on daycare. *Early Childhood Research Quarterly, 3,* 283–291.

Sroufe, L. A., Carlson, E. A., Levy, A. K., & Egeland, B. (1999). Implications of attachment theory for developmental psychopathology. *Development and Psychopathology, 11,* 1–13.

Stallings, J. A. (1980). An observation study of family day care. In J. C. Colberg (Ed.), *Home day care: A perspective* (pp. 25–47). Chicago: Roosevelt University.

Stansbury, K., & Gunnar, R. (1994). Adrenocortical activity and emotion regulation. In N. Fox (Ed.), The development of emotional regulation: Biological and behavioral considerations. *Monographs of the Society for Research in Child Development, 59,* 108–134.

Steiger, J. H., & Lind, J. C. (1980, May). *Statistically based tests for the number of common factors.* Paper presented at the annual meeting of the Psychometric Society, Iowa City, IA.

Steiner, B. (1981). *The futility of family policy.* Washington, DC: Brookings Institution.

Sternberg, K., Lamb, M., Hwang, C., Broberg, A., Ketterlinus, R., & Bookstein, B. (1991). Does out-of-home care affect compliance in preschoolers? *International Journal of Behavioral Development, 14,* 45–65.

Stipek, D., Feiler, R., Daniels, D., & Milburn, S. (1995). Effects of different instructional approaches on young children's achievement and motivation. *Child Development, 66,* 209–223.

Suwalsky, J., Zaslow, M., Klein, R. P., & Rabinovich, B. A. (1986, September). *Continuity of substitute care in relation to infant–mother attachment.* Paper presented at the meeting of the American Psychological Association, Washington, DC.

Symons, D. K. (1998). Post-partum employment patterns, family-based care arrangements, and the mother–infant relationship at age two. *Canadian Journal of Behavioral Science, 30,* 121–131.

Symons, D. K., & McLeod, P. J. (1993). Maternal employment plans and outcomes after the birth of an infant in a Canadian sample. *Family Relations, 42,* 442–446.

Symons, D. K., & McLeod, P. J. (1994). Maternal, infant, and occupational characteristics that predict postpartum employment patterns. *Infant Behavior and Development, 17,* 71–82.

Teti, D. M. (2000). Maternal depression and child–mother attachment in the first three years: A view from the intermountain west. In P. M. Crittenden & A. H. Claussen (Eds.), *The organization of attachment relationships: Maturation, culture, and context.* New York: Cambridge University Press.

Teti, D. M., & Gelfand, D. M. (1997). The Preschool Assessment of Attachment: Construct validity in a sample of depressed and nondepressed families. *Development and Psychopathology, 9,* 517–536.

Teti, D. M., Gelfand, D. M., Messinger, D. S., & Isabella, R. (1995). Maternal depression and the quality of early attachment: An examination of infants, preschoolers, and their mothers. *Developmental Psychology, 31,* 364–376.

Thacker, S. B., Addiss, D. G., Goodman, R. A., Holloway, B. R., & Spencer, H. C. (1992). Infectious diseases and injuries in child day care: Opportunities for healthier children. *Journal of the American Medical Association, 268,* 1720–1726.

Thompson, R. (1988). The effects of infant day care through the prism of attachment theory. *Early Childhood Research Quarterly, 3,* 273–282.

Tomasello, M., & Farrar, J. (1986). Joint attention and early language. *Child Development, 57,* 1454–1463.

Tomasello, M., Mantle, S., & Kruger, A. C. (1986). Linguistic environment of 1- to 2-year-old twins. *Developmental Psychology, 22*, 169–176.

Tout, K., de Haan, M., Kipp Campbell, E., Gunnar, M. (1998). Social behavior correlates of adrenocortical activity in daycare. *Child Development, 69*, 1247–1262.

Tronick, E. (1989). Emotions and emotional communication in infants. *American Psychologist, 44*, 112–119.

U.S. Bureau of the Census. (1992). *Statistical abstract of the United States*. Washington, DC: U.S. Government Printing Office.

U.S. Bureau of the Census. (1993). *Population projections of the United States, by age, sex, race, and Hispanic origin: 1993-2050*. Washington, DC: U.S. Government Printing Office.

U.S. Bureau of the Census. (1995). *Fertility of American women: June 1994*. (Current Population Report No. P20-482). Washington, DC: U.S. Government Printing Office.

U.S. Bureau of the Census. (1997, November). *Who's minding our preschoolers? Fall 1994 (Update)* (Current Population Report No. P70–62). Washington, DC: U.S. Government Printing Office.

U.S. Bureau of the Census. (1999a). *1999 Poverty statistics. www.census.gov/hhes/poverty/poverty99/pov99hi.html*.

U.S. Bureau of the Census. (1999b). *Poverty thresholds. www.census.gov/hhes/poverty/threshold.html*.

U.S. Bureau of the Census. (1999c). *Statistical abstract of the United States* (119th ed.). Washington, DC: U.S. Government Printing Office.

U.S. Department of Health and Human Services. (2001). *Adventures in parenting: How responding, preventing, monitoring, mentoring, and modeling can help you be a successful parent* (NIH Publication Number 00-4842). Washington, DC: Author. *http://www.nichd.nih.gov/publications/pubs/parenting/adv_in_parenting.cfm*.

U.S. Department of Labor, Women's Bureau. (1993). 1993 *Handbook on women workers: Trends and issues*. Washington, DC: US Government Printing Office.

Vandell, D. L. (1979). Effects of a playgroup experience on mother–son and father–son interaction. *Developmental Psychology, 15*, 379–385.

Vandell, D. L., & Corasaniti, M. A. (1990). Variations in early child care: Do they predict subsequent social, emotional, and cognitive differences? *Early Childhood Research Quarterly, 5*, 555–572.

Vandell, D. L., & Powers, C. P. (1983). Day care quality and children's free play activities. *American Journal of Orthopsychiatry, 53*, 493–500.

Vandell, D., & Wolfe, B. (2000, May). *Child care quality: Does it matter and does it need to be improved?* Report prepared for the U.S. Department of Health and Human Services, Washington, DC.

van IJzendoorn, M. H., Dijkstra, J., & Bus, A. G. (1995). Attachment, intelligence, and language: A meta-analysis. *Social Development, 4*, 115–128.

van IJzendoorn, M., Kranenburg, M., Zwart-Woudstra, H., Van Busschbach, A., & Lambermom, M. (1991, April). *Daycare and preschool: Quality of infant–caregiver attachment affects sociability in preschool*. Paper presented at the biennial meetings of the Society for Research in Child Development, Seattle, WA.

van IJzendoorn, M. H., Schuengel, C., & Bakermans-Kranenburg, M. J. (1999). Disorganized attachment in early childhood: Meta-analysis of precursors, concomitants, and sequelae. *Development and Psychopathology, 11*, 225–250.

Varin, D., Crugnola, C., Ripamonti, Ch., and Molina, P. (1994, September). *Critical periods in the growth of attachment and the age of entry into day care*. Paper presented at the annual conference of the Developmental Section of the British Psychological Society, University of Portsmouth.

Vaughn, B., Gove, F., & Egeland, B. (1980). The relationship between out-of-home care and the quality of infant–mother attachment in an economically disadvantaged population. *Child Development, 51*, 1203–1214.

Volling, B. L., & Belsky, J. (1993). Parent, infant, and contextual characteristics related to maternal employment decisions in the first year of infancy. *Family Relations, 42*, 4–12.

Wachs, T. D. (1991). Environmental considerations in studies with nonextreme groups. In T. D. Wachs & R. Plomin (Eds.), *Conceptualization and measurement of organism–environment interaction* (pp. 44–67). Washington, DC: American Psychological Association.

Wachs, T. D., & Chan, A. (1986). Specificity of environmental action, as seen in environmental correlates of infants' communication performance. *Child Development, 57*, 1464–1474.

Waite, L. J., Leibowitz, A., & Witsberger, C. (1991). What parents pay for: Child care characteristics, quality, and costs. *Journal of Social Issues, 47*, 33–48.

Ware, A. M., Barfoot, B., Rusher, A. S., & Owen, M. T. (1995). *The caregiver role in the parent–caregiver partnership: Its relationship to the child care environment.* Poster presented at the Biennial Meeting of the Society for Research in Child Development. Indianapolis, IN.

Warfield, M. E., & Hauser-Cram, P. (1996). Child care needs, arrangements, and satisfaction of mothers of children with developmental disabilities. *Mental Retardation, 34*, 294–302.

Waters, E., & Deane, K. (1985). Defining and assessing individual differences in attachment relationships: Q-methodology and the organization of behavior in infancy and early childhood. In I. Bretherton & E. Waters (Eds.), *Growing points of attachment theory and research* (pp. 41–65). *Monographs of the Society for Research in Child Development, 50* (1–2, Serial No. 209).

Weikart, D., Deloria, D., Lawser, S., & Wiegerink, K. (1970). Longitudinal results of the Ypsilanti Perry Preschool Project. *Monographs of the High/Scope Educational Research Foundation, No. 1.* Ypsilanti, MI: High/Scope.

Weinfield, N. S., Ogawa, J. R., & Egeland, B. (2002). Predictability of observed mother–child interaction from preschool to middle childhood in a high-risk sample. *Child Development, 73*, 528–543.

Weinraub, M., & Jaeger, E. (1990). The timing of mother's return to the workplace: Effects on the developing mother–infant relationship. In J. S. Hyde & M. J. Essex (Eds.), *Parental leave and child care: Setting a research and policy agenda* (pp. 307–322). Philadelphia: Temple University Press.

Weinraub, M., Jaeger, E., & Hoffman, L. (1988). Predicting infant outcome in families of employed and nonemployed mothers. *Early Childhood Research Quarterly, 3*, 361–378.

Welsh, M. C. (1991). Rule-guided behavior and self-monitoring on the Tower of Hanoi disk-transfer task. *Cognitive Development, 6*, 59–76.

Werner, E. E., & Smith, R. S. (1992). *Overcoming the odds.* Ithaca, NY: Cornell University Press.

White, B. (1985). *The first three years of life, the revised edition.* New York: Prentice Hall.

Whitebook, M., Howes, C., & Phillips, D. (1990). *Who cares? Child care teachers and the quality of care in America (Final report).* National Child Care Staffing Study. Oakland, CA: Child Care Employee Project.

Willett, J. B., Singer, J. D., & Martin, N. C. (1998). The design and analysis of longitudinal studies of development and psychopathology in context: Statistical models and methodological recommendations. *Development and Psychopathology, 10*, 395–426.

Winer, B. J. (1971). *Statistical Principles in Experimental Design* (2nd ed.). New York: McGraw-Hill.

Woodcock, R. W., & Johnson, M. B. (1989). *Woodcock–Johnson Psycho-Educational Battery–Revised.* Allen, TX: DLM Teaching Resources.

Woodcock, R. W., & Johnson, M. B. (1990). *Tests of achievement, WJ-R examiner's manual.* Allen, TX: DLM Teaching Resources.

Yoshikawa, H. (1994). Prevention as cumulative protection: Effects of early family support and education on chronic delinquency and its risks. *Psychological Bulletin, 115,* 28–54.

Yoshikawa, H. (1995). Long-term effects of early childhood programs on social outcomes and delinquency. *Future of Children, 5,* 51–75.

Zahn-Waxler, C., Iannotti, R. J., Cummings, E. M., & Denham, S. (1990). Antecedents of problem behaviors in children of depressed mothers. *Development and Psychopathology, 2,* 271–291.

Zellner, A. (1962). An efficient method of estimating seemingly unrelated regressions and tests for aggregation bias. *Journal of the American Statistical Association, 57,* 297–300.

Zimmerman, I. L., Steiner, V. G., & Pond, R. E. (1979). *Preschool Language Scale.* San Antonio, TX: Psychological Corporation.

Zimmerman, I. L., Steiner, V. G., & Pond, R. E. (1992). *PLS-3 examiners manual and picture manual.* New York: Psychological Corporation.

Zucker, S., & Riordan, J. (1986, October). *Assessing kindergarten readiness: The validity of new and revised measures.* Paper presented at the annual conferences of the National Association of School Psychologists, New Orleans, LA.

Index

Page numbers followed by an *f* indicate figure; *t*, table.